St Mary's

McGill-Queen's/Associated Medical Services (Hannah Institute) Studies in the History of Medicine
Series Editors: S.O. Freedman and J.T.H. Connor
Volumes in this series have financial support from Associated Medical Services, Inc., through the Hannah Institute for the History of Medicine program.

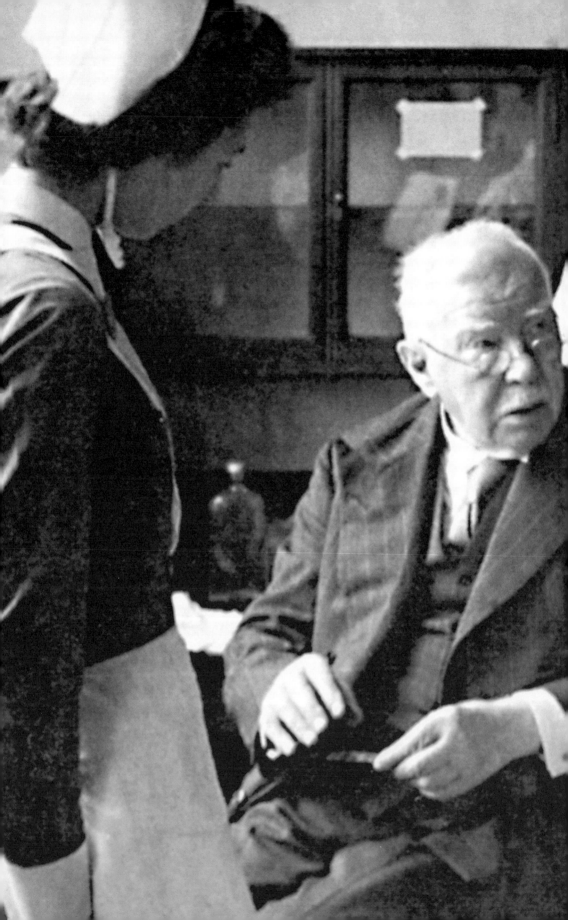

St Mary's

The History of a London Teaching Hospital

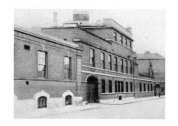

E.A. HEAMAN

LIVERPOOL UNIVERSITY PRESS

McGILL-QUEEN'S UNIVERSITY PRESS
Montreal & Kingston • London • Ithaca

© McGill-Queen's University Press, 2003
ISBN 0-7735-2513-0 (cloth)
ISBN 0-7735-2514-9 (paper)

Legal deposit fourth quarter 2003
Bibliothèque nationale du Québec

Published in the European Union by
Liverpool University Press
ISBN 0-85323-968-1 (cloth)
ISBN 0-85323-978-9 (paper)

Printed in Canada on acid-free paper that is 100% ancient forest
free (100% post-consumer recycled), processed chlorine free.

This book has been published with the help of a grant from the
Faculty of Medicine, Imperial College, University of London.

McGill-Queen's University Press acknowledges the support of the
Canada Council for the Arts for our publishing program. We also
acknowledge the financial support of the Government of Canada
through the Book Publishing Industry Development Program
(BPIDP) for our publishing activities.

National Library of Canada Cataloguing in Publication

Heaman, Elsbeth, 1964–
  St. Mary's : the history of a London teaching hospital /
E.A. Heaman.
(McGill-Queen's/Associated Medical Services (Hannah Institute)
studies in the history of medicine 15)
Includes bibliographical references and index.
ISBN 0-7735-2513-0 (bound)–ISBN 0-7735-2514-9 (pbk.)
1. St. Mary's Hospital (London, England)–History. I. Title.
II. Series.
RA988.L72S35 2003   362.1'1'09421   C2002-904759-5

British Cataloguing-in-Publication Data
A British Library CIP record is available

This book was designed and typeset by David LeBlanc
in Sabon 10.5/13.5 in Montreal, Quebec

Contents

Figures and Chart

Foreword

Sir Roger Bannister, Chairman, St Mary's Development Trust

THERE COULD BE no more appropriate time for this book to be written. It tackles the broad canvas of the evolution of over 150 years of St Mary's Hospital and Medical School. The story starts unpromisingly with the poverty-stricken navvies working on the Paddington canal and railway site in the 1850s, living up to ten in a room near reservoirs described by the medical officer as an "enormous wen." The book ends as the new Imperial School of Medicine arises, phoenix-like, from merging the existing medical schools in West London, of which St Mary's was the first. The Imperial College of Science and Technology faces some problems. It is entirely new to medicine, and its medical students, more than three hundred a year, outnumber those of all other faculties. But with its five-star research departments and more than £75 million a year in research funding, it compares favourably with America's great medical school, the Massachusetts Institute of Technology. The Imperial College's fine new preclinical building is named after St Mary's Nobel laureate, Sir Alexander Fleming.

The book also ends with the fresh start for the Paddington Basin site of St Mary's Hospital. This is now the centre of a consortium of West London hospitals, and the St Mary's Imperial College campus includes the largest infectious diseases research laboratories in Britain; later, the site is expected to become the largest cardiothoracic surgical unit in Europe, enclosing Sir Magdy Yacoub's Harefield Hospital Centre. The rebuilding project, the largest in London since Canary Wharf, involves hospitals, hotels, offices, and housing, using private and public finance. This is why it is the right moment for both Imperial College and St Mary's alumni to look back with justifiable pride on the origins of the hospital and medical school and the struggles to change medicine from Victorian methods to those of today. We know doctors will still be caring of their patients, but now they will be armoured with the results of scientific research.

The book reads at times more like a novel than pure history. There are intermingled themes, of idealists who were ahead of their time, struggling against poverty and disease but sometimes having to turn aside to fight politicians and ward off bankruptcy. The story is a metaphor, a tale of linked institutions that reflected the events from Victorian times to today, in one of the most deprived inner-city areas of London.

St Mary's Hospital arose from small philanthropic beginnings: the rich lived south of the canal, and their consciences were stirred by the poor who lived on the north side of the canal. There was also an element of self-interest. Diseases could spread through servants from the poor to the rich. At that time, half the population consisted of servants, and the other half included 526 prostitutes and 139 brothels. The author pictures for us an early scene, with diseases like cholera, typhoid, tuberculosis, and venereal disease, and, alongside them, their ineffective treatments like blood-letting and purging and surgery without asepsis or anaesthetic. As late as 1890, a nurse was reported to say, "I never seed [sic] the use of one of them temperatures." An early physician, not notably modest, boasted he could make a diagnosis without turning down the bedclothes, and another demonstrated to students the catheterisation of a woman with eyes averted in order not to endanger her modesty. The author takes us through the first glimmerings of medical science and precise diagnosis up to the present day. On the way, we meet larger-than-life-figures like Almroth Wright, the model for Colenso Ridgeon in Shaw's Doctor's Dilemma, with his vaccines and philosophy and his battle cry, "Stimulate the phagocytes!"

Dramatic change came with the National Health Service in 1948. Its inception rescued many private hospitals like St Mary's from bankruptcy as private funds dwindled and expectations of treatment rose. Dr Charles Wilson, later Lord Moran, dean of St Mary's, also president of the Royal College of Physicians and equally famous as Churchill's doctor, joined Aneurin Bevan, and they adroitly manipulated reluctant consultants and general practitioners to join the new service.

The book describes the past fifty years over which, in different ways, from student to consultant neurologist, I have been a part of St Mary's, and I can testify that the author's assessment rings true. We saw an apparently endless series of reorganizations. District hospitals were shut, often against strident public protest, and others were recreated under different tiers of political control and now under trusts. In my time as a consultant, we endured the rejection of five different rebuilding plans to replace the dilapi-

dated Victorian complex before the splendid new Queen Elizabeth the
Queen Mother Hospital rose in the 1980s. Twenty years later, this too is
inadequate for district needs. A St Mary's epidemiologist, Professor, now
Sir Brian Jarman, conclusively proved that London hospitals beds, closed
with a flourish of reorganizing zeal a few years ago, must now be reopened
or replaced. Despite the many successes of the NHS, no government has yet
been able to satisfy the public's reasonable but insatiable expectation for
free access to all the extensive treatments doctors could provide today, or
at least as much as enjoyed by comparable western democracies such as
those of France and Germany.

Paralleling the story of the hospital are the equally dramatic problems of
the medical school. When founded in 1851, it was the smallest and poorest
in London. Like the hospital, it only survived by shrewdly adapting to the
changing social needs of the district and different government strategies for
medical education. Before World War II, the dean, Dr Charles Wilson, later
Lord Moran, rescued the medical school from bankruptcy with the help of
some of his rich friends, including Lord Beaverbrook. His deanship was
marked by what some thought was the curious notion that character and
the creation of good doctors needed many of the qualities that were exemplified by the game of rugby: unselfishness, fortitude, even courage of the
kind which he had studied in soldiers as a regimental medical officer in the
trenches of the Great War. His method was entry scholarships for schools
and university scholarships for Oxford and Cambridge students. He created an atmosphere where student enthusiasm abounded, not only in every
sport but also in serious student societies, as if to make up for the narrow-
ness of the medical instruction. Staff too had to show they could join in the
student antics and fun. Professor Huggett, a burly professor of physiology,
was unpopular until he attended a fancy dress ball dressed as a snowflake!
A later dean was famous for an annual sketch in the students' soirée in
which, amidst mounting student tension, and in a dialogue of a Peter Cook
and Dudley Moore type, he eventually squirted a solemn consultant colleague victim with a soda siphon!

Over the years the high morale in the school went far beyond rugby,
though this remained first class, and the intense camaraderie and loyalty to
the school produced a certain type of doctor. Some students became research
workers, some hospital specialist consultants, but most became conscientious, caring general practitioners. During World War II, some performed
outstanding acts of bravery, one winning a Victoria Cross. Other teaching
hospitals had criticized Moran's methods, but eventually, in their own
ways, followed suit. After World War II, Moran was rightly replaced by
deans of a different mould. They expelled some of the "Doctor in the

House" superannuated students, installed IQ testing, and changed the curriculum to take in new subjects like molecular biology and social medicine. There was still the search for character more than straight cleverness, which may not be what is needed. The last dean, Dr Peter Richards, making many innovations, exposed the school to the hazards of BBC *Doctors to Be* coverage, examining the selection process itself and, later, monitoring the students and their progress as doctors. It was a bold move, but it came at a proud moment for the medical school, when the new St Mary's students, 50 per cent women, were winning more university prizes than other London medical schools and the medical school received more applicants than any other UK school, at one time twenty-five per place.

The challenge is now for the campus of the new Imperial College to recreate a sense of fellowship, camaraderie, and responsibility among the students of what is now the largest medical school in Britain. This book, with its story of adaptation and resilience in the face of successive challenges, leads me to believe that it will succeed. Reading this book gives me, as an involved insider, much encouragement. I am sure this story will inspire confidence in the wide circle of those concerned with the future of medicine and medical teaching in Britain.

Acknowledgments

THE HISTORY OF St Mary's was a team project. It was initially sponsored by the Development Trust of St Mary's Hospital Medical School and the Centre for History of Science, Technology, and Medicine at Imperial College of Science, Technology and Medicine, and subsequently funded very generously by the Wellcome Trust. I am very grateful to these sponsors, as well as to the project's two supervisors at Imperial College, Lara V. Marks and David Edgerton. Their wisdom shaped every page of this book. I am also grateful for the support and advice of a steering committee composed of representatives from St Mary's, Imperial College, and the Wellcome Trust Centre for the History of Medicine at University College London: Sir Roger Bannister, Dorothy Wedderburn, Peter Richards, Alisdair Fraser, Bill Bynum, Ann Hardy, Andrew Warwick, and Mei Sim Lei. These people and agencies encouraged me to indulge my intellectual curiosity and aim at a book that would make a serious contribution to scholarly knowledge.

At St Mary's I owe a debt of gratitude to Philip Blissett, Walter Umpleby, Jill Ascott, Malcolm Green, Andy Pritchard, and above all, Nigel Palmer, for helping me to settle in and obtain resources. Sally Smith, Dinah Aken, and Tom Berwick were also very helpful. The St Mary's archivist, Kevin Brown, who knows everything about St Mary's, generously shared his knowledge and his archives and pointed me aright when I sometimes went awrong. The archivist of Imperial College, Ann Barrett, was extraordinarily helpful and patient with my requests, as was Ann Kealey in Information Technology and Eleanor Garth in the contracts office. In the Centre for History at Imperial College, the only faculty member who was not on the steering committee was Rob Iliffe: how much more reason have I, therefore, to be grateful for his many acts of kindness and collegiality. Ainslee Rutledge, the centre's administrator, kept me sane – I think.

The Wellcome Trust Centre gave me a second home, and its staff, both academic and administrative, were extraordinarily generous to me. Thanks especially to the late Roy Porter, to Vivian Nutton, Stephen Jacyna, Christopher Lawrence, Tilli Tansey, Wendy Kutner, Lois Reynolds, Daphne Christie, Alan Shiel, John Malin, and of course, Sally Bragg. I spent considerable time at the Wellcome Library for the History and Understanding of Medicine, and at the Contemporary Medical Archives Collection which it houses, and I am grateful to all the staff there, especially Mathilde Nardelli, Sue Gold, Julia Sheppard, and Lesley Hall, who introduced me to the history of sexuality. Many other archivists and librarians opened their collections to me, and I wish to express particular thanks to the Royal College of Physicians of London, the Royal College of Surgeons of England, and the London Metropolitan Archives, where I spent long periods of time. Carol Beadle and Max Blythe at the Medical Sciences Video Archives made special arrangements for me to use that magnificent collection.

About eighty people connected with St Mary's Hospital and Medical School agreed to talk to me about their experiences, sometimes several times. Often they read over sections and helped me to get it right. Many received me in their homes with great hospitality. Without their cooperation, this book would have been thin and pallid indeed. I wish I could thank them all by name; certainly meeting them was one of the great pleasures of my work. Marion Haberhauer painstakingly transcribed these interviews.

The History Department at Queen's University in Kingston let me finish the manuscript before taking up an appointment. I remain very grateful to all my Queen's colleagues, and especially to Tim Smith and Jackie Duffin who read over the manuscript and made valuable suggestions. My two previous supervisors, Michael Bliss and George Weisz, also read the manuscript, which is profoundly shaped by their very different but, for me, equally exemplary approaches to medical history. Roger Cooter, too, crucially informed my approach to the topic and generously extended a helping hand. Keir Waddington, Geoff Rheaume, and Eileen Magnello were also supportive colleagues and friends. Gareth Rees provided expert advice on rugby football. Sushant Roy helped with the figures. Donald Akenson, Roger Martin, Joan McGilvray, Maureen Garvie, Susanne McAdam, and David LeBlanc turned a rough manuscript into a polished book. My family were, once again, enthusiastically behind me in my work. Bretia and Iain Baird bore much of that particular burden. I dedicate the book to Natalie, Piper, Sarah Bretia, and Ella Skye, learners all.

Introduction

ST MARY'S HOSPITAL began to admit patients and students in 1851, almost the same day that, across Hyde Park, the Crystal Palace opened its doors to visitors. The inhabitants of Paddington were probably no less fiercely proud of their hospital than they were of Britain's pre-eminence in the Great Exhibition, for both accomplishments spoke to a high-Victorian faith in the value of material progress through the growth of knowledge and in man's essential humanity to man.[1] St Mary's was not the first of the great London voluntary hospitals: in fact, it was at the tail end of a movement. Close by the Crystal Palace at Hyde Park Corner stood St George's Hospital, founded in 1733, shortly after the Westminster Hospital in 1720 and before the Middlesex Hospital in 1745. All of them reflected the growth of population and public philanthropy in West London.

St Mary's was the last of the great voluntary hospitals to be founded, but it was the first to be founded as a teaching hospital, with a school attached to it from the beginning. Students had walked the wards of hospitals since the previous century, but hospital governors were slow to permit formal recognition of schools. Often governors shared a distrust of scientific inquiry – of experimentation on patients – with the general population. The founding governors of St Mary's harboured no such fears, and they determined that their hospital would reflect their optimism about science as well as their concern for the sick poor. For a century and a half, school and hospital flourished side by side. But at the end of the twentieth century, the medical school was relocated to Imperial College, just south of Hyde Park, on land originally purchased with the profits of the Great Exhibition and dedicated to the advancement of science and technology.

In 1996 I was asked to write the history of St Mary's Hospital Medical School. As a professional historian, I wanted to do more than to commemorate the school; I wanted to identify the forces and influences that led to its creation, that sustained and shaped it over the years, and that made it unsustainable at the end of the twentieth century. To do that, it was necessary to venture beyond the walls of the medical school and examine the social, intellectual, and political world it inhabited. This was going to be a social history, because the whole history of St Mary's, as of contemporaneous medical institutions, rested on one simple but vital fact. Most people couldn't afford to pay a doctor for their services, as they could pay a grocer or an undertaker. Getting the ill to a doctor was always going to be a social affair. In the early years it was organized by groups of philanthropically minded well-to-do people; in later years it was done through the intermediary of the state.

The change from a voluntary, philanthropic hospital system to one mediated by the state was the result of many developments, including the changing politics of medical knowledge. Like medical practice, medical knowledge was irreducibly social. On the one hand, the provision of medicine on a mass scale, in hospitals, multiplied the trial-and-error experience of the individual doctor at the bedside by a thousandfold.[2] Some procedures were seen to be more effective than others, and medical knowledge was advanced. The process had begun to occur before St Mary's was founded, but it increased in pace over the century after 1850. On the other hand, a medical fact is always a social construct. A new observation or a new theory is always advanced within a network of social relationships – within the teaching hospital and beyond. The establishment of medical facts required the development of such scholarly forums as the medical press and professional societies. As the French experimental physiologist Claude Bernard remarked in 1865, "Art is myself, science is ourselves."[3] The construction of medical science required a complex social infrastructure that historians have hardly begun to excavate.[4] This infrastructure became all the more complex as the result of several developments within clinical medicine, including the rise of medical research and the specialization of knowledge. As a result of both these developments, increasingly formal standards of knowledge were worked out in one medical discipline after another. Furthermore, science entered medicine via the medical schools where first the teaching of nonclinical subjects and then much of the clinical teaching passed into the hands of professional scientists and academics.

Specialization, the increased use of scientific techniques and concepts, the accretion of hospital experience, and the formalization of hospital administration together led to innovations in medicine, making it more efficacious. Once basic improvements like asepsis lowered their death rates, hospitals became particularly efficacious as places where skilled knowledge and technology were centralized. The upper and middle classes, which had hitherto relied on private practitioners, began to demand access. Whereas these classes had been content to administer hospital services for the poor, for themselves they now demanded that the state mediate to ensure fair and equitable distribution. They also demanded that the state administer medical education, so that they could be certain their doctors were well trained in an atmosphere conducive to the advancement of knowledge.

The state's intervention altered traditional relationships between power and knowledge. The wealthy subscribers who governed the voluntary hospitals exercised almost no control over the consultants and no authority over the medical practices performed in the hospital. They didn't need to; it hardly mattered whether patients recovered or died, so long as proper forms of courtesy and deference were observed. This is not to say that the governors didn't try to save people's lives, but only that they were more likely to hear complaints of discourtesy than of therapeutical inefficacy. Once the state became involved, it had to ration medical care in a way the governors had not. One way of doing so was to dictate terms to doctors. To accomplish that, the state had to redefine knowledge so that it served power better, a process that required that the state wrestle from the doctors the power to define knowledge. This it did, by invoking both efficacy and social justice. But the doctors were always close behind the state, making sure that their own power – political, administrative, clinical – never quite got lost in the shuffle.

This, crudely stated, is the argument of the book before you. It is divided into five parts. The first outlines the social context within which St Mary's was founded and the standards of medical practice and medical knowledge prevalent in mid-nineteenth-century London. The second, examining the turn of the twentieth century, signals the beginnings of change; successive chapters describe the growing efficacy of hospital practice and "medicalization of the hospital," the early appearance of scientific research in the pathology department, and the attempts by the traditional clinicians running the medical school to keep up with the growing demands of science. The third section, which concentrates on the interwar period, outlines the pressures (viewed both locally and nationally) leading to the National Health Service, and the re-organization of the pathology research institute and the medical school, both of which teetered on the brink of scientific and pedagogical modernity.

In the fourth section, which focuses more narrowly on the medical school from the 1940s to the 1980s, modernity arrives with a thump.

These three chapters chart the institutionalization of science in the clinical departments, the academic departments, and in the student's life. The fifth section looks at the social and political consequences of scientization, with one chapter showing the confrontation between the state and the hospital under the NHS and another showing the confrontation between the state and the medical school at the end of the twentieth century. The final chapter in the section, which concludes the book as a whole, returns to the matter of social relationships. The emphasis on social history draws attention to the vast impersonal forces buffeting doctors, patients, and lay officials alike, but it also emphasizes that medicine remained first and foremost a relationship among people. It was never *just* about power and knowledge; there was always another, intangible element of concern for the well-being of others, along with an appreciation of the essential complexity of people and of the fact that they have psychological needs as great as their physical ones.

If this book makes a contribution to the existing historiography, it is by insisting that no history of a medical institution can be complete that does not explore both the science and the politics of medicine; here power and knowledge were always intertwined. Oddly enough, no one has ever attempted such an account of any of the great London teaching hospitals. Existing institutional histories tend to commemorate scientific advances rather than probe the conditions giving rise to them.[5] Zachary Cope's history of St Mary's Hospital Medical School, written for the school's centenary, exemplifies this tradition. The book contains a wealth of details, but Cope's decision to organize the book around individual biographies precluded serious analysis.[6] This is not to suggest that there are not some very fine histories of the London teaching hospitals, only that they are not informed by recent work in the history of science.[7] This is a serious lacuna in the historiography because the London teaching hospitals were for much of the period the primary institutions for creating and distributing medical knowledge in England. Without studies of this sort, we have little idea as to how medical practitioners knew what they knew. The present study tries to convey the changing texture and content of medical knowledge over the last century and a half, by surveying hospital practices, textbooks, lectures, informal mechanisms of communication, and above all, scientific controversies, both notorious and obscure. St Mary's provides a useful case study: home to some of Britain's most celebrated and notorious medical scientists and practitioners, it has always been at the centre of debates about medical science and medical politics.

How representative was St Mary's? Some of the forces shaping it were common to all the London teaching hospitals; others were peculiar to it.

Without similar studies of other institutions, it is hard to distinguish the local from the general. Moreover, I'm not convinced that developing a calculus of representativity is a useful activity. Instead, I have conceived of this account as illustrative in the way a biography can be illustrative without being representative. In its very peculiarities, the history of St Mary's Hospital and Medical School serves as a reminder that power and knowledge always have a local, human face. At St Mary's that face was sometimes brilliant, sometimes comic, sometimes joyful, sometimes tragic, but it was never boring.

FOUNDATIONS

The Cornerstone
Paddington

FROM THE BEGINNING, St Mary's was slightly out of step. London's general hospitals were mostly built in two waves, one associated with medieval Christian piety and the other with "Georgian philanthropy" among the enlightened patricians and bourgeoisie. The first to be founded on voluntary subscriptions was the Westminster Hospital in 1720.[1] By the mid-nineteenth century, voluntary hospitals were becoming unfashionable, and St Mary's, in a suburb which in 1851 was characterized by social relations still reflecting eighteenth-century paternalism as much as nineteenth-century industrialism, was the last of the great London voluntary hospitals to open.

Paddington

For centuries Paddington had been a sleepy village on the outskirts of London, most of its inhabitants clustered in a few dozen cottages around the junction of Harrow Road and Edgware Road. The land, formerly monastic, was held by the See of London, which used it for grazing. Consumptives and farmed-out babies were sent to benefit from the healthy airs, and during the Great Plague of London many people were evacuated there.[2] One indication of both Paddington's popularity as a resort for the ill and their blighted hopes for health is a burial rate several times that of the baptismal rate. In 1702–11 there were more than ten births a year on average and more than thirty-three burials. By the end of the century baptisms were in double digits and burials in triple digits.[3] In 1730 a philanthropic medical man named Rees, with the help of some colleagues, set up wooden sheds in the fields of Paddington to cater to travellers and gypsies. Local residents who were unable to pay for medical care also began to attend.[4]

Paddington's other claim to fame was as a way station with some notorious inns. Edgware Road was a major thoroughfare from the north and midlands, carrying goods and livestock for the London markets. Cattle, sheep, and even geese were herded down Edgware and then along Oxford Street to Smithfield, bringing traffic to a standstill. In the 1750s a group of entrepreneurs built a New Road from Paddington to Islington that would circle London, avoiding the paved streets. The New Road, now Marylebone and Euston roads, still carries much of the London traffic away from the densely packed West End. The old cottages at the Paddington terminus at Harrow Road were torn down, and Tyburn gallows, which were at Bayswater and Edgware (where the toll booth was then erected), were moved to Bryanston Street and Edgware. A few years later in 1783 the triple tree was pulled down, first replaced with a portable gallows and then moved to Newgate gaol. This marked the end of "Paddington Fair," or "Paddington Dance," as these hangings were called. The processions from Newgate to Tyburn were too raucous and apt to turn violent.[5]

Property values in Paddington rose, and the prosperous classes of London migrated westward. First Marylebone, and then, as that parish filled up, Paddington drew these rich settlers. The bishop of London and his two hereditary lessees, recognizing the possibilities, obtained an act of Parliament in 1795 that would permit building on a long leasehold (ninety-nine years rather than the traditional "three lives"), and they divided the ground-rents, with one-third going to the See of London. They planned Paddington as a suburban town, with houses for artisans and wealthy bourgeois. But the transport revolution transformed the quiet village into a teeming industrial centre.

First came the canal. The Grand Junction Canal to Birmingham was built during the early 1790s, coming into London at the Thames. Its path was indirect, adding days to the journey, so a branch line was added, terminating in Paddington. The head of the canal interest was William Praed, MP, a Cornish banker who gave his name to the street connecting the canal with Edgware Road. The Paddington branch was inaugurated 10 July 1801, and a crowd of twenty thousand people turned out to Westbourne Green Bridge to watch the spectacle.

Business on the canal basin was slow at first – water was in short supply, the canal banks frequently caved in, and the company failed to build promised roads. But soon it began to flourish, and the Canal Company raised the wharf rents from £50 to £300. One early wharfinger, Augustus

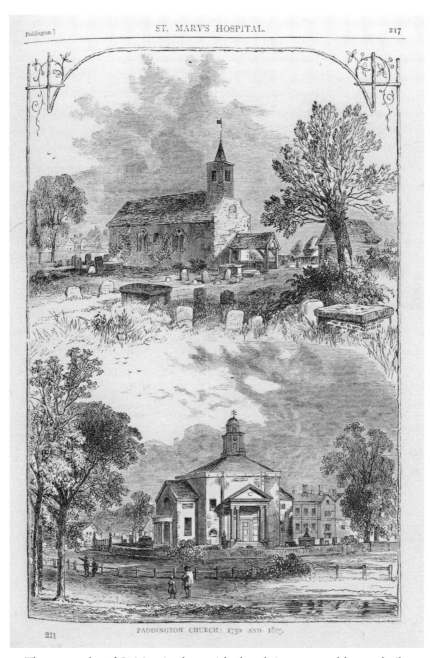

PADDINGTON CHURCH: 1750 AND 1805.

211

The namesake of St Mary's: the parish church in 1750 and later rebuilt.
British Library

Cove, moved his family and business to Chapel Street, Paddington. Unhappily for him, Thomas Pickford, a large carrier, coveted his wharfage and with the Canal Company's connivance assaulted Cove and destroyed his buildings. Cove sued, and he published Paddington's first newspaper, the *Paddington Gazette Extraordinary*, which appeared in ten numbers in 1808, emblazoned with such headlines as "A Trial Now Pending: Goliath against David; alias the Grand Junction Canal Company against Augustus Cove." He posted copies on a board on Chapel Street, where Paddingtonians read them with relish.[6]

Despite Cove's best efforts, the Paddington canal terminus prospered for two decades. Imports included building goods, especially bricks, stone from Leicester quarries, and salt from Cheshire. Exports included waste products from across London, notably ashes and manure.[7] Cattle, sheep, poultry, cheeses, and other foodstuffs were traded at a market that sprang up near the canal basin. In 1820, however, Regent's Canal opened, connecting the main branch of the canal directly to the docklands and bypassing Paddington.

A plan for developing the Paddington estate. Guildhall Library, Corporation of London

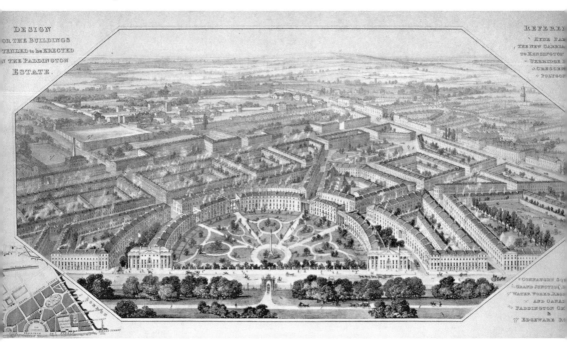

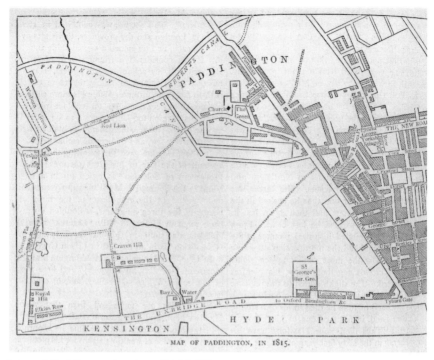

Map of Paddington in 1815. British Library

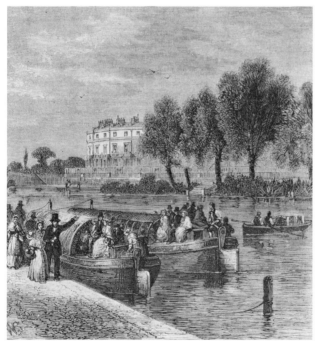

Paddington Canal in 1840. British Library

Even the new canal's conveniences failed to ward off the railways. In 1833, despite desperate opposition from canal interests, the Birmingham & London Railway bill passed. The railway closely followed the Grand Junction Canal, with bridges over the waterway that canal company employees tore down until the railway got an injunction to stop them. While the canals lost the fast-moving traffic, they maintained their share of the heavier traffic. There was still considerable activity around the canal basin into the twentieth century. Meanwhile, the Grand Junction Canal Company had developed the lucrative sideline of providing London with water, although its reservoirs on Praed Street were soon too polluted to serve as the source.

The growth of railways gave Paddington its second wind when the Great Western Railway (GWR) built its eastern terminus there. Paddington was an obvious choice, being at the edge of the built-up area of London with green fields still to the west and north, and the canal handy for ease of shipping across London. The first station, installed under the brick arches of Bishop's Road, couldn't contain the ever-increasing traffic from the west country and Wales, so a larger terminus (which still stands on Praed Street) was erected in 1854, with five platforms and a soaring metal and glass roof modelled after Paxton's Crystal Palace. Fronting it was the Great Western Hotel, the first big railway hotel in London.[8]

Under these influences – road, canal, railway – Paddington developed a growing population of artisans, shopkeepers, and navvies. The green fields disappeared to developers at a staggering rate. The census in 1811 indicated 4,609 people living in the parish, but only one-quarter of the houses were subject to poor rates, "the rest being miserable huts occupied by paupers and very poor people."[9] Many of these were wooden shanties erected near the canal by Irish navvies who planted potatoes around them.[10] Twenty years later in 1831 the population stood at 14,540, and the number of houses had doubled to nearly 2,000; by 1851 these figures had tripled. Growth was especially intense in the northern part of the parish, St Mary's district, where it was over 250 per cent – that is, ten times faster than the metropolis as a whole during the 1840s. One observer estimated the influx of inhabitants over that decade at 1,600 to 1,700 annually.[11]

The rich had drifted westward to escape the worst elements of the "enormous wen." Now they found themselves living in an industrial suburb. Side by side were extremes of wealth and poverty, the "city of palaces" that overlooked Hyde Park serving as a facade for the swarming slums a few blocks further north. On Harrow Road could be found both mansions and almshouses. From the 1840s it was the site of the Lock Hospital and the parish workhouse, but also the address of the likes of James Beatty, Esq., who made his fortune as engineer-in-chief of the Crimea railways. When

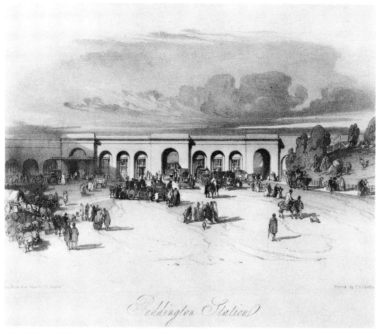

The first railway station in Paddington. National Monuments Record, English Heritage

Beatty died in 1856, his belongings were put up for sale at his premises, 13 Blomfield Terrace, Harrow Road.[12] The auction list reveals what could be found in a well-to-do businessman's house in Paddington in the mid-nineteenth century. There were three floors of bedrooms, with the servants' furniture mostly japanned (lacquered in black), and the family bedsteads in mahogany and damask. The drawing room was furnished in rosewood. The dining room had a Turkish carpet, mahogany chairs and sideboards, and a dinner set for twenty-five. *The Bridgewater Treatises* and *The Builder*, Byron, Clarendon, Dickens, Gibbon, Shakespeare, and Whewell nestled together on rosewood bookshelves.

In contrast to these large, airy houses were the dark and damp homes of the poor, many in the mews between the broad avenues, often atop stables. Censuses and rates assessments showed that the tenements were growing increasingly crowded through subdivision. Poorer families crowded into single rooms, their rents too low to be rateable, so that the parish vestry saw its receipts decline and demands for relief grow.

Poverty wasn't new. The parish maintained seventeen almshouses from 1714 and a small workhouse a century later.[13] But these facilities could not

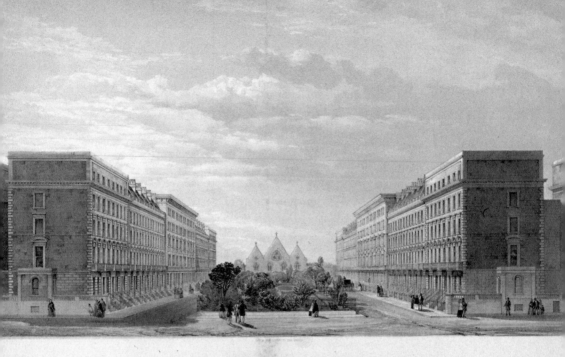

NORFOLK SQUARE, HYDE PARK.
NEAR WESTBOURNE TERRACE.
HOUSES TO BE LET OR SOLD. APPLY TO Mr LINDFIELD, AT THE OFFICE.

Agent's advertisement for properties in Norfolk Square, Paddington. Guildhall Library, Corporation of London.

meet growing demand. In 1820, a year of hardship, dozens lived in the workhouse, and hundreds more clamoured for casual relief. A select vestry, essentially a special committee of leading citizens, was named to investigate and overhaul the system. Reporting two years later, it found 824 people claiming relief from the parish, of whom 635 were indeed legally settled on the parish and entitled to it. The rest were removed to other parishes or refused. At that point, casual and outdoor relief payments amounted to a total of about £37 weekly. The outdoor poor were visited weekly in their homes by the overseer, who would determine their "character and conduct" as well as their needs.[14]

Some of those relieved had been reduced by illness. In July of 1820 the Paddington vestry allotted five shillings weekly to the mother of six children, two of whom had smallpox; they admitted another woman into the workhouse for medical relief after she lay in the fields for two days. Still another pauper was sent to a lunatic asylum.[15] The parish maintained a surgeon who attended the paupers on the order of the Select Vestry or its successor, a "Board of Guardians."[16] In 1837 the surgeon, F.G. Girdwood, had to defend himself against a charge of unskilfulness when he bled a girl whose arm festered. The guardians also subscribed to the Fever Hospital, the Smallpox Hospital, the Humane Society, the Middlesex Hospital, St George's Hospital, the Queen Charlotte Lying-In Hospital, and the Truss Society.

The Poor Law of 1834 ushered in an unhappy new regime for the paupers of Paddington. Prior to its introduction, the guardians tolerated high numbers of outdoor paupers as preferable to "the abuses almost inseparable from such establishments" as the workhouse, and in 1833 they spent nearly three times as much on outdoor as indoor relief – £2,644 as compared to £907.[17] They tried to keep outdoor numbers down by publishing the name, age, and address of every outdoor pauper. The indoor poor, housed in the workhouse, the county lunatic asylum, and a farmhouse in Islington (for "refractory" paupers), numbered between about sixty and eighty, depending on seasonal employment and the weather. Most were women and boys.

The New Poor Law was designed to end the provision of relief to the able bodied by refusing them outdoor relief and requiring that they enter the workhouse. At the same time it would streamline administration by vesting it in groups of parishes, called unions, so as to counter any "unduly narrow local interests."[18] By 1837 outdoor relief costs in Paddington had halved from 1833, while indoor relief remained stable.[19] In 1837 Paddington was made a part of the Kensington Poor Law Union, along with Chelsea, Hammersmith, and Fulham, against the protests of the Paddington vestry who preferred to maintain local control of relief and rates. It formed one of the smallest parishes in the union, and there were frequent financial quarrels. Under the union the number of Paddington paupers rose in 1838–39 to around a hundred, maintained in the Chelsea workhouse. Costs rose as well: in 1839–40, the Paddington vestry paid £3,199 to the Kensington Union. The average stay of a Paddington inmate was sixty-six days.

Sometimes the chain of responsibility broke down, as in the case of an unnamed woman who had two children and no means of support. Her mother took her in, and the four of them, plus another grandchild, occupied a small back room on Kent Place, Wharf Road, near the canal basin. When the woman fell ill, William Ley, surgeon at the Western General Dispensary, was called in and, diagnosing typhus fever, he wrote a certificate for parish relief, which the mother immediately took to the workhouse, but her daughter was not removed for four days, at considerable risk to the surrounding community.[20] In April 1844, following a fatal incident, the Marylebone guardians wrote to Paddington urging "the necessity of some house of reception in this parish for sick and destitute Poor."[21] Probably the Marylebone workhouse on Paddington Street received some of the urgent cases, along with the Western General Dispensary in Lisson Grove with its six beds.[22] The Paddington guardians could do little, for the union workhouses were overflowing.

By the mid-1840s pressure from below and above dissolved the union, and the Paddington Board of Guardians was made responsible for poor relief in the parish. It hired a physician and a surgeon, Dr Mackenzie and Mr Harper, at salaries of £50 apiece. The guardians bought land from the bishop on the canal at Harrow Road and started building, borrowing £9,000 from the Treasury to do so. On Michaelmas Day, 1847, the Paddington workhouse opened.[23] The guardians hired a chaplain and head nurse and arranged for Mackenzie to doctor the inmates. The nursing was done by pauper inmates. The vestry established a gravel pit on the grounds, and the men were put to work breaking stones. Conditions were unpleasant. In January 1848 Mackenzie advised that the diet of porridge, soup, bread, and pudding was causing skin disease, so vegetables and salt pork were added. In February the bedding ran out. Washing facilities were so scarce that inmates washed their hands and faces in their chamber pots.

The Poor Laws increased the distance, social and economic, between the wealthy and the poor. But long before its introduction, Paddingtonians had already begun to emphasize these distinctions. In 1824, taking advantage of Sturges Bourne's Act, designed to reduce relief payments by a process of de-democratization and ensure the hegemony of the propertied, the vestry assigned multiple votes to propertied residents. The change placed parish business in the hands of developers. One local radical, aggrieved by the sudden and steep increase in the rates in the 1840s, wrote, "I am of opinion, after the most careful and impartial investigation of this subject, that the *bona fide* government of this parish is, and has been for years in the hands of the bishop and his lessees, (through their agents in the parish) and a few builders."[24] During the 1840s the main response to problems in Paddington would be the erection of impressive new public buildings: not only the workhouse but also a new vestry hall, a succession of churches, and the voluntary hospital.

In 1848, pointing to the green fields, the guardians congratulated themselves on the "comparative healthiness and cleanly State of this Parish generally."[25] If one counted the death rate by the square yard, Paddington looked healthy, but calculated on a per capita basis, it looked less so. The London death rate was twenty-four per thousand for the six years ending in 1853. In Paddington it was eighteen per thousand, but in poorer North Paddington it was twenty-three per thousand. As for epidemic diseases, while figures for Paddington were below London as a whole (18 per cent of mortality versus 28 per cent for London), some areas were repeatedly struck by cholera, smallpox, scarlet fever, measles, whooping cough, diarrhoea, typhus, and typhoid fever.[26]

The causes of disease seemed obvious: "It is now all but universally known that wherever there is an accumulation of decaying vegetable and animal matter, there will arise from it effluvium offensive to the senses and injurious to health." This was published in 1847 as the considered opinion of the Metropolitan Working Classes' Association for Improving the Public Health (its motto, "We can be useful no longer than we are well").[27] Open sewers festered, including the Bayswater, once a charming brook, finally covered over as Ranelagh sewer at mid-century. Sewage was a burning issue, the sort of thing an MP would loudly berate.[28] Then there was the canal basin, where bloated animal carcasses bobbed while the rubbish of London awaited transhipment on the wharves. Horse manure spilt into the basin as barges were loaded. In 1856 the medical officer of health, John Burdon Sanderson, described it as "a stagnant and fetid pool" with "a large quantity of animal and other organic impurities, and from its surface every breeze carries noxious emanations."[29] Charles Murchison, a physician at the London Fever Hospital, invoked Sanderson's remark and the clinical records of St Mary's when he blamed the canal basin for outbreaks of typhoid fever.[30] Private builders used the rubbish to build foundations for houses. As people poured into these dark, damp jerry-built cottages, which were poorly drained, poorly ventilated, poorly lit, and surrounded by stagnant, fetid bodies of water, disease became endemic in Paddington.

The well-to-do of Paddington began to worry about the slums. Early pamphlets published to raise support for a new hospital warned, "It is in the abodes of poverty and wretchedness that contagious diseases always spring up, and it is there that they acquire, if concentrated, the virulence which enables them to bid defiance to art, and finally to extend their ravages to the houses of the wealthy and the great."[31] One aspiring medical investigator in Paddington, Graily Hewitt, observed, "Many of the best streets in the parish have deaths set down to them, which there is reason to believe would not have occurred had not disease been present in, and been propagated from, close ill-ventilated streets, or mews in immediate proximity to them."[32]

There were also less tangible, more volatile threats posed by these warrens. In 1842 Edwin Chadwick's *Report on the Sanitary Conditions of the Labouring Population* declared that disease of the body could lead to disease of the social body, that is, to social disorder: "The noxious physical agencies depress the health and bodily condition of the population, and act as obstacles to education and to moral culture; that in abridging the duration of the adult life of the working classes they check the growth of productive skill, and abridge the amount of social experience and steady moral habits in the community: that they substitute for a population that accumulates and preserves instruction and is steadily progressive, a population that is young, inexperienced, ignorant, credulous, irritable, passionate, and dangerous."[33] As England experienced severe social disruption during the 1840s, Chadwick tried to tap into prevalent fears, insisting that sanitary reform could prevent social unrest.

Looking around them, drawing upon the newly discovered science of social statistics, the Victorians saw considerable evidence of social decay. Indictable crime rose sevenfold between 1805 and 1842.[34] The crime wave came home to Paddingtonians when the headless, limbless body of a woman was found on a building site on Edgware Road in 1836. (Girdwood's forensic skills were tested when her head was found in Stepney and her legs in Brixton.[35]) The perceived crime wave was one reason for the state's newfound aggression in attacking pauperism. Another was the cholera epidemic of the early 1830s, which stirred up social tensions as across Europe the rich blamed the poor for creating the filth and the poor blamed the rich for poisoning them.

One response was philanthropic action. Several orphan schools opened. In 1838 the Paddington Visiting Society was formed "to promote the religious and moral improvement of the poor, in co-operation with the parochial clergy, to relieve distress and sickness, to encourage industry, frugality, and provident habits, and generally, to cultivate a friendly intercourse between the poor and the wealthier and more educated classes of society." The society sponsored a provident dispensary on Star Street, as well as a lending library and a savings bank.[36] Other charities were rationalized, as in 1838 when the age-old parish custom of throwing bread and cheese from the church steeple on the Sunday before Christmas was abandoned, having become "a sort of fair-day for the sturdy vagabonds of London, who came to Paddington to scramble over dead men's bones for bread and cheese." Instead, the funds were put towards parish relief.[37]

During the 1840s such concerns took on urgency. It was during this time that Paddington assumed its modern character as a place of endless motion, "an unconscious synonym for all that is *restless* in a man."[38] The Great Western Railway terminus made it a natural stopping place for the country folk who during the "hungry forties" were driven from their farms to seek a livelihood in the city. The bishop of Nassau later recalled: "The people in that parish were for the most part country-born, too often they had been utterly disappointed in the expectations which had brought them to the great city, but whether prosperous or not, they were nearly always destitute of what is so much better than success in business, the gracious influence of a Christian home, brotherly love, examples of faith and piety among their neighbours."[39]

If social bonds were weak among immigrants, they seemed even weaker among transients. Henry Mayhew's survey, *London Labour and the London Poor*, which was serialized before it appeared as a book in 1851, began by observing that society consisted of two races, those who settled and those who did not: "the pickpockets – the beggars – the prostitutes – the street-sellers – the street-performers – the cabmen – the coachmen – the watermen – the sailors and such like. In each of these classes, – according as they partake more or less of the purely vagabond, doing nothing whatsoever for their living, but moving from place to place preying upon the earnings of the more industrious portions of the community, so will the attributes of the nomad tribes be more or less marked in them." This wandering race was more animal than moral, more improvident, cruel, pugnacious, and irreligious than the settlers, and disinclined to labour or to respect either property or female honour.[40] Such vagabonds teemed in Paddington, especially the sailors, cabmen, and prostitutes who, indeed, each became special objects of charitable attention. Before mid-century there was a special bargeman's chapel run by dissenters, and after mid-century a sick benefit society for the cabmen of Paddington.[41]

Prostitutes had a special presence in Paddington once the Lock Hospital with its attached hostel for Magdalens was moved from Hyde Park Corner to Harrow Road in 1842. They also lived and worked around Paddington, spilling over from the West End into Tyburn, then Paddington itself. Again, the problem came to public attention in the 1830s, as Michael Ryan in England and Parent Duchâtelet in France published lurid investigations of the women.[42] In 1837 Paddington vestry received complaints against "disorderly houses" in Tichborne Street, and in August 1838 the residents of Frederick Street, off Connaught Square, complained that houses numbered 1, 4, 5, 6, 9, 12, 13, 14, 16, 19, and 21 were serving as brothels. By 1841 Berkeley Street and Cambridge Street were added to the list. In 1857 it was estimated that Marylebone and Paddington contained 139 brothels, and 526 prostitutes.[43] Prostitution entered into local middle-class culture. Thomas Hardy wrote his poem "The Ruined Maid" while living in Kilburn during the 1860s. In 1865, at a sermon to mark the consecration of St Mary Magdalene Church, the Reverend J.E. Bennett remarked that the choice of saint was very apt for such a place, a reminder of "the infamous lives, the degrading scenes, the horrible profanations of all that is decent and virtuous which are daily enacted in the streets of the people here surrounding you."[44]

Thus by the 1840s Paddington was seen to be assuming the burden of advanced urban society. More than that, the parish seemed to be concentrating some of the worst features of London life within its boundaries. The well-to-do launched an offensive aimed at repressing social disorder and relieving misery. This offensive was spearheaded by Christians and Christian priests. Of the 106 earliest supporters of St Mary's Hospital, fourteen – more than 13 per cent – styled themselves "Reverend."[45] The church-going public expanded enormously during the 1830s and 1840s, and the old parish church of St Mary's, consecrated in 1791, could no longer contain them. A Baptist chapel opened in Praed Street in 1827, and a Methodist chapel on Queensway in 1829. The Anglican church fought back with district chapels and new churches. The parish church of St Mary's was moved after it found itself on the "wrong" side of the newly built railway tracks and in a neighbourhood – Paddington Green – that was fast declining. ("The glory and grandeur of Paddington is removed further west, and Paddington Green might now just as well be 'over the water,' a district your real west-ender will never admit having visited, and only rarely confess that he has even heard of it."[46])

A new parish church was established in 1845 off Sussex Gardens, and six more churches followed over the next decade. All this building work cost a small fortune. In the nine years ending in 1852, more than £20,000 was raised through church rates, made compulsory at a vestry meeting chaired by the bishop himself. The rates tripled between 1838 and 1859, rising from £14,418 to £41,895. Even the Anglican rate-payers began to protest. In 1834 a Paddington Parochial Association for the Reform of Abuses was formed, and through the 1840s and 1850s protests grew, amplified by a new local journal, *The Ratepayers' Journal for the Parishes of St. Pancras, Marylebone, and Paddington*. There were further protests at shady land deals: repeatedly, aiming to improve land values, the bishop donated waste land for churches and the hospital on streets ravaged by canal and railway works.

The churches, like the hospital, demonstrated the prevalence of Christian and genteel values. The same values were pronounced weekly in sermons, some of which have survived. During the early 1830s the Anglican Reverend Archibald Campbell preached on the text "Stand in Awe, and Sin Not," and he counselled terror, admiration, and love to the parishioners of St Mary's. He remarked, "We naturally feel a certain degree of respect for those that are above us, whether they are above us in station, or in wisdom, or in goodness ... We naturally feel respect for everyone who can help us ... We naturally think and speak with respect of those upon whom our fate depends – who are to try us, to condemn us, or to acquit us."[47] Campbell saw this as an argument for respect of God, but it was equally an argument

for respect of social and political elites, especially when these behaved philanthropically. Joseph Toynbee, the first aural surgeon at St Mary's, remarked in a letter to his daughter in 1860, "It seems strange that the
working people cannot afford to educate their children, provide themselves
with proper homes or pay for medical attendance without assistance from
the rich. But, doubtless, the kindly feeling this induces is a boon to both
rich and poor."[48]

The well-to-do were told variously that the poor should be treated with
sternness and with kindness; that they were, deep down, just the same as
the respectable, and that they were a race apart. Social boundaries were not
inviolate. Economic insecurity was widespread throughout society. Some
men and women rose on the social ladder, others tumbled downwards.
George Morland, a landscape artist who lived opposite the White Lion Inn
in the early 1790s and kept eight saddle horses and livery there, styled himself as a horse dealer and mingled with gentry as well as the pugilists who
fought on Paddington Green. Later he had to decamp from Paddington to
escape his creditors and died in a debtor's prison.[49] Thomas Payne was a
respectable man on the borderline between the labouring and middle classes when he was hired by the Grand Junction Canal Company to superintend their warehouse and wharf at Whitefriars at the turn of the century.
But when he crossed Thomas Pickford, refusing to give Pickford's barge the
right of way in the wet dock, he was speedily fired, his papers seized, and
his accounts not settled. He died in the poorhouse in 1814.[50] Half a century later one pauper called upon to testify about conditions at the Paddington workhouse was a badly crippled woman named Mary M'Donnell. In
the course of her testimony, the "Commissioner remarked that the witness
seemed well educated, and she began to cry very bitterly, and said her father (now dead) was a gentleman by position."[50] M'Donnell's case merits
attention because her illness may have been responsible for her poverty. Increasingly after 1834, historian Ruth Hodgkinson remarks, sickness was
seen to be not just *a* problem of poverty, but *the* problem of poverty.[51] This
fact slowly worked its way into state policy.

The Poor Law of 1834 made no provision for illness.[52] Traditionally
many vestries granted medical relief to the sick poor without imposing the
humiliating legal burdens of pauperization. However, under the New Poor
Law, illness was not a mitigating circumstance. Only paupers were eligible
for free care by vestry-paid medical officers. Therefore, anyone ill and unable to pay for a private practitioner or a nurse was legally obliged to sell
the family possessions, break up the household, and enter the workhouse.
In 1840 the Poor Law commissioners reaffirmed the principle when they
determined that medical relief was to be offered but only when "absolutely
necessary" so as to prevent medical relief "from generating or encouraging

pauperism." In Paddington the guardians relaxed the rules so far as to erect a shed for storing the furniture of those who entered the workhouse through sickness.

The refusal to distinguish between the healthy and the sick reveals the intended strengths and ultimate weakness of the system. The reforms introduced into the Poor Law in the 1830s aimed to make it more impersonal and thus more certain in its workings. In this they paralleled reforms to the justice system, which Bentham and his followers tried to make more visible, predictable, and educative so as to deter wrongdoing and build character.[54] The Poor Law was intended to reinforce the discipline of the marketplace, which dealt bouquets to the industrious and brickbats to the idle. The early Victorians, especially the middle classes, believed that this was justice at work. If an improvident pauper could wheedle a pension from the parish, then there would be no reason not to be an improvident pauper, and the natural justice of the marketplace would be thwarted. By centralizing in the Poor Law Board the power to determine who would be relieved and how, and centralizing in the unions the application of these rules, local circumstances would be prevented from thwarting the course of natural justice. Illness, being a mitigating circumstance considered locally, was lost in the process.

Sickness became the Achilles' heel of the Poor Law. In 1854 a parliamentary select committee remarked that there would be less pauperism if there were more medical relief. In case after case disease caused poverty in otherwise independent families. The Poor Law was supposed to make the relationship between habits and economic status a stable and predictable one; but disease was unpredictable, striking rich and poor, industrious and idle, innocent and guilty alike. Families who had to enter the workhouse because illness had struck a husband, a wife, even a child, were being penalized for something they could not control. And if the poor law system did not serve justice, then it did not teach justice. It might even persuade workers that there was little point in working, if the result of a lifetime's effort could be swept away overnight and the situation exacerbated by an unfeeling government.

One example of an unhappy case, and the kind of social conscience it aroused, was provided by Edward Sieveking to a gathering of "ladies" at a working-man's college in the summer of 1855. Sieveking spoke of a carriage painter he had seen at St Mary's with such severe rheumatism in his wrists that he could not work:

Not long after, having been struck by the pitiable condition of the man, I visited him, and found him in a small room at the top of a house, surrounded by four young children to whom he was doling out a scanty afternoon meal. His wife had died at the Hospital; he was, consequently, ill as he was, required to nurse and tend four children, one of whom was an infant; and, at the same time, there was no possibility of earning the daily bread. What could medicine effect under such circumstances? and is it to be wondered at that the poor man soon fell a victim to such an accumulation of mental and bodily suffering? The four children, of necessity, became inmates of the parish-workhouse; deprived of parental care and affection, what happiness is there for them in childhood, what prospects for their after-life?

Sieveking denounced the philosophy of deterrence: "Let no one venture to say that improvidence is at the bottom of all such misery. My experience would lead me to deny it most emphatically – not that improvidence exists, but that improvidence is the essential cause of excessive suffering and premature death among the labouring-classes."[55]

Paddington's gentry might not worry about such inequities for their own sakes, but their servants were another matter. In 1848 servants were the first to be granted medical relief without a workhouse test. Servants were usually young, poor, and alone, without the means for medical care. Being country-born, they were ineligible for parish relief in the city. Coping with sick servants quite literally brought home to the genteel classes the problem of working-class health. And Paddington was awash with servants. In 1833 they made up nearly half the total population. With a general hospital in the vicinity, on the other hand, the distressing problem of sick servants became a pleasant exercise in benevolence. For a few guineas a year an employer could recommend servants or poor acquaintances to the care of celebrated Harley Street consultants.[56]

A stately new public building would also beautify the neighbourhood and improve the value of nearby properties. Those with the most to gain were among the most enthusiastic founders of St Mary's. At a public meeting called to promote the new hospital, the bishop of London offered the provisional committee a three-quarter acre site near the canal basin (worth £3,885). The Grand Junction Canal Company waived its freehold rights in return for a municipal water contract. The company was represented on the committee and later on the board of governors. Thomas Thistlethwayte, the bishop's hereditary lessee, donated £1,000 towards the new hospital. These were handsome donations, but they were a pittance compared to the rents that the Paddington Estate produced, around £25,000 per year at mid-century.

There were other financial considerations. At the workhouse infirmary the guardians had to pay for medical attendance. At a voluntary hospital, by contrast, physicians and surgeons offered their services for free. Whereas indoor relief increased the rates, a voluntary hospital reduced them, and the costs were distributed among those most able and willing to support it. Paddington paid as many pence on the pound as other ratepayers paid shillings. In 1858 at St George's-in-the-East, the rate was three shillings ninepence in the pound; in Paddington it was four pence.[57] Moreover, "it was a mark of social status to subscribe to, or govern, a voluntary hospital."[58] The *Lancet* observed: "If the millionaire of Belgravia bestows ten guineas on a hospital, where he can send his servants for gratuitous medical relief, his name is advertised in the daily papers as a benevolent patron of charitable institutions. The struggles of the poor ratepayer, whose family is pinched to support the workhouse, are unrecorded and unhonoured."[59]

Then there was the matter of autonomy. The Poor Law was designed to undermine local initiative and to subject the overseers of poor relief to centralized control. Hospital governors, by contrast, enjoyed complete independence. The *Lancet* reflected in 1856 that the British mind was rooted with a "love of governing." This ruling passion was easily and cheaply satisfied by a subscription to a hospital where governors could "enjoy very extensive powers of governing," including dictating terms to doctors.[60] St Mary's Hospital was designed to cater to this ruling passion to the fullest possible extent because rather than by an appointed board as elsewhere, government was by all the governors who cared to attend the weekly meetings.

On this matter of parochial responsibility, it should be noted that the hospital was originally intended to provide for both Paddington and Marylebone and was provisionally named for the two parishes. In 1852 the Reverend J.H. Gurney urged his Marylebone congregation to support the hospital,[61] but though Marylebone's poor patronized the hospital, Marylebone's rich did not. They could look to the Middlesex Hospital and just beyond it to University College Hospital. Thus, when the Reverend Elliott spoke to a Marylebone congregation in 1847, urging the claims of the poor and especially the sick poor ("No real congregation of really faithful people would willingly permit the honest and industrious man to be pulled down by sickness to greater poverty"), he could add, "As to hospitals or dispensaries, this district or its neighbourhood is well provided."[62]

The medical profession also had a founding role. It was commonly said that St Mary's was established by doctors, with the help of benevolent lay persons.[63] The virtual founder of St Mary's was Samuel Lane, a surgeon who had trained at St George's Hospital. Finding his way there blocked by a powerful clique, he rallied support for the erection of a new teaching hospital. Nonetheless, the medical men were only one of the springs of action; the involvement of the well-to-do was crucial. In 1827 a surgeon named Wardrop had tried to establish a hospital off Edgware Road in a small way, renting some houses, but the scheme failed. It was precisely because St Mary's was projected as a large-scale enterprise, one that appealed to the civic pride, benevolence, and self-interest of the ruling classes in Paddington, that the project was successfully accomplished. The early hospital reflected above all the aspirations and the concerns of the Paddington bourgeoisie.

Ab Initio: The World the Governors Made

In 1842 a committee of 106 gentlemen printed an appeal for a new hospital. As well as fourteen clergymen, there were nine "captains" (the neighbourhood attracted returning India men[64]), and six knights or baronets; peers and physicians were absent. Lane was not on the original provisional committee of 1842 but joined it later. This committee pointed out that the district stretching from Oxford Street and the Uxbridge Road to Kilburn and Regent's Park housed a flourishing population of 150,000, with an annual mortality of 4,500. Most of these deaths – 3,000 – were among working persons "who depend on the labour of their hands for maintenance" and who could not support themselves during illness. It had therefore become "the duty of this wealthy and increasing district to provide against casualties and serious illness occurring among its poorer population."[65] In March 1843 a meeting was called in the parochial schoolhouse on Tichborne Street, off Edgware Road, with B.B. Cabbell, MP, in the chair. Seventy men and two women subscribed £1,200, and a provisional acting committee was elected, which included Samuel Lane and several of his family. After the committee supported the creation of a maternity department, women composed 20 per cent of subscribers. By June, subscriptions totalled £4,371, and peers were in attendance. It was resolved to begin building once £15,000 had been collected and to abandon the project if three years did not suffice to collect it. Four trustees were named: the Reverend Campbell, B.B. Cabbell, vestryman Henry Kemshead, and Captain Madan. Henry Tatham was both secretary and lawyer, as well as a generous benefactor. The first chair of the hospital was the genial Duke of Cambridge who dispensed his patronage and his guineas freely among dozens of charities, including fifteen hospitals.[66] He occasionally chaired meetings and presided over fund-raising dinners. When he died in 1850, the seventy-two-year-old Earl of Manvers succeeded him.

Three years did suffice to collect £15,000, including the value of the land donated by the bishop. The provisional board of governors had decided that 380 beds were needed in the district, but that they should begin by

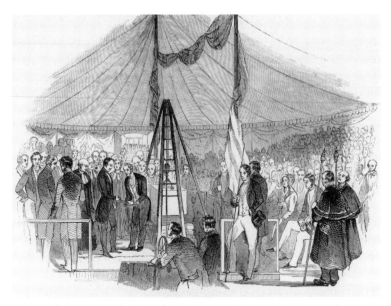

Prince Albert laying the foundation stone of St Mary's Hospital in
1845. St Mary's Hospital NHS Trust Archives

erecting one wing of the hospital to accommodate 150 patients, with the
rest to follow as subscriptions permitted. (Subscriptions, unfortunately,
never permitted.) The architect Thomas Hooper tendered his services gra-
tuitously, designing a stately public building more like a Bayswater palace
than a hospital, with soaring ceilings and a splendid staircase. In June 1845
Prince Albert laid the foundation stone, and the building work began, at an
agreed price of £33,787. The course of construction did not run smoothly.
One contractor died, another went bankrupt, and the work had to be halt-
ed when the governors ran out of money. All these problems led to pro-
tracted legal disputes. Further disputes centred on the quality of
workmanship: the fireplaces, for example, were built on wood and had to
be redone after a fire broke out. There were endless problems with drains
and ventilation. All the board members had their own opinions on ventilation which they aired volubly at meetings.

During the late 1840s, even as the building works stalled, the governing
committee met regularly to plan the management of the hospital. Hospitals
have been described as inward looking,[67] concerned with patients only
once they set foot on hospital grounds and only with cure rather than prevention. But from the beginning the founding governors of St Mary's tried
to incorporate new epidemiological practices by registering the patients.
Vested interests and hidebound routine prevented older hospitals from
pursuing such inquiries, but at a new institution like St Mary's, the gover-

nors announced, such innovations were possible. They laid down the program in their first annual report in 1852, promising that it would permit them to trace epidemics throughout the neighbourhood and, one day, perhaps, throughout the country:

If, therefore, a correct registry were made, incipient cases of such epidemic diseases as Fever, Diarrhoea, and Cholera, occurring in a neighbourhood, might be traced by the hospital records to a particular street, house, or family from which they originate. Such a register would also contain the records of the development, progress, and subsidence, in the locality, of all such diseases; – circumstances of the utmost importance in the study of their causes. So again, as respects another large class, – the hereditary diseases – such a registry, if kept with ordinary care, would contain the records of the diseases affecting the different members of the same family, and of different families related by consanguinity, both direct and collateral, and must very soon furnish to the enquirer some data to distinguish between the cases of disease transmitted from parent to offspring, and those acquired by anti-hygienic influences, and thus lead to a better knowledge of the laws of transmission.[68]

St Mary's was thus a pioneer in health statistics. Prior to this, none but Poor Law medical officers were competent to make such inquiries, but the guardians kept them too short of time and money. In 1859 when Florence Nightingale began her long campaign to reform the London hospitals and asked the registrar general how she might obtain statistics of their work, he advised her that "St Mary's is a more likely institution to supply this information than any other."[69] It seems more than coincidental that, fifty years later, Paddington workhouse would pioneer the use of case files for outdoor relief cases.[70] The fact that the poor were physically engulfed by the well-to-do in Paddington made them more susceptible to middle-class curiosity.

Medicine was the point of St Mary's, but to consider it as a medical project is too limiting. In many ways medicine at St Mary's was subordinate to social and political principles. The idea of an institution organized around medicine was unthinkable. It is thinkable now in a secular age when the principle of the division of labour prevails everywhere,[71] but in the mid-Victorian period other concerns trumped the purely medical. Historian Stefan Collini has argued that moral considerations had priority over all others, including religion, art, and politics.[72] Every medical intervention had also to be considered from the point of view of its moral effect. Even the medical profession was to be moralized at St Mary's, by the provision of a residential college, supervised by the hospital chaplain. As early as 1846, the governors planned the college (modelled on Oxbridge) to reduce "disorderly conduct," thus "elevating the character" of the medical profession.[73]

Medical influence over the hospital was curtailed in several additional ways. It was strictly limited in the first mass hiring (as seen below) and subject to the governors' veto in subsequent years. Every purchase of equipment or medication also had to be approved by the governors. The physicians and surgeons were kept out of the all-powerful House and Finance Committee.[74] Within their own sphere of diagnosis and treatment, admission and discharge, the medical staff were given a great deal of autonomy, save that certain types of patients were prohibited and the governors tried to restrict hospital stays to two months. Autopsies were not always permitted, for fear of offending the patients. Thus the early hospital was largely shaped by the lay governors' sense of propriety and was designed as a constitution or charter for social relations more generally.

The Hospital as Moral Universe[75]

Becoming a hospital governor was easy, so long as you had a few guineas to spare. Subscriptions earned governors the privilege of recommending patients for admission. Discharged patients were given a letter to take to their patron to express their gratitude. The second privilege afforded governors was that of governing. As seen, the provisional committee that drew up the constitution for the new hospital tried to make it a fully public and fully accountable institution by distributing the power of governance among the general body of subscribers, rather than conferring it upon a committee: "The Sub. Com. could not fail to observe that the hospitals in this country have too much the character of private institutions, and they find that there is a growing opinion that at no distant time, amid the social and sanitary improvements which must force themselves upon the legislature, such improvements in the management of hospitals must be included, as will tend, by correct statistics and otherwise, to render them more generally available for the advancement of the sciences of medicine and hygiene."[76] The governors showed remarkable prescience in predicting that publicity and the development of statistics together would eventually make hospitals scientific and public institutions. Still, to ensure that power was not too diluted, the governors also created "permanent and independent" closed managing subcommittees (House and Finance, Medical, Building, and Medical School). They also limited access to the hospital to subscribers and, despite protests from liberal-minded governors, barred reporters from the board meetings. Journalists were all too apt to be cynical and sneering about the work of governance. When one of the governors of St Mary's was caught selling spirits to the hospital at an inflated price, for example, the local press (under headlines of "The Scandal at St Mary's Hospital") commented,

"The governing body contains a large proportion of people who are without any intrinsic ability, character, or position, and who therefore seek to purchase a little social position and consideration by the small subscription requisite to constitute them 'a Governor of St. Mary's Hospital.'"[77]

The founding governors believed that St Mary's could transform their community for the better. It would be a microcosm of the whole, catering to the mind, body, and soul: "The most imperative of our Christian duties, and the most worthy objects of our philanthropy are comprised in this great undertaking, – to comfort and heal the sick, to promote the advancement of medical science, to open out new sources of hygiene, to improve the moral and religious habits and increase the intellectual acquirements of youth destined to follow the medical profession – thus not only to provide for the necessities and to alleviate the miseries of the poor, but to subserve the dearest interests of the rich, are the beneficent objects sought, under Divine Providence, to be fulfilled by the establishment of St. Mary's Hospital."

Not all the governors agreed on all points. Several argued for a closed board of management. One Dr Gairdner submitted his opinions in writing, along with his resignation, maintaining that "popular Government, whether by open Boards or any other similar device, is the fruitful parent of vulgar brawls, great public scandal and total neglect of the real business of a Hospital." Gairdner added that wealth didn't bring "skill" or "experience" in hospital administration, and he insisted on the need for "vigilant inspection and powerful controul not to be obtained from open fluctuating popular Boards."[78] The open-board principle prevailed, and voting rights were, on a majority of five, extended to subscribers of one guinea a year or ten guineas life membership. St Mary's was, then, from the start a liberal establishment. By way of compensation, it was agreed on a majority vote of one that the actions of the weekly board were not open to discussion at annual meetings. Other governors were more interested in the religious aspect of the hospital: the duties and nomination procedure of the chaplain. If a new chaplain was to be elected, the governors attended in legions.

The governors also developed rules of conduct for patients, nurses, and domestic staff. Patients were kept on the grounds, because if let out, they tended to return drunk. The nurses, who began work at 6 A.M. and were in bed by 10 P.M., were ordered to "conduct themselves with tenderness to the Patients and with Civility and Respect to Governors and Visitors."[79] The governors had an endless battle keeping their staff in order. Within a month of opening they had discharged the messenger boy for going AWOL; and within six months they fired one nurse for "inefficiency" and an assistant nurse after "repeated admonitions for insolence and disobedience and promise of amendment." A third nurse went in January 1852 for drunkenness.

The governors visited other hospitals to learn what was needful. They chose iron beds over wooden ones and were spared the bedbug infestations of Paddington infirmary. Medical instruments included a complete amputation collection for £10, a trephining set for £4.10, a post-mortem case for £21, and splints, trocars, midwifery speculums, forceps, catheters, and so on, all for about £100. Within a couple of weeks a chloroform apparatus, stomach pump, enema pump, dental instruments, and a small electromagnetic apparatus had been added. The operating theatre was fitted with a railing for the "visitors and gentlemen" who came to watch.

The governors bought brooms, brushes, buckets, bedpans, beer cans, and bug traps. Every six months they took tenders for provisions. The first order included beef for roasting for fifty every Sunday and "Clods and Stickings of Beef without Bone for Beef Tea"; also eggs, butter, cheese, lard, bread and flour, milk, tea (black, green, finest black, finest green) sugar, sago, arrowroot, mustard, pepper, salt, vinegar, and salad oil. Initial weekly costs for fifty beds were about £20 in provisions, and another £13 went in wages. Butcher's bills were the highest, followed by bread, butter, and beer. In November the governors decided it was improper for the hospital to buy wine, beer, and spirits each day from a local pub, so they put these up for contract. They hired a surgeryman to dole out beer, work the lift, clean the windows and the morgue, make bandages, shovel coal, and attend coroner's inquests. They also took in donations, ranging from pennies inserted into the poor boxes placed round the hospital to Bibles from the Society for the Diffusion of Christian Knowledge to flannel petticoats donated by a surgeon's wife.

Early in 1851 officials from the Great Western Railway asked if they could use the newly constructed hospital as a hotel during the Great Exhibition. The governors refused, insisting that the hospital would then be open, and on 13 June 1851, the momentous words appear in the governor's minutes: "Three Patients were admitted." The first operation was not performed until July, when William Coulson removed a stone from the bladder of a nine-year-old boy by lithotrity – that is, by surgical incision through the perinaeum. John Snow administered the anaesthetic. Little blood was lost, and the patient did well. According to the *Lancet*, "At the conclusion of the operation Mr. Coulson addressed the numerous medical friends who had assembled on the occasion, and in very impressive language and tone dwelt on the difficulties the original projectors of the institution had had to overcome; and he hoped that 'what he had done this day would be the commencement of a long line of services which he and his colleagues would render to the poor.'"[80] By the end of 1851 St Mary's had admitted 348 patients into the wards, of whom half were cured and one-tenth had died. Overall medical, salary, and other costs were about £2,800.

Initially, fifty beds were opened; the next year, the number was raised to 150.

In 1852, the first full year of operation, St Mary's admitted 1,114 patients into the wards. John Burdon Sanderson, who was both medical officer of health and medical registrar, did a statistical survey of these patients which illustrates the early work of the hospital. Most – 57 per cent – were men; women were less liable to industrial accidents and more likely to be treated at home. A third of the patients came from Paddington, another third from Marylebone, and the rest from London and beyond. Half the patients were cured, another third were relieved or convalescing at the end of the year, seventeen were discharged incurable, eighty-eight died, twenty-six discharged themselves, and four were dismissed for bad conduct. Injuries, especially to the head, and fractures made up nearly a quarter of admissions. Disease of the lungs, fever, and rheumatism each accounted for ninety-four cases, or 8 per cent. Around the 4–5 per cent mark each were heart disease, dyspepsia and constipation, anæmia and debility, abscesses, cancer, stricture, and uterine cases. There were a handful of venereal cases, epileptics, erysipelas, hysteria, paralysis, fistula, poison, scrofula, and ruptured perineum. Burdon Sanderson also recorded the occupations of in-patients, dividing them into servants (24.4 per cent), labourers (23.5 per cent), traders and artisans (19.3 per cent), those doing household work (9.2 per cent), cabmen and drivers (3.4 per cent), needlewomen (3.5 per cent), and the rest various, unknown, or children.

The outdoor department, including casualty and maternity, treated 5,067 people in 1852. Casualty patients did not need a letter of recommendation, and there was no means test, so the occasional aristocrat, perhaps run over by a hackney, was seen. In order to continue attendance in the out-patient department, however, one needed a letter. The secretary usually kept a list of benevolent subscribers with a letter to spare, or he might give one himself. At first nearly half the outdoor patients were casualty cases. Fifteen years later, casualty accounted for 58 per cent of all out-patients, but by 1880, another fifteen years later, the numbers were again almost equal. The most acute patients were usually admitted to the wards, so letters were of less importance there, accounting for only 31 per cent of patients in 1865 and 20 per cent in 1880.

St Mary's inherited the Paddington Lying-In Charity, founded in 1843 by female subscribers as a stopgap after the Bayswater Lying-In Hospital moved up in the world to become Queen Charlotte's Hospital in Marylebone. A guinea subscription earned the right to recommend three women for midwifery care. The funds were used to pay local accoucheurs and provide the mothers with linen, groceries (sugar, soap, tea, wine, and arrowroot), and prayerbooks. It was a successful and popular charity, which had raised and spent over £700 in its seven-year life, delivering 1,448 women.

There were no maternal deaths at all, though sixty-eight of the infants died. St Mary's incorporated the charity as it stood; the district accoucheurs were reappointed, and the lady governesses continued to subscribe their guineas to a separate fund. Indeed, so successful was the maternity program that the governors often poached on its funds.

What the patients had in common was poverty, though they might try to hide it. In 1867 Caroline W., a nineteen-year-old servant, came in with "great weariness, palpitation of heart and breathlessness on any exertion; pain in head," as well as heavy menstrual bleeding and a venous murmur. She improved on being treated for anaemia and, nearly a month later, the physician recorded, "It was now ascertained that she was living very poorly (this she had refused to acknowledge before) and dinners were ordered for her from the St. Mary's [soup] kitchen. With this assistance the improvement was still more rapid."[81] Some patients had to be fed up to survive an operation or a malady. One unmarried pregnant woman with persistent vomiting received a spoonful of nourishment every half hour and "injections of beef tea."[82] In 1858 a woman suffering from puerperal fever asked to leave the hospital but was persuaded to stay with a regime consisting of one pint of stout, nine ounces of wine, four ounces of brandy, two eggs, and one pound of beef jelly daily – as well as a full diet and tonics.[83]

In 1860 senior physician Thomas King Chambers admitted a teenage girl who suffered from fever, boils, and abscesses, including a purulent infection of her entire left thigh, which gave two pints of pus daily:

Her state of debility was such that she could not in the least help to feed herself. Yet all this time her stomach was in a state that a gourmand would regard as the seventh heaven. She was literally always hungry. As she swallowed her last bit of beef-steak she would feebly ask when she was to have some more, and what would be her dinner to-morrow. And the way her eager eyes followed any particle of victuals that passed her bed was quite affecting ... So we allowed her wonderful appetite full swing, and fed the delicate puny maid like a gigantic gladiator. The consequence was, that she recovered from an amount of purulent disease which it would have seemed impossible for the human frame to support, and recovered perfectly, for I saw her in the April after looking as healthy and walking as briskly as if she had never been ill.

It is not clear how much good the hospital did apart from bolstering nutrition. On the surgical side, until asepsis improved chances of survival, there was very little exploration of the body apart from its surface and crevices. The recollections of Edmund Owen, who came as a student in 1863 and joined the staff in 1872, were not flattering to the surgeons. Except on op-

eration day, the surgeon hadn't much to do; he superintended a few dressings, inspected a fracture or two, and lectured. Operation day was Wednesday in the afternoon, and all the surgical staff gathered for it. The operating
table was a large pine table with a mattress stained by many dark sinister
blotches. The seniors began with the serious operations such as amputation
or mastectomy, and then the juniors would perform lesser procedures.

Operations included amputation for compound fractures or tuberculous
joints or necrosis from osteomyelitis, joint excisions, jaw resections, litho-
tomies, and colostomies. The students were ignored and watched in silence.
There was no preparation, not even washing of a limb before amputation,
though a very hairy one might be shaved. The same instruments were used
again and again, and the same bloody operating coat was worn by the surgeon, usually a threadbare frock coat. If the wound filled with pus, each
ward had its own sponge to swab it out, the sponge being passed from
wound to wound.[84]

Two St Mary's physicians, one at the end of a long career and the other
just beginning, testified to the limits of medicine. In 1873 senior physician
Francis Sibson confessed to the British Medical Association that whereas he
had been taught how to cut short fever, "Every physician now knows that
fever cannot be shortened by one day," and so he treated only the effects of
the disease, not its cause. Sibson drew an analogy with the accoucheur:
most times labour went well enough without him, but there might be fatal
complications that he could avert.[85] W.B. Cheadle, appointed to the staff in
1867, warned students of the failings of physic: "We confess that we cannot stop continued fever, or acute disease, but we have learnt how to guide
the patient through the mortal crisis, how to sustain the flickering life, how
to ward off the fatal accidents which threaten at every stage. We can arrest
syphilis, check diarrhoea, modify phthisis, relieve or cure epilepsy. We can
control or direct the course of morbid action in a hundred different ways,
prevent secondary lesions, remove pain, relieve distress. And, thus, suffering is lightened, and lives saved or prolonged every day."[86] Unfortunately,
St Mary's did not normally admit syphilis, phthisis, or epilepsy. Still, on the
wards these physicians were not powerless. They could ease pain and provide food and nursing. The out-patient department was another story.
Here, one surgeon admitted, patients deteriorated because they couldn't get
the food and bed-rest they needed, and treatment was "generally a compromise, and not that which the patients properly ought to have."[87]

Poverty was a problem, writ large, that the hospital shared with the patients. Funds were never sufficient to the ambitions of the governors. They
hurried into opening 150 beds in 1852 before they could fully support
them. In 1853 the maintenance deficit was £737. In 1854 it was £2,422,

compounding the original debts on the building. With subscriptions below subsistence, the governors relied increasingly on legacies, which were uncertain. At the end of its first decade St Mary's cost about £7,000 a year to run and brought in only £4,000 in subscriptions. The governors called a public meeting to meet the crisis and heard arguments for and against closing beds, with the former finally prevailing.

The meeting also heard of complaints from unhappy subscribers.[88] The year 1861 saw an unprecedented number of complaints, fourteen in total, aired before the governors, ranging from premature dismissal of a sick patient to insolence among the nurses to medical mismanagement. The register of complaints reveals much of daily life at St Mary's because it indicates expectations of behaviour. Certainly, the governors attached great importance to the full airing of complaints. The early regulations stipulated that all patients be asked upon leaving whether they had any complaints to make. The governors wished to resolve problems in-house before they could become public scandals. Complaints were mostly of two sorts: discourtesy and malpractice. Discourtesy was much the more troublesome to the governors.

Of a total of 139 complaints heard within the first twenty years, seventeen were directed against patients, for insolence to hospital staff or to other patients. One of Chambers's prize patients, a prostitute without a uterus (admitted with advanced syphilis after fainting in the Lock's chapel), was discharged after displaying the "violent temper" typical of her "unhappy class."[89] Drunkenness has been mentioned; other patients were caught smoking in a closet. In October 1862 Eliza Whiteman was sent out to the parish infirmary for persisting in "begging their diets from other patients, in committing nuisance on the floor of the Ward, and wilfully upsetting the whole of the patients' Tea when cautioned not to interfere with it."[90] Quite a different sort of misdemeanour was reported in 1852 when one patient alarmed another with religious importunings. The governors reprimanded the woman "upon the impropriety and inhumanity of her conduct and informed her that she would never again be admitted into the Hospital except under circumstances of extraordinary urgency."[91]

More worrying was rampant insolence among the hospital staff. Honours were equal between domestic staff and nurses: each group earned sixteen complaints from 1851 to 1871. Porters would insist on insulting and even assaulting not only patients but also their patrons. The nurses were said to be unkind or callous towards patients, ignoring their deathbed calls for attention, insulting them (one boy complained that a nurse said he "was the child of a dirty mother and was suffering from starvation"), or filching their eggs. Usually those charged were exonerated. Other breaches of decorum committed by nurses included drinking beer in the ward and sleeping on the job.[92] In 1853 the governors ordered that tell-tale clocks be installed to keep the night nurses from sleeping, but the nurses found a way to fiddle the instruments with a bent pin.[93]

Until the 1870s St Mary's was staffed by pre-Nightingale nurses lacking professional training, but at least one consultant remembered them fondly as efficient, kindly, and unsentimental. Sister Kavanaugh, for example, was a clever cupper and a poet, who "kept her men patients in capital order"[94]; she left St Mary's to become matron of Coventry Hospital. Nonetheless, turnover was high: in July and August of 1854, six nurses were fired for inefficiency, neglect of patients, improper language, and misappropriating hospital blankets. Matron Alicia Wright, the self-taught daughter of a Greenwich practitioner, was twice threatened with dismissal for inefficiency and failure to maintain discipline, but she served till compulsory retirement at age sixty-five in 1876. This may have been because she was well connected: her sister was Lady Lethby. Many nurses persisted until their retirements, and as late as the 1890s one "ancient" nurse was heard to say, "I never see'd the use of them temperatures."[95]

Junior house officers were sometimes rough and rude with their out-patients, either for lack of experience or because they were callous and callow young men. They could be easily chastized, but qualified medical men could not. In April 1853, after a reprimand for tardiness, the entire out-patient staff denied the imputation of neglect and haughtily asserted that being "from the nature of our Offices continually exposed to the complaints of individuals," they rather than the patients should be believed.[96] Later that year the confrontation between position, expectation, and credibility was even starker. A maternity patient living in Kensal New Town complained that the accoucheur, Dr H.A. Aldred, stayed only for five minutes and told her "that the Child's head was pitched for the world," and they must manage for themselves. Aldred defended himself vigorously: he had been attentive, but when he told the woman that he wouldn't be needed for several hours, she and her supporters "began to launch out into the most insulting invectives against me and threatened that the husband would lay a stick about my back &c that I thought it was only becoming to me as a Gentleman, and a duty incumbent upon the dignity of the Hospital that I should refuse farther to attend her."[97] Over time, doctors' attitudes towards patients softened. In 1897 one surgeon observed, "Formerly it was fashionable to treat them roughly, to disregard their feelings, even to swear at them."[98]

Medical malpractice accounted for twenty-one of the 139 complaints heard in the first two decades. Most were made between 1861 and 1865 and may reflect a wider dissatisfaction with the medical profession, which had newly secured legal privileges over irregular practitioners.[99] Doctors blankly denied charges of malpractice, and the governors usually backed them up. If an eye became abscessed or a hand wound scarred badly, the surgeons blamed the patient's unhealthy lifestyle. The only cases that did result in censure votes were those where the doctor or surgeon had failed to see the patient, delegating the work to someone unqualified. A boy named Lindon had his arm treated as a fracture and bound up for two months and was then dismissed by Ure as incurable, but when he was then found to have a dislocation, the medical staff insisted that there had also been a fracture.[100] Twice, patients undergoing eye surgery who lay in bed with bandaged eyes for several days complained that they were neglected by the surgeon. Both complaints were shown to be unfounded and probably speak more of the mental state of the patients, alone, blind, and helpless in a strange and frightening place.

Most complaints made by patients and governors as well as hospital staff (not least the chaplain, who had a strong sense of the respect due him) reflected anxieties about personal relations within the hospital – and beyond. According to eighteenth-century social theory, society was bound together by shared manners.[101] In the nineteenth century, the people who met face to face in the new industrial cities and jostled one another on the streets seemed to lack these shared manners, and it was not clear in what sense they formed a community. The founders of St Mary's Hospital worried about the quality of life in that part of West London where they lived. They believed that it needed a hospital to show the world that Paddington could muster those civic amenities that brought prestige and comfort, and to show one another that the spirit of community continued to flourish amongst the palaces and slums.

Historians may doubt whether a nineteenth-century hospital could improve the health of the sick poor. Regardless, it was essential that the community find some way of accommodating illness among its poor, that is to say, of recognizing its presence and its special needs. Hospitals provided attention – medical, surgical, and spiritual and emotional. People were not reducible to their physical ailments, and much of the hospital apparatus was directed at acknowledging and indeed celebrating this fact. In subsequent years all this was to change. In the face of confirmed social problems, the moral tinkering came to seem less effective, while the medical tinkering became more so. The world that the governors created was to be swept away.

Becoming a Consultant
The Founding Staff and Their Activities

ARRANGEMENTS ON BEHALF of the sick poor in Paddington were determined as much by social pressures as by medical ones. The foregoing chapter emphasized the civic purposes of St Mary's Hospital, as conceived by the lay governors, with only glancing references to the practice of medicine on the wards. This chapter surveys mid-nineteenth-century hospital medicine as a system in its own right, viewed from the perspective of its practitioners: the consultants. A complex interplay of social, epistemological, and technical factors went into the making of mid-century medicine as a pattern of knowledge and practice. By treating the founding staff of St Mary's as a cohort and examining their clinical or laboratory activities and their career trajectories, it is possible to identify the main features of hospital medicine in mid-Victorian London.

The physicians and surgeons of St Mary's were not a cohort until they had been appointed to the staff. Before that, they were collections of individuals. Some were apprenticed, some university educated; some studied abroad, while others practised in the provinces. There was no certain route to success because medicine was very much in a state of flux, with multiple, competing licensing bodies – the royal colleges, the Society of Apothecaries, and the universities. This condition persisted for decades after state registration was achieved in 1858. What the physicians and surgeons did ultimately share was prominence, in the guise of a London consultancy. This chapter describes their paths to St Mary's.

Mid-nineteenth-century medical hierarchies were deeply controversial. The elite hospital consultants studiedly distanced themselves from the mass

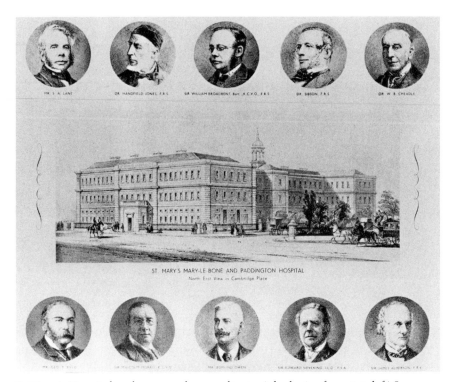

St Mary's Hospital and some early consultants: (*clockwise from top left*) Lane, Handfield-Jones, Broadbent, Sibson, Cheadle, Alderson, Sieveking, Owen, Morris, Field. St Mary's Hospital NHS Trust Archives

of general practitioners, and they dominated the Royal Colleges of Physicians and Surgeons, leaving the rest to be licensed by the Apothecary's Society. By mid-century a large mass of general practitioners demanded licensing reform, higher educational standards, registration, and their own Royal College of General Practice. In West London they formed a "Medical and Surgical Association of Marylebone," to demand a unified education in medicine, surgery, and obstetrics so that, they said, the English public could be treated by well-qualified men.[1] The general practitioners levelled a critique of the medical establishment that has become orthodoxy among historians. Above all, the hospital men stand accused of gaining and exercising power without reference to medical knowledge. S.E.D. Shortt asserts that before the mid-nineteenth century, "Clinical acumen, research publications, and teaching ability were extraneous to the criteria which determined status."[2] Ivan Waddington argues that the status of the physician was "based overwhelmingly on his claim to be a gentleman rather than a technical expert."[3] Geoffrey Rivett maintains "Personal influence rather

than achievement" was "the key to advancement."[4] Jeanne Peterson claims
that appointments were based not on expertise but on educational affinity;
from 1800 to 1850, Guy's and St Bartholomew's only hired their own students, while St George's and St Thomas's did so in six of seven hirings.[5]

Some blamed the emphasis on connection rather than knowledge upon
the lay governors who appointed consultants. The problem permeated not
only medicine but also other would-be sciences, not only proprietary hospitals and schools but also universities. In 1845, when the chair in botany
at Edinburgh went to a local candidate rather than to the eminently qualified Joseph Hooker, Charles Darwin complained, "What a disgrace it is to
our Institutions, that a Professor should be appointed by a set of men, who
have never heard of Humbolt and Brown."[6] But Hooker did enjoy a successful public career. In botany as in medicine, conditions began to change
around the middle of the nineteenth century. Historians of medicine have
signalled this change, but they have not studied it in any detail. How and
why did lay governors alter their hiring practices? *Pace* Darwin, appointment by laymen could be an important guarantee of scholarly credentials.
Samuel Lane convinced the governors at St Mary's to preserve lay control,
warning that if medical men made appointments, aspirants would become
toadies: "If, in our medical institutions, the governors delegate their elective powers to the medical officers without any reservation of private
judgement, they must not be surprised if young men are induced to trust to
their advancement, rather to the favour of those in power, than to their
own talent and industry in the acquirement and improvement of professional knowledge."[7] Thus it wasn't simply a question of doctors obtaining
autonomy from meddling governors so that they could then install modern
medicine. The process was more complicated. British political tradition
privileged recourse to a broad-based public opinion as the best preservative
from faction and corruption. In this respect medical knowledge was no different from medical charity: both required public scrutiny.

The governors at St Mary's spent months discussing the criteria of appointment because they were determined to fill the sixteen vacancies on the
staff according to general principles. A competitive exam was ruled out
since senior men would consider it beneath their dignity to be examined.
While the grounds for each appointment were never made explicit, it is possible to see guiding principles at work in the choices made. One-quarter
were Fellows of the Royal Society (FRS), suggesting a preference for scientific credentials.[8] Half had taught, one-quarter of them at Samuel Lane's
School of Anatomy, suggesting another appeal. Many of the early consultants and governors had liberal and reforming credentials. Three founding
governors and lecturers, Henry Ancell, James Bird, and Isaac Baker Brown,

figured prominently in both the Marylebone Medical and Surgical Association and the National Association for General Practice. Two others, James Alderson and Edward Sieveking, were in the liberal wing of the Royal College of Physicians. Joseph Toynbee and Francis Sibson helped found the Provincial Medical and Surgical Association (later the British Medical Association, or BMA). Whether political affiliation or surgical skill or scientific accomplishment was decisive in any particular appointment is impossible to say. John Rose Cormack was a liberal and a scholar; above a dozen statesmen of medicine testified to his "great scientific acquirements." Yet Cormack's application to St Mary's was unsuccessful, perhaps because he had earlier quarrelled very publicly with the governors of the Royal Edinburgh Infirmary and resigned his position.[9]

If individual cases cannot be determined absolutely, nonetheless a survey of the men who were appointed does permit some general remarks about career-making in London in 1850. In particular, it reveals the growing value but also the danger of resorting to publicity to advance one's career.

The traditional avenue to advancement was by personal recommendation. These informal relationships were not simply nepotistic old-boys' networks, for they also helped to create the preconditions for objective communication. In the early days there was no way to be certain of anything, whether the skill of a house surgeon up for hire or the reliability of an autopsy finding, unless one trusted the person who made the claim. The character and accomplishments of that person served to guarantee what he was claiming. Those with the most honour and prestige were the most credible. Some historians have argued that objectivity evolved from these forms of gentlemanly trust.[10] Genteel status was not a sufficient guarantee of truthfulness (for gentlemen did, after all, disagree), but it helped.

Of course, true gentlemen were amateurs who did not need to earn a living. Doctors earned their living. But by established tradition, medicine, along with the church and the law, was one of the few professions open to gentlemen. Physic was the more gentlemanly, because physicians acquired a university degree; but by the end of the eighteenth century, surgeons too were elevating themselves successfully to the status of gentleman, with Sir Astley Cooper being one outstanding example.[11] Some were more gentlemanly than others: two of the early St Mary's staff "dropped their aitches." By contrast, James Alderson, the senior physician who wore his silk hat and plum-coloured greatcoat in the wards, was touted as a suitable candidate to preside over the Royal College of Physicians (RCP) in 1857, being "a physician of distinguished reputation, a man of science, a liberal, a scholar, and a gentleman."[12]

At mid-century the medical press agonized about how to keep up gentility in the profession. Insisting on a general preliminary education was one way. In 1845 the *Lancet* declared, "We would send forth our students from this great metropolis to the ends of the empire, fit companions for the squire and clergyman of the parish, the nobleman and gentleman of the district, and therefore, if their inferiors, not absolutely ignorant in literature, and well-versed, and far their superiors, in science."[13] A social distinction was admitted, but the goal was to make it as small as possible, especially intellectually. What mattered to the *Lancet* was not whether the lord of the manor would marry his daughter to his physician but whether he would accept the physician's credentials. It was easier for the physician to stand upon his knowledge of physic if he could show a wider cultural competency.

Social and epistemological status went hand in hand. James Alderson sought to transmit to St Mary's students those same genteel qualities that served his own career so well. As he announced during an early clinical lecture (in a long, formal "period" that was itself a demonstration of high literary culture): "The perfection of medical acquirement to be hoped from the opportunities so wisely and carefully afforded – the adoption of a high standard of medical ethics – and the practice of increased refinement of manners, both professional and social, which may be expected from the certain degree of discipline necessarily included in a collegiate system, the want of which has been so often felt in *mere* schools of medicine – are amongst the anticipations which we venture to indulge in; and much good is also to be looked for in the correct and sober views which may be here imbibed, of the true dignity of the profession, and the course which is most likely to extend its useful bearing on society, and sustain its position in the social state."[14] Not just medicine but society itself was to be improved by the change.

As the profession expanded, personal acquaintance became less useful, especially as the graduates of medical schools applied for jobs far afield. Medical societies helped to bridge this problem; here men of different schools could meet and listen to one another. Many of these gatherings were very convivial – social intercourse was still vital to the cultivation of fellow-feeling among the medical men. But along with the journals that reported on their activities, these gatherings also introduced new ways of assessment and new forms of relationships, characterized by increasing impersonality.[15]

The nineteenth century was a golden age for medical societies and medical journals that provided ambitious men with new tools for self-advancement. A phenomenal number of new medical journals came into publication at this time, on average one every seventy-seven days, with boom periods before and after mid-century. *The Lancet* and the BMJ were read by thousands.[17] Most societies published their transactions in some form, while the general medical press printed summaries of the papers and discussions that followed

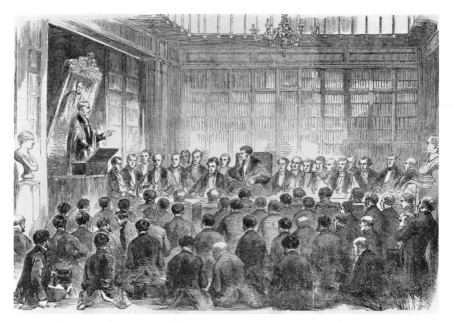

James Alderson delivering the Harveian Oration to the Royal College of
Physicians of London, 1854. The Wellcome Library

them. Controversial topics drew huge crowds, as in November 1851 when
an advertised discussion on ovariotomy at the Royal Medical-Chirurgical
Society drew 145 members and seventy-five visitors.[18]

William Tyler Smith, the physician accoucheur and lecturer on midwifery
at St Mary's, spoke to students in 1860 about the significance of the medical press:

[It] was to the body medical what medical men were to the public. The press,
more than any other influence, moulded the profession as a body politic. By its
agency, extravagances were checked, grievances hunted out and redressed, discoveries made known, and abuses prevented. In a word, the press, as a whole was
an embodiment of the public opinion of the profession, and when it ceased to be
this, it failed in its influence. It was perfectly democratic, as open to the voice of
the youngest student as to the utterance of the highest persons in the profession.
It was a great educational instrument, modifying the laws, institutions, opinions,
habits, and manners of the profession, more than any other single agency. In
consultation, two or three might meet; in Societies medical men might gather by
hundreds, but in the press alone could they all, as it were, stand face to face,
and enjoy the privilege of an exchange of thought. It alone could deal with the
thousands of the profession as with one man.[19]

For Tyler Smith, the profession was an "imagined community" knit together by print culture. But publicity seeking could be carried too far. Medical men were expected to behave like gentlemen, not like Phineas T. Barnum. Physicians who let their names be published by puffing pill-pushers risked deregistration. The frontier of acceptability was always in motion, however, so that what shocked one year could become a well-established genre within a generation.

The Staff Roster

The co-existence of different ways of building up a career, through traditional avenues as well as through the new print culture, can be seen in the life patterns of the senior staff at St Mary's and especially in senior surgeons Samuel Armstrong Lane and William Coulson, both born in 1802. The doyen of the founding staff at Mary's was Samuel Lane, a man of humble origins – the son of a tailor – but lofty ambitions. Lane set out to work his way through the medical profession by teaching and by personal relationships maintained at his school, St George's, as well as in a post at the nearby Lock hospital. Surgical skill and a certain flamboyance helped – Lane was one of the first to attempt an ovariotomy in the early 1840s, and he performed a successful blood transfusion around the same time. He estab-

---

Consultant staff at St Mary's Hospital in 1851

SENIOR STAFF
Surgeons to in-patients: Samuel Lane, William Coulson, Alexander Ure
Physicians to in-patients: James Alderson, Francis Sibson, Thomas King
  Chambers

JUNIOR STAFF
Surgeons to out-patients: James Lane, Henry Spencer Smith,
  Henry Haynes Walton
Physicians to out-patients: Edward Sieveking, Charles Handfield-Jones,
  William Markham

SPECIALIST STAFF
Ophthalmic surgeon: William White Cooper
Aural surgeon: Joseph Toynbee
Surgeon accoucheur: Isaac Baker Brown
Physician accoucheur: William Tyler Smith

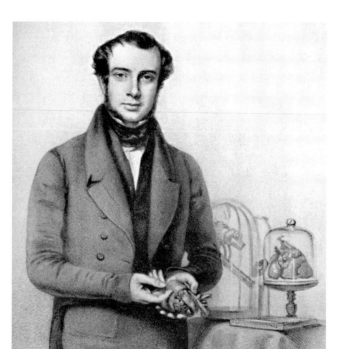

Samuel Lane.
Heinemann and
St Mary's Hospital
NHS Trust Archives

lished at Grosvenor Place a School of Anatomy (modelled after the famous school at Great Windmill Street where he had undergone his early studies), which was intended to provide preclinical education for St George's. But his partner in the enterprise fell out with a clique at St George's that founded a rival school within the hospital, and as a result Lane became unappointable. Thwarted in that direction, but enjoying popularity and prestige by reason of the school and his lucrative West End surgical practice for the bladder stone, he was able to gain professional and lay support for the foundation of a new general hospital – St Mary's – where he and his followers made splendid careers for themselves.[21] He accomplished this almost without publication: in 1841 he began a series of articles on venereal disease in the *Lancet,* but stopped abruptly for fear of being stereotyped as a venereologist. After this he published no more, although letters and speeches occasionally appeared in the medical press, and he edited and updated a classic surgical text. His nephew, James Lane, followed him in all things: the Lock, the School of Anatomy, St Mary's, and the objection to publishing.

The Lanes contrasted greatly with the Coulsons. William Coulson was the son of a Benthamite master painter in the Devonport dockyard. Apprenticed to a surgeon in Penzance, he then studied in St Thomas's Hospital, and in Paris and Berlin during the 1820s. Returning to London, he was

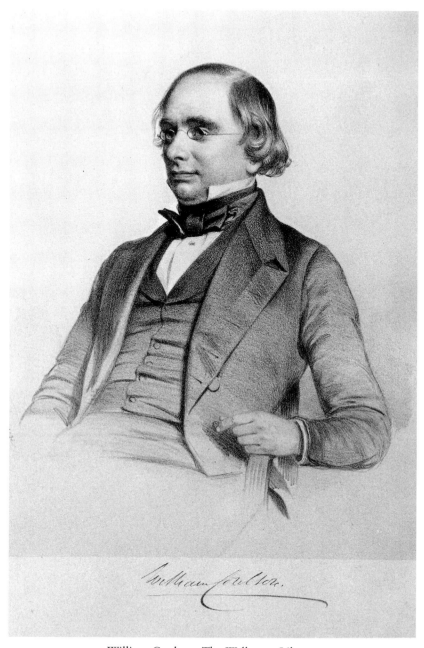

William Coulson. The Wellcome Library

from 1828 to 1832 attached to the Aldersgate Dispensary (which he left
during a dispute about the sale of offices) and from 1830 to the City of
London Lying-In Hospital. Like Lane, Coulson made his name for geni-
tourinary surgery, though his practice was based in the City, so the two
were not rivals. He was a flamboyant performer and would triumphantly
wave a removed stone sixty seconds after making the incision, to a spatter
of applause (though some said that it had been up his sleeve).[22] Celerity reduced both pain and risk of infection. Coulson also introduced to England
lithotomy, an operation to crush the stone without incision. His skill at this
most lucrative of specialities earned him a fortune so that he retired early
from St Mary's to become a sheriff.

Coulson's brother was the editor of the *Morning Chronicle*, and William
(who shared his brother's political liberalism) also began to write for the
medical press and especially the *Lancet* from its establishment in 1823. He
helped the new paper to infiltrate the teaching hospitals and expose them
to public and professional scrutiny, a controversial act at the time. A prolific writer, he was the author of several monographs, most of them first serialized in the *Lancet*. When elected president of the Medical Society of
London in 1861, on taking the chair, he urged his colleagues to publicize
their findings: "Science, gentlemen, in one respect resembles commerce. It
can flourish only in a social state, and under an interchange of produce. We
may produce individually; but to accumulate wealth, we must meet and exchange our products."[23] In 1875, when Samuel Lane voted to exclude the
press from hospital board meetings, Coulson voted to admit them.

Coulson raised a son to follow him, but Walter Coulson lost his place at
St Mary's in 1865 when he took a position at the new Hospital for the
Stone. New specialist hospitals were cropping up, many founded by men
who could not obtain a general hospital position. Older specialty hospitals
restricted themselves to diseases barred from general hospitals – such as
syphilis and lunacy – but the newer ones encroached into general medicine
and surgery.[24] A "hospital for the stone" was the last straw. It threatened
the private practices of surgeons, because the specialists credibly claimed
greater expertise based on the concentration of cases. St Mary's felt the
threat directly when the Marquis of Townshend, having read a piece in the
Morning Post about the mortality of stone cases in general hospitals, asked
for an account of the St Mary's practice.[25] Thus, Walter Coulson was told
he must choose between St Mary's and the stone hospital. He decided to
give up the Mary's position and then run for it again, believing that his supporters outnumbered his critics. When he lost the election, the experience
set back the cause of specialization a full generation at St Mary's. Junior
staff who were advancing themselves through specialized appointments

were forced to give them up: Edward Sieveking his position at the National Hospital[26] and James Lane his position at St Mark's Hospital for Diseases of the Rectum, while another junior physician, William Markham, became the voice of anti-specialism within the BMA. Into the twentieth century St Mary's was a bulwark of generalism.

Like the senior surgeons, the three senior physicians at St Mary's were also studies in contrasts. Two of them, James Alderson and Francis Sibson, practised in the provinces, Hull and Nottingham respectively. They sent papers to the medical and scientific societies, notably the Royal Society (to which both were elected fellows), before coming to London in 1848 in search of greater prominence. Alderson was the son of Hull's leading physician and a Cambridge wrangler, as well as an Oxford DM. In 1847 he published a work on stomach disorders, closely describing a few cases to diagnose indigestion and cancer respectively. While the distinction could not influence outcome (cancer patients usually starved to death), he admitted, a surer display of prognosis would better distinguish orthodox practitioners from the quacks who promised miracle cures. The *Lancet* described the book as the "production of a mature physician, who, after many years of provincial practice, makes his debut in London as an aspirant for metropolitan professional fame, the present volume being one of the means chosen for introducing himself to the profession."[27] Alderson's "urbane manners and pleasing presence" earned him a succession of posts in the Royal College of Physicians, culminating in a four-year stint as president as well as a knighthood and royal patronage.[28] Clinical work was of less interest to him, and he abandoned it in 1867. He "belonged to the old-fashioned physicians who prided themselves on diagnosis by instinct. Dr. Alderson said he could say what was the matter with three-fourths of the patients in a medical ward without turning down the bedclothes."[29] In one of his two Harveian orations to the Royal College, Alderson insisted that medicine was a science, using that term loosely to mean something like organized knowledge. His own medico-scientific writings, on lead poisoning, for example, were bookish and, according to his obituarist, contained nothing of permanent value.[30]

By contrast, Francis Sibson was bursting with scientific curiosity. It was whispered that he was disappointed if his cases, especially the aneurysms, didn't end in a post mortem, and he toiled at the dead house morning and night. He told one student waving a freshly cut kidney in his face, "Look at it, dear Owen, as if you *loved* it."[31] Sibson was apprenticed to an Edinburgh surgeon, studied at Guy's briefly, and then spent thirteen years attached to the Nottingham General Hospital. In 1848 he came to London, obtained an MD from the University of London, and began to teach at

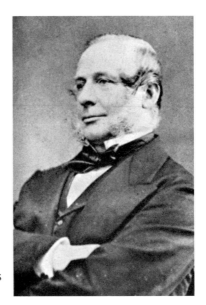

Francis Sibson. Heinemann
and St Mary's Hospital NHS
Trust Archives

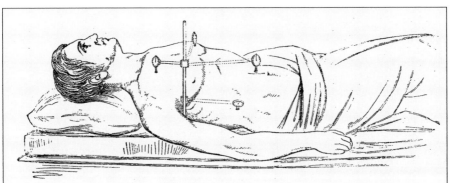

CHEST-MEASURER APPLIED.

By placing the instrument in the manner here represented, the patient lying
on the flat plate forming the basis of the instrument (see fig. at p. 3), the
rack and dial, by a little adjustment, can be successively applied over the various
parts of the chest and abdomen without disturbing the patient.

The patient should be desired to look at the ceiling, that his attention may not
be directed to the dial, by watching which his inspiratory movements are inevitably
disturbed.

The instrument should be steadied by the hand holding the slide carrying the
rod and dial, the finger and thumb having hold of the outer rotating tube of the
horizontal rod (see fig. at p. 3).

To make a complete examination, the rack and dial may be successively applied
over the different parts of the chest and abdomen, in the manner detailed in the
note in the opposite page.

Sibson's chest measurer. The Wellcome Library

Lane's School of Anatomy, where his demonstrations on visceral anatomy were well attended. At Mary's he was remembered as an outstanding clinical teacher. At the time of his appointment in 1850, he was engaged in a mammoth map of human anatomy and was applying this anatomical knowledge to problems of diagnosis – for example, by measuring diminishment in lung capacity, to which end he designed a "stethometer."[32]

The third senior physician, Thomas King Chambers, was also making a splash in London in 1850. A graduate of Oxford, Chambers participated in a movement to reform medical studies there, advising successive regius professors of medicine on the curriculum.[33] He gave the Gulstonian lectures at the Royal College of Physicians in 1850 and had just published a landmark collection of medical statistics, accumulated by examining ten years of post-mortem records at St George's, where he trained. This enabled him to compile figures on the incidence of diseases in the wider population and to discover which were likely to coincide – for example, showing that Bright's could cause heart disease. Here was a body of evidence that anyone could turn to for confirmation, which made it seem more objective than stories by individual practitioners. But use of this source soon became bogged down in a controversy about frequency of uterine ulceration. If some people saw it often and others rarely, then once again the data was only as good as the person doing the post-mortem. Nonetheless, in 1850, Chambers seemed a good choice both as a researcher and as an educational reformer, and he too enjoyed royal patronage.

The governors also hired four specialist physicians and surgeons: an ophthalmic surgeon, an aural surgeon, a physician, and a surgeon accoucheur. Two of them, William White Cooper, the ophthalmologist, and Joseph Toynbee, the aural surgeon, assisted Robert Owen at the Hunterian Museum. Cooper had a position at the North London Eye Institution, and his study of impaired vision went into its second edition in 1850. He died just before receiving a knighthood in 1886. Toynbee is a more memorable character, the first aural surgeon to obtain a position in a general hospital. The son of a large tenant farmer in Lincolnshire, he was apprenticed to a London practitioner and studied at Little Windmill Street, St George's, and University College Hospital. He was elected surgeon to the St James and St George's Dispensary but continued his anatomical dissections and was elected FRS in 1842 for demonstrating the non-vascularity of auricular cartilage. In the late 1830s he took up aural surgery, vowing to make it a field of academic study. He performed thousands of dissections and collected hundreds of ears. His important contributions to the field included a prototype artificial eardrum as well as some anatomical discoveries.[34] Toynbee was also a champion of better education and living conditions for the

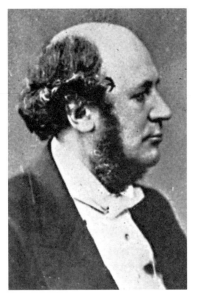

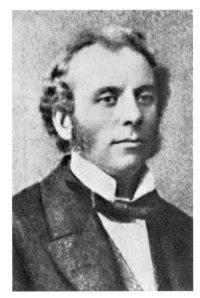

Thomas King Chambers.
Heinemann and St Mary's
Hospital NHS Trust Archives

Joseph Toynbee.
Heinemann and St Mary's
Hospital NHS Trust Archives

Isaac Baker Brown.
The Wellcome Library
and British Journal
of Obstetrics and
Gynaecology

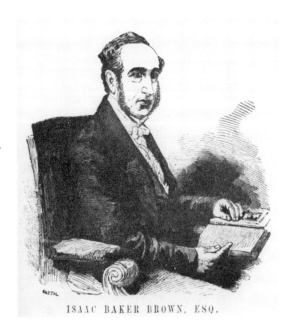

ISAAC BAKER BROWN, ESQ.

working classes, and his son was a man of the same mettle, an early advocate of the university settlement movement that became Toynbee Hall.
Joseph Toynbee died a martyr to experimentalism in the chemistry lab at St
Mary's when he inhaled some prussic acid and chloroform that he thought
might cure tinitis.

The two accoucheurs were equally remarkable figures. Isaac Baker
Brown, the surgeon accoucheur, was a nephew of Samuel Lane, but his career was in the Coulson mode, marked by great showmanship and inces-
sant publication. Hardly a month went by without a paper trumpeting the
latest results of his latest surgical technique. He had considerable success
repairing ruptured perinaeums and, with Spencer Wells, helped to make
ovariotomy a practical technique. The operation was a drastic one, a last
resort for women who had not been relieved by tapping or pressure (Baker
Brown favoured *The Life of Nelson* strapped to the belly) and would die
without it. He made enemies at St Mary's, and these colleagues threatened
to call in the coroner if another patient died from the operation.[35] Consequently, he opened his own small hospital in Bayswater, the London Surgical Home for Women, and when it proved a success, resigned from St
Mary's in 1858. William Tyler Smith, the physician accoucheur, who had
been among Baker Brown's foremost critics, finally began to perform ovariotomy himself. St Mary's did not, therefore, hire a surgeon accoucheur to
replace Baker Brown, and as a result became an institutional base for gynaecological physicians, as opposed to surgeons. A successor to Tyler Smith, Alfred Meadows, helped found the British Gynaecological Society.[36]

Tyler Smith was of humble origins and he earned his way with his pen
when he came to London, writing for and sub-editing the *Lancet*. He was
the author of two important works on obstetrics, the first one in the realm
of high science, seeking to apply to parturition physiology and reflex theory (which he learned from his friend, the physiologist Marshall Hall), and
the second one a simple and popular manual. Tyler Smith's mode of ovari-
otomizing was rather different from Baker Brown's. However, like Baker
Brown, he was a ceaseless innovator, developing, for example, a new way of
stanching postpartum haemorrhage (with a flow of water) and a new bougie
that permitted the first therapeutic intervention on the fallopian tubes. He
was an advocate of publicity: at the inaugural session of the Obstetrical
Society of London in 1859, he remarked that publicity and intellectual
progress went hand in hand: "Silence was not progress. As iron sharpeneth
iron, so in the collision of mind with mind, true doctrines were brought out
and sustained. Discussion had well been said to be the very life and soul of
science."[37] For Tyler Smith, textual representation could be preferable to
actual presence. To perform his ovariotomies, he had a cottage erected on

the hospital grounds and kept visitors out so as to prevent infection (he was an early convert to Semmelweiss's theories of infectious transmission). Those who wanted to know his results had to read about them.

By contrast, Baker Brown invited crowds to come watch him operate. When he gave a paper on vesico-vaginal fistula repair at the Medical Society of London in November 1859, he described one operation at which a physician and four surgeons, Jones, Nunn, Hemphill, Harper, and Edwards, all assisted. In the ensuing discussion others mentioned that they too had attended the operations: Dr Hall Davis remarked that "having been a lecturer on midwifery for many years, and having been obliged to speak of the incurability of these lesions," he had, "during the past two or three years, been extremely gratified, in witnessing, both at St. Mary's Hospital and at the 'London Home,' Mr. Brown's great success in the operation for their cure." Likewise, a Dr Gibb "bore testimony to the success of the operation as practised by Mr. Brown at St. Mary's Hospital."[38]

Baker Brown kept up the publicity so as to attract referrals. But some colleagues accused him of publishing prematurely or hiding unfavourable results. He would claim to have cured a cyst with injections only weeks after the operation, and the cyst might refill some months later; or his plastic operations might leave the patient incontinent. Hostile speakers levelled these accusations at paper after paper, and when his former house surgeon at St Mary's, H.H. Vernon, corroborated them, Baker Brown was further embarrassed.[39] His already vulnerable position became entirely untenable when he began to perform clitoridectomies in order to relieve hysteria and epilepsy, which he believed were brought on by masturbation.[40] In 1867 the Obstetrical Society of London (founded in 1858 by Tyler Smith) held a discussion on clitoridectomy and voted to drum Baker Brown out. Forced to emigrate, he died impoverished and insane.

Gynaecological Contentions

The clitoridectomy incident reveals the limits, social and epistemological, imposed upon scientific curiosity in mid-Victorian London. It is ironic that Baker Brown probably did more to publicize his surgical work than any man of his day, and yet he was ostracized by polite medical society for performing "secret" and "unpublishable" work. Faced with this charge at the Obstetrical Society, he responded with perfect truth that no man had been "so open in his practice as I have."[41] He also argued that others beside himself were guilty of similar operations and "secret quackeries." He was right, but no others had gone to such lengths to publicize their work. Baker

Brown was thrown out of the society ostensibly on moral grounds, for having failed to obtain consent from patients and their husbands (he insisted he had and that they were lying for modesty's sake), for having advertised his work to the public, and for having lied to the Lunacy Commissioners about the presence of lunatics in his Home.

Though Baker Brown called for a scientific investigation of clitoridectomy, none was carried out. Even if others tried the operation and failed, this non-replicability would not be decisive, for few had such good ovariotomy results as Baker Brown. They might watch what he did, but they could not so easily do what he did. There was also concern about the entire process of innovation. The Marylebone Manifesto of 1844, which the youthful Baker Brown had signed, denounced qualified men who gained a clientele by "promulgating and adopting a novel and absurd theory" and perpetrating "an experiment upon the health and lives of his fellow creatures, to which experiment many may fall victims." But the manifesto could only give vague assurances that these men were few in number with limited scope for action, that a good hospital education created "established principles of practice," and that medical science was after all improving.[42] That the manifesto invoked the advancement of science suggests that experimentation and innovation were, so to speak, hard-wired into hospital medicine, despite its assurances to the contrary. The idea of experimentation and research was fraught with ambiguity.

Even more important was the fact that it was *gynaecology* at stake. The female body remained a last outpost of mystery, even of enchantment. Obscure emotional and mental forces were thought to connect the uterus to the rest of the body, subjecting even the brain to its influence. The peculiar status of women in society – the fact that they were governed by shame[43] – made their reproductive organs taboo, to themselves and to the rest of the world. Even in the name of science, medical men could not stare at the vagina with impunity, as Tyler Smith told the Medical-Chirurgical Society in 1850: "No man has the right to go, speculum in hand, amongst the generative organs of living women, just as he would go amongst the dead specimens of a pathological museum."[44]

Tyler Smith made these remarks during a debate about the use of the gynaecological speculum. The obstetric physician at the Western General Dispensary in Marylebone, J. Henry Bennet, believed that uterine ulceration was extremely common among women, and he claimed to have observed it thousands of times. Tyler Smith objected that, while the speculum had a legitimate and proper use (in cases of obstinate discharge), it was abused when applied to sick women, some young and unmarried, who came into a public charity for help. Bennet's applications of it, done "in a spirit of experiment, and not from the conviction of their necessity in each particular case, were 2000 *immoralities* altogether unjustifiable." Bennet tried to reply that it was only by overcoming an excessive modesty that women came in for necessary examinations and treatment.[45] But the dispute ruined his chances of becoming physician accoucheur at the new Paddington hospital. Tyler Smith's chivalry was the surer path to professional advancement, at least in the eyes of the lay governors who overlooked his lack of clinical experience and appointed him. When the chivalry had outworn its use, Bennet complained in 1856, Tyler Smith abandoned it and began himself to use the speculum for research, that is, "for purposes of study and investigation as well as for treatment."[46]

Medical men who sought gentlemanly status had to live up to lay standards as well as scientific ones. In the case of gynaecology, this meant they must exercise a certain discretion. Thus Tyler Smith's manual of obstetrics described how to catheterize a woman without looking at her genitalia, "a matter which, of course, should always be avoided, if possible."[47] His operations were performed privately. He opposed the use of anaesthetics in childbirth for reasons of modesty.[48] And, in 1867, it was he who urged the expulsion of Baker Brown from the Obstetrical Society. The charge of secrecy stuck against Baker Brown because women, guided by their (so-called) natural reticence, "dare not for their honour" mention the unspeakable things done to them. Brown's true crime was in being a latter-day Bichat whose slogan might have been "Open up a few vaginas!" He exposed to the light of science what was most dark and secret. Gynaecology was caught between scientific and lay standards of accountability, which would continue to divide medical knowledge so long as lay governors appointed hospital consultants.[49]

The clitoridectomy incident reveals that consensus could be reached about acceptable standards of medical practice. There were not yet full-fledged paradigms in medicine, but medical public opinion could become the basis of an orthodoxy. As much morality as objectivity went into the making of these opinions, but that showed the need for agreement around basic epistemologies, such as the fitness of corpses or vaginas as objects of knowledge, before there could be serious debate about the evidence in a particular case. This accords with the findings of other historians who have shown that controversies over therapeutics in mid-nineteenth-century France and America could lead to consensus.[50] It tends, on the other hand, to disprove the claim that while French and American physicians looked for "for cognitive and technical tools that would transform knowledge and most especially practice," the "English reformers looked more to legislated, structural solutions to the profession's problems."[51] Professional solidarity was always as much a problem of shared knowledge as it was of politics.

Still, the forms of knowledge generated and circulated at St Mary's in the 1850s and 1860s were primitive, as an examination of research practices shows. Research practices are not the sort of thing one expects to find among the London medical elite. According to a recent survey of medical knowledge, "British medicine was dominated throughout the nineteenth century by physicians and surgeons whose chief pride was their lucrative private practices. They did not see themselves as medical scientists; they taught bedside skills that would prove useful when their protégés set up as general practitioners."[52] The author of this statement conflates science with research.[53] The founding consultant staff of St Mary's did not participate in generalized research paradigms, of the sort that Thomas Kuhn identifies with modern science.[54] But they did routinely perform research-like activities. In 1850, introducing the Gulstonian lectures, Thomas King Chambers clearly enunciated (albeit in flowery Victorian phrasing) a philosophical attachment to the advancement of knowledge, achieved through reading and observations derived from practice:

The time spared by us from the active duty of applying our knowledge to the benefit of mankind cannot, I think, be better spent than by engaging our minds in a retrospect of the advances made in science by those whose mission it is to search out pure truth, and to whom pure truth is a final object to live for. To us, knowledge, how good and lovely soever it be for its own sake, must always be a by-end, a step merely towards the still better and lovelier goal of "good-will towards men."

Our object, then, in reviewing these researches, and in adding to them such observations as our own sphere of actions supplies, should be to deduce from them rules of practice, to gather from the tree of knowledge fruit for the solace and refreshment of mankind.[55]

We now turn to the knowledge-generating practices of the founding staff at St Mary's. As sociologist Steven Shapin has remarked, we need to know, quite practically, "What did people *do* when they made or confirmed an observation, proved a theorem, performed an experiment?"[56]

Did Mary's Consultants Perform "Research"?

Today the term "research" usually suggests coordinated investigations performed by teams of workers who receive research grants. This modern sort of research could be seen in some continental universities by the mid-nineteenth century, but not yet in English academe and even less so in the English medical schools.[57] Here the gentlemanly tradition was still strong. Those hired as lecturers, including Burdon Sanderson and chemist A.J. Bernays, did have foreign and thus stronger research credentials than the hospital staff. Original research was invoked by hiring committees during the 1860s as grounds for an academic appointment. The record for the honorary consulting staff is more mixed.

Another of the founding senior consultants was the surgeon Alexander Ure, son of the chemist and philosopher. He inherited his father's interest in chemicals and experimented to find ways of dissolving the kidney stone that might rival Coulson's operation – but without great success.[58] Ure published monographs on several topics, and he was the first to observe "biotransformation," the chemical combination of drugs in the body (in this case, the combination of benzoic acid and glycine to create hippuric acid).[59]

James Lane and Henry Spencer Smith, two of the three junior surgeons, were protégés of Lane and were not at the forefront of either publication or medical politics. Spencer Smith came from Lane's school and became dean at St Mary's, devoting his life to establishing the school rather than practising or doing research, but he did translate Schwann's cell theory in 1851. The third assistant surgeon was Henry Haynes Walton, who already had a position with a small specialist institution, the Central London Ophthalmic Hospital. He eventually became the ophthalmic surgeon at St Mary's. Haynes Walton wrote monographs, sent reports of recent operations to the weekly press, and overstepped the bounds of acceptable publicity more than once. Posters for the ophthalmic hospital were criticized by the *Lancet*, and so was a conversazione Haynes Walton held in 1858 which he enlivened with microscopic displays and a demonstration of the ophthalmoscope, performed on patients from his eye hospital. Worse yet, the affair was publicized in the lay press, as a puff for the institution. The rest of the St Mary's staff hastily denounced the action and dissociated their hospital from the wrong-doing.[60]

The assistant physicians were active in both the medical press and medical politics. Charles Handfield-Jones became a fellow of the reformed Royal Society in 1848 for a piece he wrote on the liver. He spent the 1850s in the out-patient department at St Mary's observing a great number of domestic servants with vague nervous symptoms such as flushing, insomnia, and fatigue. From this clinical material he constructed a theory of "malarial" nervous influences (blamed on the canal basin) to account for nervous disorders in the general population. By 1859, drawing on vivisection experiments as well as clinical observations, he had developed a full-blown theory of nervous inhibition as causing a variety of ailments from rheumatism to pneumonia.[61]

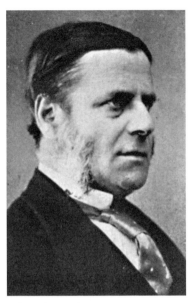

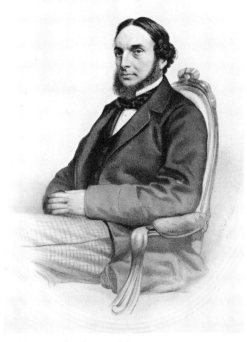

Edward Sieveking.
Heinemann and St Mary's
Hospital NHS Trust Archives

William Orlando Markham.
The Wellcome Library

Edward (later Sir Edward) Sieveking, was versatile and eclectic in his interests, though he styled himself a generalist before all else.[62] The son of a German merchant, he studied and practised in England and Germany and translated Rokitansky, the greatest dissector of his day. He also wrote for and edited the *British and Foreign Medico-Chirurgical Review*. Shut out of the wards, he and Handfield-Jones studied corpses and produced a manual of pathological anatomy.[63] Sieveking tabulated the incidence of tubercular lesions in consecutive corpses, a project that would have been useful to his second career in insurance advising.[64] He participated in medical reform movements, including a campaign to train pauper nurses, and was a member of the Epidemiological Society. He was also a physician to the Prince of Wales, albeit an unpopular one, named by the queen and avoided by the prince.[65]

The third junior physician, W.O. Markham, was an iconoclast. His adherence to a "rational scepticism" earned the opprobrium of the old guard. According to one reviewer, "To have contemplated almost at the beginning of one's professional career writing upon the pathology, diagnosis, and treatment of diseases of the heart, in the face of the clinical experience of Hope, Stokes, Walshe, Latham and Corrigan, was a bold idea, though a very conceited one," and not supported by the results.[66] In the great debate about bloodletting of the late 1850s, Markham took the view that the old

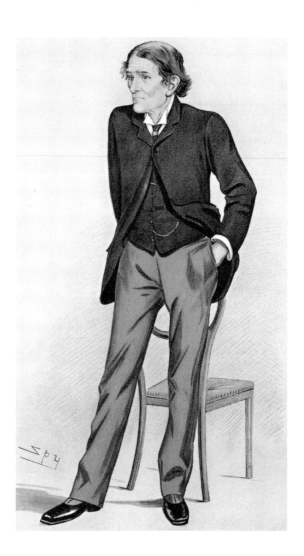

John Burdon Sanderson.
The Wellcome Library

masters had been wrong to think that venesection worked at all. Apparently Markham had his finger on the pulse, because soon afterwards he became editor of the *BMJ*, where he enjoyed a wide audience for his sceptical theories.

John Burdon Sanderson disagreed with Markham and attributed the decline in bloodletting to a decline in inflammatory diseases. He insisted that clinical experience, not pathology, drove the change. Despite this insistence that the bedside was the decisive realm of knowledge, Burdon Sanderson was a pioneer of laboratory-driven medical science. All his life he straddled bench and bedside, beginning as a physician, then becoming a professor of physiology, and finishing as the regius professor of medicine at Oxford. He qualified in Edinburgh in 1851 and then studied experimental physiology under Claude Bernard in Paris. On his return to London, he served as reg-

istrar and medical superintendent at St Mary's Hospital, and when the
school opened, taught botany and medical jurisprudence. As medical officer of health (MOH) for Paddington from 1856, he produced reports that
drew the attention of John Simon, who found further contracts for him, enabling him to gain income from research. Meanwhile he began to perform
experiments on anaesthetized dogs, testing the effects of curare and other
drugs. There were no jobs available at St Mary's, so Burdon Sanderson
joined the Brompton in 1859 and the Middlesex in 1860. In 1870 he gave
up hospital work for physiology, first with a laboratory at the Brown Sanitary Institution (a veterinary centre at University College sponsored with
private funds), then as professor of physiology at UCL, and then as Wayn-
flete Professor of Physiology at Oxford. With Michael Foster at Cambridge,
he spearheaded the "laboratory revolution," by teaching many future physiologists, publishing a practical manual of experimental physiology, and
taking a leading role in the defence of vivisection.[67]

Burdon Sanderson's testimonials reflect the fact that he straddled science
and medicine.[68] The earliest letters, by his premedical teachers, described
him as an assiduous student of medical science. Those sent to the Western
General Dispensary in 1855 added the recommendations of the clinicians
at St Mary's. Alderson praised his acquirements, assiduity, and talent;
Chambers commended his moral and intellectual worth, skill, and benevolence; Sibson described him as "an able, judicious, and untiring investigator of disease, and most kind in his manner to the patients." Four years
later, in an application to the Brompton, Burdon Sanderson had new references with a new emphasis on scientific research. The senior staff of St
Mary's – Sibson, Tyler Smith, Coulson, Samuel Lane, and Ure – still insisted upon his "honourable gentlemanlike character," but the junior staff –
Handfield-Jones and Sieveking – emphasized his research credentials, describing him as "a truly scientific as well as a practical physician, well
versed in physiological and chemical enquiry, and therefore well qualified,
not only to employ the existing stores of medical knowledge, but to enlarge
and increase them by the results of his own work."

Taken as a group, the majority of the staff at St Mary's publicized their
work and actively expanded the medical-public sphere. For 1849, future
Mary's men gave at least sixteen papers before the medical societies; in
1850 the number was thirty-two. At the end of the 1850s the numbers remain fairly high: twenty-one papers in 1858, fifteen in 1859, and fourteen
in 1860. They had their preferred societies, with senior figures like Toynbee, Alderson, Sibson, and Lane more active in the statelier societies like
the Royal Medical-Chirurgical and the Royal Society, and at the annual
meeting of the British Medical Association. Toynbee and Coulson were also

frequent contributors to the new Pathological Society, along with their juniors Handfield-Jones and Burdon Sanderson. The Western Medical Society and the Medical Society of London (the two merged in 1850) often heard from Coulson and Baker Brown, while Sieveking and James Bird were particularly active in the Epidemiological Society. These men also served on the executives: Sibson presided over the Harveian Society in 1854 and Alexander Ure in 1857; Lane presided over the Western Medical and Surgical in 1856, Coulson the Medical Society of London 1861, Sibson in 1862, and Baker Brown in 1865, while Tyler Smith took the chair of the Obstetrical Society of London during the early 1860s. Spencer Smith served for several years as secretary, then as vice-president of the Med-Chi. If a Mary's man occupied the chair of a society, other Mary's men were more likely to present papers.

Whether or not the content of these papers – the lesions counted, the drugs tried, the feline splenic nerves cut – constituted a radical departure from traditional consultant activity, the sheer quantity of publicity was new. Friendly alliances were still necessary for self-advancement, but so, increasingly, was a public display of knowledge or skill. The early staff at St Mary's illustrate this change and perhaps helped to bring it about. To pursue a position at a hospital where one hadn't trained required publicity. At Guy's, for example, there was a flourishing internal community: a large crowd of students, a medical society, and mechanisms for advancement and self-publicity within the hierarchy. St Mary's had no such community in 1850. It is true that a large part of the Grosvenor Place School was simply transported across Hyde Park to initiate the school at St Mary's. This school-within-a-school did form an internal community, and it tended not to publish. Lane accomplished the move by his outstanding personal qualifications and by promising the governors rents from the school. But few of the incoming staff could rely on internal patronage, and so had to publicize their accomplishments. Staff-student organizations like a medical society and a rugby club could not be sustained until the mid-1860s, and a journal not until the 1890s. It was only in 1897 that the St Mary's staff and alumni collectively wielded enough patronage to elect a candidate to the council of the Royal College of Surgeons. Thus, the early Mary's staff had necessarily to be active in the wider medical public sphere outside the hospital, both before their election and for years afterward.

Students and successors followed the same pattern. William Broadbent, who came to St Mary's in 1858 as resident obstetric officer, published widely, spoke often, and became Sir William, senior physician.[69] Ernest Hart began his studies in Lane's school, then came to St Mary's in 1854, and in 1863 obtained the first new consultancy opening at Mary's on the resignation of White Cooper. By this time he had made a name for himself, scientifically with his treatment of popliteal aneurysm by means of flexion, and politically for founding the Junior Medical Society of London. In the early 1860s Hart wrote for the *Lancet*, then became and remained for thirty years editor of the *British Medical Journal*. He turned the small struggling journal into the powerful professional organ it has been ever since. Once again, not all of the newer generation published. George Gascoyen became assistant surgeon in 1864 almost without publishing – but he was another protégé of Samuel Lane.

Most of the consultant staff at St Mary's Hospital performed activities that can only be described as research. Sibson and Handfield-Jones vivisected, while Ure, Alderson, and Chambers experimented with chemicals. T.K. Chambers's fascination with digestion led him to reproduce this process chemically in the school's lab and in the classroom. Several made anatomical discoveries and gained an FRS for their pains. Surgeons proposed or adapted new operations and designed new instruments. There were therapeutic trials of various sorts, as when Sibson gave rheumatic patients enormous doses of opium and then drew up tables to show the results. Sieveking, Chambers, and Toynbee also tabulated statistical results –

Sibson's statistics: coffins represent deaths. The Wellcome Library

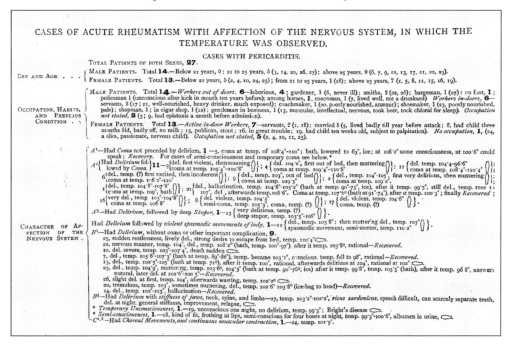

therapeutical, pathological, and anatomical. Handfield-Jones even suggested that the BMA be used to collect therapeutical statistics from practitioners across the country.

All in all, these men worked to advance scientific knowledge in a myriad of ways. They also experimented on themselves, as a story, doubtless about Sibson, reveals: "A late physician to the Hospital was a most enthusiastic scientist. This question of incompetence of the mitral valve was brought forward in private discussion amongst the senior and junior physicians of the Hospital many years ago. It was decided to see what the effects of running around Hyde Park would be upon the hearts of the individuals present. They accordingly ran around Hyde Park – Sir William Broadbent was one of the juniors – and when he came back his heart was as good as when he started. The late physician referred to, an older man, came back in a state of collapse, breathless, and with a systolic murmur at the apex due to over-exertion and fatigue of muscular tissue in his left ventricle."[70]

A snapshot of the gentlemanly approach to scientific investigation is provided by the preparation Chambers undertook for the Gulstonian lectures on obesity he presented to the Royal College of Physicians in 1850. He determined to base them on pathology, treatment, and physiology but, as he told Henry Acland, anatomy lecturer and future regius professor of medicine in Oxford, he wasn't certain how to pursue physiological analysis. He didn't do much laboratory investigation, but he did produce laboratory-style demonstrations, floating tallow dust on water and borrowing samples of injected fat to show to the audience. As for clinical evidence, Chambers and Acland speculated freely on the meaning of their encounters with patients. Chambers noted to Acland: "Your idea about the great extent of capillaries developed in fat people, came just in time to hitch in with my own notions. I have been scribbling on the use of fat in giving the power of resistance to disease, when developed in proper quantity; and am beginning to speculate on the causes of why that power of resistance is lost when the fat exists in excess. Your explanation is a much more sensible one than any I have thought of – It chimes in moreover with Hippocrates view of the subject, who attributes the ill health of corpulent persons to the smallness of their sanguineous organs compared with the size of their bodies."[71] For Chambers, medical knowledge was a glorious and eclectic melange of ancient ideas, laboratory investigations, and clinical observations, all put together into a pleasing literary and dramatic form. The clinical observation – that it is healthier to be well nourished than to be either obese or undernourished – was hardly the evidence-based medicine of today, but it was a true and an important observation nonetheless. "Research" was bricolage: one made do with the tools to hand, rather than setting out to create conditions for inquiry. While Chambers's physiological knowledge was rudimentary and bookish, it was enough to earn him the position of physiology examiner to the University of Oxford.[72]

Francis Sibson made good use of the facilities afforded by the hospital to perform research. He was particularly interested in rheumatic diseases and carried out what would now be recognized as therapeutic trials and cohort studies, for example, by dosing rheumatic fever with opium. He identified the sex and occupation of his rheumatic patients and tallied the incidence of the disease and its complications among a series of one hundred consecutive patients. Many were young women working as domestic servants. "They are growing, their frame is not yet knit, they are sensitive to cold and wet, and they are subject to palpitation..." he observed. "Then the labour of these poor girls, especially in hard places of service, is great and constant; they carry weights up and down stairs, often in lofty houses; they are constantly on foot, standing rather than walking, so that full pressure is continuously made on the joints; or what is worse, they are kneeling, sometimes on cold and even wet stone floors, hard at work, scrubbing and brushing."[73] Another rheumatologist of St Mary's, W.B. Cheadle (who replaced Alderson in 1867), also made important observations based on his patients. With a second appointment at Great Ormond Street, Cheadle developed a large paediatric practice among the middle classes as well as the poorer hospital cases. In an outstanding piece of medical detection published in 1878, he discovered scurvy afflicting some of his patients who were fed on milk substitutes of dubious value. His work helped to place infant feeding on a sound basis, rooted in physiology.[74]

Even where there was a conception of research and an attempt to perform carefully considered experiments, innumerable practical difficulties stood in the way. A paper given by William Broadbent to the Clinical Society in 1869 illustrates some of them.[75] Broadbent developed a simple, clear, and testable hypothesis, that "substances closely allied chemically must have an analogous action on the system, or the diversity in their operation should be capable of explanation on chemical principles." Iron was known to cure anaemia; therefore, related minerals should have a like effect. Broadbent decided to experiment in the St Mary's out-patient department (OPD), an ideal place to see anaemic domestic servants. One such, Emma B., did recover when given chloride of manganese, but an accompanying dose of quinine, he admitted, diminished the value of the case. Another improved under the influence of manganese and dinners ordered from a soup kitchen, but when she began to talk of taking another position, he had to add iron to the regime: "She was by no means well when I gave iron with the manganese; but it seemed likely that I should lose sight of her, and I thought it my duty not to deprive her altogether of the known good influence of iron, lest the improvement should be only temporary." A third case did well on manganese, but twice in his absence his clinical assistant gave iron. In the fourth case, manganese did no good, and the patient had to be admitted to the wards, "where she recovered under the usual treatment." Of patients on whom Broadbent tried nickel, he remarked, "I had many of those cases which make out-patient practice so unsatisfactory, the patients discontinuing their visits after one or two weeks. In some of these there seemed to be marked improvement, in others not. One patient gave me time to try manganese, nickel, and iron in succession, and derived no benefit from any of the three metals."

In short, work could be done, but patients and assistants were often uncooperative, and it was difficult to disaggregate other causes for improvement or relapse. The OPD was especially treacherous to young researchers because they had so little control over patients. The problem wasn't wholly resolved by promotion to the wards. In 1875 Broadbent admitted a forty-year-old woman "of irregular habits and engaged in hard work," with a visibly pulsing aortic aneurysm. During his holiday she was given ergot (Sibson's treatment of choice), but when Broadbent returned he prescribed ninety grains of iodide of potassium per day. The woman improved enough to wander about the hospital but was so abusive and violent towards hospital officials that she was dismissed; she died six months later.

If these isolated observations show the difficulties of medical fact-gathering, nonetheless Broadbent's career as a whole demonstrates how much could be done by a determined investigator.[76] The son of a Nonconformist woollen manufacturer, he studied in Manchester before moving to London to complete an MB. He entered Mary's at the lowest level, resident obstetrical officer, doggedly worked his way through house jobs, a curatorship, a registrarship, and lectureships, and in 1865 became assistant physician. As Cope remarks, he was an outstanding clinical observer, a quality that earned him an MD, FRCP, and FRS. Broadbent claimed he learned to observe from Sibson. His paper on bilateral association of nerve nuclei, which advanced what Hughlings Jackson called the "Broadbent hypothesis," was a classic piece of neurology. Broadbent explained why some volitional movements, such as deep respiration, persist in paralysis, noting that they only occurred in nerves acting on both sides of the body, so that the combined nerve nucleus could be excited even if only one set of fibres functioned. Broadbent was also a leading cardiologist of his day; his wealthy patients donated thousands of pounds to the hospital.

Students and colleagues took up Broadbent's work, but it would be inaccurate to see a research paradigm at work. Broadbent didn't perform "re-

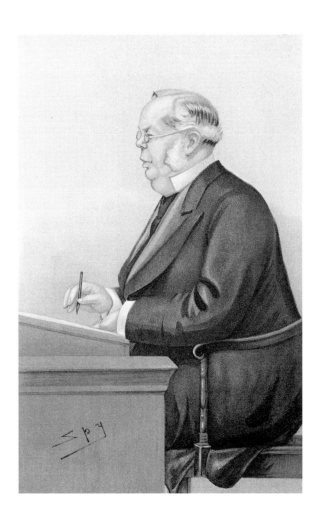

William Broadbent.
The Wellcome Library

search" so much as he made clinical observations.[77] His virtuosity lay above all in diagnosis, which he tried to make scientific by urging colleagues and students to penetrate beyond superficial diagnoses such as "valvular disease" to deeper causes operating according to laws of cause and effect. But this sort of knowledge was not easily taught. Broadbent's lectures did not provide pat answers to propel students through exams. One student, describing a ward round of the 1890s, remarked: "He gives no detailed exposition of all the possible signs and symptoms of aneurysm in text-book style, which no doubt accounts for the remark of a third-year student that 'he is not a good teacher,' but he lucidly and impressively demonstrates the special features of the particular case." For example, Broadbent observed that aortic sounds were "very difficult to describe"; in an aneurysm, "the sound is more drum-like and voluminous than normal."

Other Mary's men tried to depict cardiac disease more objectively. Sibson made extensive measurements and diagrams of the chest in health and sickness and used a tuning pipe to show the pitch of a murmur. Later, David Lees made tracings of the heart to show enlargement. But there was much distrust of these new diagnostic tools among the elite London consultants.[78] Lecturing on a case of mitral stenosis in the 1890s, Broadbent remarked of a sphygmographic tracing of the radial pulse done by a clerk that it exaggerated the oscillations, and he insisted on the advantages of the educated finger over instrumental aids.[79] The physician who had trained his senses to an extremely high degree of acuity tried to teach this acuity; but students wanted simple, objective methods to get them through exams. A sphygmograph was not as good a diagnostic instrument as a Sir William Broadbent, but it was more generalizable.

A comparable confrontation over objective measurements appeared in the *St Mary's Hospital Gazette* of 1907–08. A recent rash of chloroform deaths had blamed upon careless administration, mostly by students. A former student advocated a new apparatus that measured the exact quantity of chloroform administered. Honorary anaesthetist Rowland Collum defended the older, subjective methods and insisted that the safety of the patient depended not on a knowledge of the exact amount of chloroform administered but on the watchfulness and experience of the administrator. Dosimetric methods might answer in the laboratory, but "dogs and cats are as a rule strict teetotallers and non smokers, and do not vary much in their degree of neurosis, or in their general mode of living." However, the pressure for quantitative methods that worked well for the many and not just the few was irresistible. That same year, the physiology lecturer at St Mary's, N.H. Alcock, developed his own dosimetric machine which he tested in the anaesthetic department. Later anaesthetists remembered Collum as an arch-conservative.[81]

The tension between objective and subjective measurement was heavily informed by the mid-Victorian hostility to specialism in medicine. During the 1860s, William Markham, also a cardiologist, confronted this problem squarely during a dispute with Edward Smith of the Brompton concerning the existence of a pretubercular "diathesis" or predisposition which Smith claimed to detect.[82] Markham argued that there was no such diathesis: there was only health or flagrant disease identifiable by symptoms and lesions. Smith replied that Markham could not detect the changes in breathing because he was not sufficiently skilled with the stethoscope. Markham rejected any practice so highly refined as to be, like the cult of Isis, reserved for the few: "Experience has satisfied me that when the ausculatory signs, in any given case, are such as not to present, to any ordinarily skilled person, clear and distinct indications of deviations from health, they are worth nothing as indications for treatment. It surely, indeed, would be wiser to abandon the stethoscope altogether, than to submit to the conclusion that only one man in a thousand is able to use it effectually"[83]

The sceptical Markham was bound to defend medical knowledge as accessible to all capable of reasoning and listening. Truth could only be guaranteed by universality of access, as philosopher Jürgen Habermas has remarked of the nineteenth-century political public sphere.[84] The logic of the argument led Markham almost to a position of philosophical relativism, the view that "truth" is merely agreement among observers: "That which alone can give to a particular fact in the treatment of disease the stamp of genuine value, is the wide and uncontradicted assertion of its truth by competent observers. A true experience in medicine, I would define as the result which is arrived at through the observation of numerous fitting observers; who, after due investigation, arrive each at a like conclusion – the conclusion not being contradicted by the observation of other equally capable observers."[85] According to this theory, knowledge required a community of "fitting" knowers. Mechanisms of sociability were no less valuable in proving one's case than empirical evidence. Clinical knowledge was unambiguously true because so many respectable generalists believed in it.

A further obstacle to the development of clinical research was, of course, the fact that hospital consultants were entirely unpaid and had to support themselves by private practice. This reduced the number of hours that they could spend at the hospital. Broadbent's ward round, careful and searching though it was, lasted only an hour and a half. Sir William Osler, a cardiac authority himself, felt keenly the contrast between traditional British clinical medicine and the new and encroaching forms of systematic scientific research. At a speech given at St Mary's in 1911, he rebuked the hospital pathologist, Sir Almroth Wright, for his contempt of clinical knowledge: "Think of what would have happened if a man of Sir William Broadbent's wide sympathies, clear judgement, and enthusiasm had had a great modern clinique at St. Mary's Hospital, such as those of Leyden or of Kraus at Berlin – do you suppose the bacteriological tail would have wagged the clinical dog? Far from it!"[86]

To conclude, in the mid- and late-nineteenth century, there existed a great deal of systematic knowledge of medicine. Some things were known to be true, others speculated about, others hotly disputed. The clinicians, broadly speaking, tried to enlarge the common pool of knowledge about the body, disease, and therapeutics, often with great enthusiasm and scientific habits of mind. This was especially true of the early staff, who had by and large to earn a name for themselves in order to get a consultancy. Some made important contributions to the advance of medical knowledge. Their successors were not under the same pressure because most of them trained at St Mary's and needed only to impress their teachers. William Broadbent and Charles Handfield-Jones produced original work of sufficient quality to obtain an FRS; John Broadbent and Montagu Handfield-Jones, their sons, who also became consultants to St Mary's, lacked the stature of their fathers, and neither published as extensively. By the time these men came of age, it was more difficult for the gentleman-physician to dabble in scientific research, which was becoming a much more organized and demarcated field of activity. While they might still participate in a wider and somewhat vague "pursuit of knowledge" it was harder now to describe what they did as serious research.

There was little agreement on the identity of research in medicine. The Royal Commission on University Education in London, which sat between 1910 and 1913, heard long and detailed evidence on the relationship between science, medicine, and research. Several distinguished clinicians testified that hospital clinicians performed research. J.H. Fisher, a former dean of St Thomas's, argued, "I should have thought that every teacher is interested in research work, and all our clinical teachers are at the present moment taking advantage of the opportunities which our laboratories and the officers in charge of them afford to advance Medicine." Wilmot Herringham of St Bartholomew's maintained that almost every hospital in London contained at least one man eminent for research and able to organize a research team. He added of research, "We all do it when we are young, we do not get on the staff unless we do; it is because we are known to be men who are working in that way that we are selected."

But when the commission asked the pathologist at St Thomas's for his opinion, L.S. Dudgeon replied that, outside of neurology, little true advancement of knowledge was made by physicians. "I do not know a physician who is famous, apart from the neurologist, for his original work ... If you want to advance research, you must do it by the pathologist."[87] The pathologist at St Mary's, though he had no truck with the Royal Commission, held similar views and did much to discredit the notion that hospital consultants had ever performed anything like research. Nonetheless, when one looks beyond the debates to examine what hospital consultants actually did in 1850, it is evident that they did perform research. Whether or not they did so in 1910 will be discussed in a later chapter.

3

The School

BY 1850 SCHOOLS were cropping up at hospitals across London, actively encouraged by hospital governors. Schools provided prestige, cheap labour on the wards and an income from fees. Lane's school had prospered, and Mary's might do the same. The founding governors proclaimed, a "Hospital without a School is sadly crippled in the noble work which it is founded to accomplish."

Elsewhere, some still opposed letting students onto wards. At the same time as St Mary's was being planned, a governor at the Leicester Infirmary objected to proposals to permit students there, saying he "did not like to acknowledge any object of the Infirmary but what was for the benefit of the poor." As a result, a reference to the goal of promoting knowledge was expunged from the minutes.[1] A local government board order some years later excluded students from all Poor Law infirmaries. In Paddington Infirmary in 1892 the overly keen medical superintendent was firmly told "that there is no intention of making the Infirmary a School of Medicine."[2]

At St Mary's, by contrast, the school was run as a private fiefdom by the consultants and lecturers. They raised start-up costs by selling debentures to local practitioners. They also paid 20 per cent of the school profits to the hospital governors, who nominally controlled the school but usually rubber-stamped the decisions of the Medical School Committee (MSC). Disputes only occurred when the clinicians tried to tailor hospital administration to pedagogical ends.

Nor were many professional controls imposed from without. Before the General Medical Council was created in 1858, the school had only to ensure its curriculum met the lax licensing standards of the royal colleges and the Society of Apothecaries. Courses varied widely: in the 1850s only five of eleven London medical schools taught courses in clinical medicine and surgery, only five taught histology, and one did not even teach pathology.[3] Standards gradually improved, with new classes introduced and attendance on the old ones enforced. The process gained momentum in the 1880s when the royal colleges created a conjoint licence.

Still, examinations were hardly objective. Rather than teaching uniform standards, exams and textbooks taught the students to negotiate the idiosyncrasies of authors and examiners. In 1848 a practitioner named Edward Crisp complained that he failed an RCP examination because he hadn't read a book on stomach cancer by Alderson, who examined him.[4] In 1861 W.B. Cheadle almost failed his Cambridge MD because he adopted the new ideas from Edinburgh and Paris against drugs for pneumonia, advocating only rest and fortifying liquids. The examiner, regius professor Sir George Paget, gave him a sharp look and asked some pointed questions but let him through.[5] Some examiners trotted out pet specimens to display their virtuosity. As an examiner for the Royal College of Surgeons (RCS), the forensic surgeon at St Mary's, Augustus Pepper, always brought his favourite relic, a decomposed skull disinterred from the moat of a farmhouse. The "Moat Farm Murder" made Pepper famous when he identified the skull by dental records as a missing Miss Holland and the murder weapon as a service revolver belonging to her bailiff, who was convicted of the crime. Mary's students knew the relic well, but they happily pretended otherwise until "one cheerless afternoon, a high-spirited youth did not do the preliminary stuff, but on being shown the skull and asked 'What is this?' replied at once, and brightly, 'Miss Holland's skull.' After that, alas! we saw the skull no more."[6]

For three years St Mary's Hospital provided informal clinical teaching to about forty students who paid to walk the wards. In 1854 the school formally opened, having secured the approval of the licensing bodies. When the Royal College of Surgeons criticized the scanty pathological museum, Samuel Lane donated his splendid personal collection. The staff added interesting specimens they came across – pieces of a patient struck by lightening, for example. New staff usually cleaned out the old junk, as in 1873 when violin bows, an elephant caecum, and other items were sold and a spectroscope was purchased with the profit. The first microscope was donated by Spencer Smith, in lieu of an unclaimed sessional prize.

The hospital provided a mortuary or dead house where the students learned dissection. At first the mortuary was housed in the basement, but after complaints of bad smells, a new one was built on the hospital grounds. This, however, created the problem of conveying dead patients there discreetly. In July 1855 the hospital president, Earl Manvers, donated £100 to pay for a covered passage "with a view" (he said, the pun probably unintentional) "to putting an end as soon as possible to the scandal & outrage upon Common decency which at present prevails at Saint Mary's Hospital."[7] Another requirement was a chemistry laboratory for practical teaching, and a trained chemist rather than a dabbling physician. The routine hospital lab was designated the analytical teaching lab and placed under A.J. Bernays, one of a select group of British chemists who trained at Liebig's outstanding laboratory in Giessen.[8] Bernays engaged in research, published textbooks, and soon moved to the older and more prosperous school at St Thomas's Hospital.

The Curriculum

Teaching posts were of several sorts: prestigious and sought-after lectureships in general medicine and surgery, ancillary clinical lectureships, preclinical lectureships, and a roster of low-level practical tutoring or coaching positions. Usually senior staff gave the general lectures, and assistant staff taught the practical and ancillary courses, with the exception of Samuel Lane who taught anatomy (but left practical and comparative anatomy to Haynes Walton and James Lane). The elder Lane's lectures were very popular, and students complained when he gave them up. At a time when these courses were usually taught in desultory way, Samuel Lane was an acknowledged master. Handfield-Jones taught physiology with Lane, Markham taught morbid anatomy, and Sieveking was lumbered with materia medica for sixteen hapless years. These were the core courses.

Specialist staff taught their subjects in the out-patient clinics. Mental disorders were added in 1867, using the Maudsley Asylum. Histology was added in 1864, first as part of the physiology lectures and later as a full course. Hospital governor James Bird taught a course in military medicine when the Crimean War raised interest in the subject. Natural history was taught by the hospital dispenser, who also took in a few dispensary pupils on his own account, as the hospital dentist did dental students. In the 1860s, special classes for higher exams (the MB of the University of London and the FRCS) were added. Morbid anatomy was taught informally until 1860 when a lectureship was created. It appeared in the school calendar as "the elementary structure of diseased tissues, the structure and pathological significance of tumours, and the various lesions to which the internal organs of the body are liable. The morbid conditions of the urine and the different kinds of vomited matter, sputum, &c. will likewise be described. The course will be illustrated by recent specimens from the post-mortem

Theatre, Microscopic Demonstrations, and Specimens from the Museum."
This was all very modern for, as Russell Maulitz shows, pathological anatomy had only recently and precariously established itself on the curriculum,
lagging behind continental schools.[9]

Students could complete the requisite courses in two and a half years, in
part because there was no strict separation of dissection and surgical work.
Lecturers gave the same course year after year, while much of the direct
examination coaching was done by registrars or, from 1870, by tutors.
Changes were made only when the licensing bodies demanded them, as in
1870 when physiology and surgery were split into general and practical
classes, while practical chemistry, pathological anatomy, and forensic medicine were made compulsory.

Whereas hospital governors appointed consultants, the MSC determined
the academic appointments. Consequently, the preclinical lecturers were
chosen on academic grounds. Bernays's replacement, Augustus Mattheissen, was appointed because he was of "very high order both as regards scientific attainment and original investigation." Like Bernays, Mattheissen
soon left St Mary's for a bigger field at St Bartholomew's (where he caused
a scandal by seducing a technician). The dispenser, Lindsay Blyth, was
hired to teach natural philosophy by reason of his "scientific acquirements,
as well as his great zeal and aptitude for teaching others."[10] His successor,
St George Jackson Mivart, came on the recommendation of Thomas Huxley, a leading Darwinian. Mivart turned against Darwin and towards
Catholicism, becoming an isolated and unhappy man. Happily, he was ap-
preciated at St Mary's and given a silver bowl on retirement.[11]

Another academic appointment was Henry Charlton Bastian. A graduate
of University College London, Bastian had completed an MD on the specific gravity of the brain when he was appointed lecturer of pathological
anatomy and curator of the museum in 1866. The hiring committee described him as "the author of many scientific papers of value and importance"[12] (including a piece on nematoids in *Philosophical Transactions* that
very month). A month later, the physicians convinced the governors to hire
him as a supernumerary physician. Sibson was delighted with the appointment, seeing it as a turning point in Paddington, as he confided to a friend:
"In Bastian our profession has a true engineer and worker who, by his
concentrated research, has already advanced science, and will do much to
develop the science of Pathology. I count his accession to St. Mary's as the
most important addition our staff has yet acquired and I feel that it will add
to the growing prosperity of the school, which last year stood fifth in point
of numbers, as regards the new pupils."[13] Bastian, however, left St Mary's
for UCL in December 1867. He too fell out with Huxley and the other Dar-
winians. Among his critics was the St Mary's physiologist, Henry Lawson,

a prolific journalist. Nonetheless, Bastian's appointment at St Mary's reveals that the academic staff could influence the governors. Lawson and
Walter Pye similarly taught physiology in the medical school before they
were appointed to the clinical staff of the hospital.

Researchers made desirable colleagues, but the education purveyed was
distinctly unacademic. Above all, the teachers prided themselves on offering a "practical" education. In 1856, reporting on the school's progress, the
dean and Sibson insisted on this point: the goal at St Mary's was "to make
an eminently clinical and therefore practical school of medicine and surgery; to train up a class of sound and well-educated – because thoroughly
practically educated, medical men."[14] Clinical teaching was still new in
1850, but the English medical schools took it up as their emblem. "Practical" was the highest accolade that British medicine awarded itself, in contrast to the "systematic" or "theoretical" or "bookish" learning seen on the
continent. Generations of inaugural lecturers at St Mary's enjoined practi-
cality onto the incoming students, as William Shepherd did in 1873, calling
book knowledge "the most hateful of all knowledge." Said William Gow
in 1897, "It will require a large amount of learning to conceal the fact that
you find it difficult to remove a foreign body from the eye."[15]

The system of "practical" education had its critics, who complained that
the standard was too low and that it created a medicine with little intellectual content. The GP might know what paces to go through when confronted with the body of the patient, but he wouldn't read medical journals

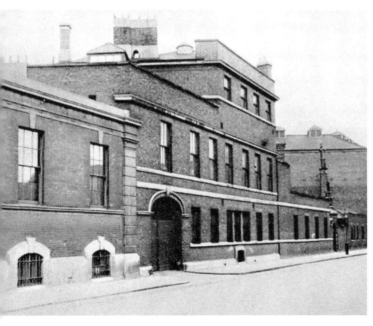

The early medical school
building. Heinemann and
St Mary's Hospital NHS
Trust Archives

to learn of new treatments, let alone contribute anything. Once he had qualified, the GP's intellectual growth was at an end. There was some evidence that Mary's men were among the worst offenders. Edmund Owen, an examiner for the RCS, remarked in 1899 that St Mary's students tended to fail on their written work: "I should think that some of our men have never written a paper, by way of practice, in their lives." Six men had failed a recent RCS exam on their papers.[16]

Attempts were made to spur students to higher efforts. The dean, Spencer Smith, sponsored book prizes awarded annually from 1854. Exams were introduced for the lecture courses. Students wrote answers to questions in six subjects: anatomy, physiology, medicine, surgery, chemistry and materia medica, and midwifery. Practical tests in chemistry and anatomy were added a few months later. In 1860, in keeping with the "practical" emphasis, clinical prizes were introduced, awarded to the students who provided the best case report and the best anatomical preparation. Sibson admitted that "the few books on offer" to St Mary's students couldn't compete with rich prizes at older hospitals.[17] At the same time, the students were regularly bombarded with speeches praising original inquiry. When Sibson urged this ambition upon the students at Lane's School in 1851, his remarks were already such a cliché that they could be summarized rather than repeated verbatim in the press: "Dr. Sibson concluded his address by urging the student to aim high, to prosecute original research, to scrutinise all his cases, shunning routine, whether they be among the rich or the poor, and to extend the boundaries of medical knowledge by adding to its common stores."[18] Such high aspirations met with disappointment: in 1862 even Sibson, though an ardent dissector, complained that students were neglecting their ward work in order to dissect.

Student Culture

The wards, along with the dissection room, were quintessential places of identity formation. It was a relief for students, and sometimes a shock, to be working with living people rather than the books and bits that had occupied them for two years. As one lecturer remarked, it was easy enough to perform a diagnosis when told that a child in the next room had suffused eyes, fever, a rash, sneezing, and siblings with measles, but it was less easy when actually confronted with a two-year-old crying shrilly and hiding his face, while his mother uttered "strange yiddish sounds" or produced a flow of irrelevant information about her eldest child having died of croup the previous year.[19]

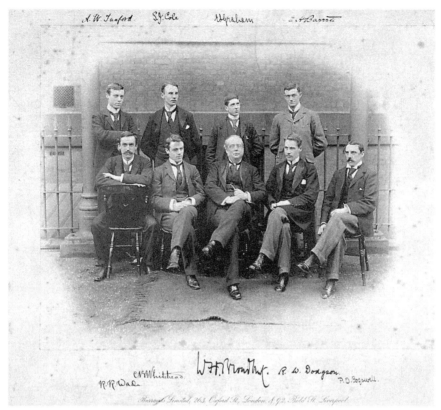

Sir William Broadbent and students in 1896.
St Mary's Hospital NHS Trust Archives

The library. St Mary's Hospital NHS Trust Archives

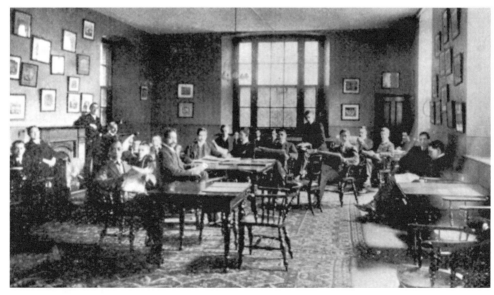

All students were required to follow ward rounds. The "most diligent" became eligible to serve as clerks and dressers, first in the wards, then the OPD, and then the special departments. All students did at least one three-month stint, but the top students completed three stints before being eligible to compete for house jobs. Clerks and dressers took case histories and performed simple tasks, including follow-up attendances.[20] The resident medical officers (RMOs), on the other hand, were qualified. They admitted patients and provided most of the routine medical and surgical care, following courses of treatment prescribed by the consultants. RMOs provided continuity of care between the twice-weekly visits of the senior staff. They were supposed to call in their seniors for difficult cases; Edward Parker Young made a stir when, as a newly qualified houseman, he amputated both legs of a man crushed by a train. The housemen also administered anaesthetic for their seniors, though various unfortunate incidents finally ended that policy.

Just how much *teaching* went on in the hospital is difficult to know. Students learned surgery by watching their seniors operate and by cutting up corpses, neither of which experiences could be called a genuine initiation. There was little supervision in the wards: consultants visited twice weekly, spending only a couple of hours at their rounds or clinics. In 1871 a medical tutor was hired to supervise the students more closely and give them hands-on practical training in preparation for the revised examinations. A medical superintendent was named in 1881 to supervise the RMOs and co-ordinate hospital practices. Nurses also taught medical students; a good casualty nurse could prevent students from making serious errors. It was said of old Grannie Colbeck, who claimed to have taught all the surgeons in St Mary's between 1887 and 1919, that under her boisterous management there were "no cerebral haemorrhages sent home as drunks to die, no broken limbs turned away without support or an x-ray."[21]

Working with living bodies was the second rite of passage for the doctor; working with dead bodies was the first. The corpse was a quasi-sacred and taboo object. Many patients objected to having their bodies sliced open after death.[22] Sometimes autopsies were performed without permission and relatives were horrified to receive back a naked body coarsely sewn up with black twine. By entering the dissection room and picking up knives, the students were flouting social conventions, and sometimes they went too far. In 1866, there was a newspaper scandal when, during a coroner's inquest, a student flipped the sheet of the corpse with his cane, discomfiting the jurors. In 1871 the dissection room had to be closed on Saturday afternoons because the students were running amok. In 1876 someone broke in and overturned body parts into the sawdust.[23] Old students later recalled gruesome pranks played in the dead room, such as the time they parcelled up the pickled heart of a murderer from Newgate and mailed it to a shop-keeper who refused them credit. On another occasion during the 1880s the students played a prank on the dissection-room porter, who turned their stomachs by gnawing on chunks of meat as they dissected. One day they substituted a slice of human flesh for his veal sandwich. The porter took a bite, paused, looked at the sandwich, and then shrugged and went on eat-ing. Leonard Rogers, later Sir Leonard, just managed to cry, "No, Bill!" be-fore leading a rush to the slops pail. When told the story, the porter's reaction was "an angry demand for the return of his purloined veal."[24]

Students occasionally ran wild in the classroom as well. In 1877, when Lawson complained of "great disorder" in the physiology classes, the MSC investigated the matter and found that all the students, even the better ones, had participated in the disturbances. The MSC blamed Lawson, and had he not died soon afterwards, he would have been fired.[25] In 1910 a letter in the *Daily Mail* signed by "Henry Nash, late of St Mary's Hospital" com-mented that the ragging of lecturers in Oxford was nothing compared to the amusement that London medical students derived from their lecturers: "I have known the latter to be bombarded with blotting-paper and india-rubber during what appeared to the students an uninteresting lecture."[26]

Occasionally students were hauled up for bad behaviour. Serious because it became public was the behaviour of students Arkle, Farquharson, and Roberts, who were "in the habit of stretching their heads & bodies half out of windows & pelting & hooting at all the passers by, especially at young & unprotected women." They set upon the landlord, who had them up in police court. When the defence tried to suggest they were studious young men, the landlord replied that the three "were in the habit of roaming about the streets until five o'clock in the morning, and then lying in bed until twelve o'clock in the day. He did not know whether these were stu-dious habits." The magistrate set a fine of £3 and commented, "It was most disgraceful that gentlemen connected with the medical profession should behave in such a manner."[27] Two of the three were rusticated. Being con-victed in court for theft was a sure path to expulsion. So was a drunken assault on a teacher. Sometimes the misbehaviour was purposeful. In No-vember 1893 six students attacked a local medical man who had been tak-ing some of the OPD throat cases, preventing the students from seeing them. They bandaged him from head to foot to immobilize him, soaked him in spirits, and bound him to the railings near his house.[28] The six were suspended for two weeks.

Paying students trickled in slowly, with seventeen the first year, thirteen the next, and only eleven in 1856. Were the students at St Mary's repre-sentative of the general run of London students? An early student described many of them as former apprentices who had never studied any anatomy and physiology. They called themselves "practical men" who could bleed, set a broken leg, and prescribe for bronchitis or gout, but never completing their preclinical studies, they wound up as unqualified assistants. Even Sibson found it difficult to explain cardiac sounds to men who had never dissected a heart and who often had to be told, "Don't say you can hear it if you don't."[29] But things picked up; the first Oxford clinical student came in 1856. In 1860 the intake of twenty-five was "unprecedentedly good."

Some of the early students achieved some prominence. The first two to enter St Mary's, both of whom transferred from St George's, were George Gascoyen, who joined the surgical staff, and Henry Cook, who became surgeon-general of the India Medical Service and dean of the Faculty of Medicine at Bombay University. Others became pillars of their local communities. Thomas Linington Ash, who qualified in 1858, built up a large consulting and private practice in Holsworthy, Devon, and served as a justice of the peace and a county councillor. J.H. Prosser Staples, whose father was a cupper, practised in Burwood Place and served as vice-president of the Harveian Society. His son, another Mary's man, inherited his practice. Two men who settled in Paddington, Stamford Felce and Edward Parker Young, became vestrymen and governors of St Mary's Hospital, with Felce rising to become vice-president. In 1863 the school attracted an exceptionally able cohort, including George Field and Edmund Owen, both of whom joined the St Mary's staff, and Henry Franklin Parsons, who became chief medical officer for the Local Government Board. According to Field, Parsons was the top student that year, while Owen got a good second – and Field played cricket. Owen began to dissect with the enthusiasm of a Vesalius, became prosector at the RCS, and eventually consultant surgeon at St Mary's.[30] Less remarkable as a student, Field received a less prestigious appointment as aural surgeon.

Not everyone did well. One of the school's failures was Murrough O'Brien, the son of a deputy commissioner in India. Coming to St Mary's in 1886, O'Brien learned cardiology from Broadbent, forensic science from visiting lecturer Arthur Conan Doyle, and midwifery from Braxton Hicks and the local midwives.[31] He remembered a half-blind, ornery old surgeon who wouldn't let anyone speak up to point out he was amputating the wrong leg. (This was probably Haynes Walton: too vain to admit his eyesight had faded, he surreptitiously donned and doffed his pince-nez immediately before and after operating.[32]) O'Brien was an athlete who began the day with a dip in the Serpentine and won the mile race for three years in a row. But when he failed his exams and his family refused to pay for a resit, he had to leave the school. On the advice of a student who had failed the year before, he emigrated to Canada, acquired a degree from the Manitoba

Medical College, and had a long and eventful life as a "saddlebag surgeon" on the prairies.

In 1878, when Robert Farquharson inquired into the current status of the early Mary's graduates, he found that four had joined the hospital, one hundred were in practice in London, 168 were in the country, and fifteen were abroad. Twenty-two had joined the army, four the navy, and fourteen the India Medical Service. Fifteen had abandoned medicine, and twenty-nine had died.[33] Farquharson thought these "a very useful addition to the number of the profession." In 1908 the students of 1888 had a twenty-year reunion and took a survey of their standing. Five had dropped out. Of the rest, two were lecturers, four were medical superintendents, and four were consultants (including Mitchell Bird, Dolamore, and Collier at St Mary's). Five had become GPs, four joined the services, and three had died.[34]

New Growth

By 1858 the school had paid for itself, and in 1859 it was turning a profit. The spoils were annually divided according to a complicated formula that out of each £100 allocated £17 to the three surgeons, £14 to the three physicians, between £5 and £6 each to the lecturers in anatomy, physiology, medicine, surgery, material medica, and lesser sums to the rest, with as little as 10s. going to the aural surgeon. Nobody would get rich on this income. Still, the profits did rise, to above £1,000 in 1866, when the intake was twenty-four students, providing about £50 each for the senior staff. By the end of the 1860s, however, the profits were slipping, with only thirteen preclinical and three clinical students coming in, and a grand total of fifty-six in the school. St Mary's was now the second-smallest school in the metropolis, with only 4.5 per cent of all the medical students in London; only the Westminster had fewer. The lecturers elected an energetic new dean, W.B. Cheadle, who coaxed the intake up to thirty by the mid-1870s. Cheadle persuaded the hospital to relinquish its fifth share of the school's profits and spent the money on entrance scholarships and a medical tutor.[35] Numbers continued to rise. In 1875 profits reached nearly £1,600, and in 1880 they peaked at £1,900. However, that figure reflected a higher tuition fee; the actual number of students had declined. In 1879 St Mary's had the smallest intake in London. Profits declined rapidly to £1,210 in 1882.

The 1850s had been a good time to found a teaching hospital, as student numbers in London rose between 1850 and 1875 from around 1,000 to 1,750. Then the honeymoon ended. It is perhaps significant that the last of the founding senior staff at St Mary's retired in 1870. The assistant staff were mostly still teaching, but few were prominent clinicians. Sieveking

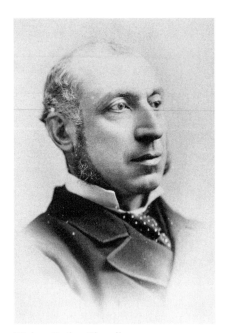

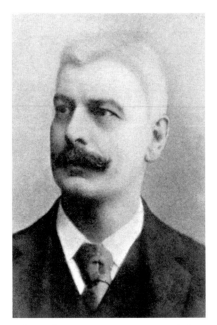

Walter Butler Cheadle.
The Wellcome Library

Edmund Owen. Heinemann and St
Mary's Hospital NHS Trust Archives

was occupied with insurance advising; Markham, once a fiery young Turk, had left to become a reactionary public health inspector. The newer hirings tended to be unfortunate or short-lived. Among the surgeons, George Gascoyen (on staff 1864–76) died early of lung trouble, Walter Pye (1877–91) went mad, and Alfred Wiltshire (1871–85) was struck by paralysis; among the physicians, Bastian (1866–67) left, Henry Lawson (1866–77) died, F.B. Nunneley (1868–70) took religious orders, Robert Farquharson (1877–79) entered politics, and Walter Pearce (1887–1890) shot himself one day at the hospital.

Some hirings, particularly in surgery, were successful. Edmund Owen, who was educated at St Mary's and hired as a surgeon in 1870, was, according to Cope, who would have heard him, "probably the best surgical teacher that St. Mary's has ever known." His lectures were forceful and clear, and he humiliated wayward students mercilessly.[36] His stature was not merely local, for Owen was also on the staff of the Great Ormond Street Hospital, and an examiner at the Royal College of Surgeons, then sixteen years a councillor and finally vice-president, as well as president at various times of the Harveian Society, the Medical Society of London, and the council of the British Medical Association. He published several monographs and lectured widely. Another successful appointment was Herbert

Page in 1875, the first non-Mary's-trained surgeon, who came in as a locum for Owen. Part of his appeal may have been an expertise with railway injuries, having worked for the London & North West and the Great Western lines. Page was the first Mary's man to become a successful legal expert, his exactness of expression much loved by judges. A graduate of Edinburgh, he came to London the same year as Lister, whose theories on sepsis he shared. In 1877 the hospital purchased a carbolic spray for the operating room. (Listerian methods had been attempted earlier: in 1873, Owen treated a two-year-old girl whose wrist was opened by a chaff-cutter. He sutured the wound with "carbolised catgut ligature" and then wrapped it in dressings soaked in weak carbolic acid. The precautions did not ward off erysipelas and an abscess which set in at three weeks, but the child finally recovered.[37])

During the 1880s a wave of new hospital hirings, almost none recruited internally, reinvigorated the medical school. They included two UCH-trained surgeons, A.J. Pepper (hired in 1882), the first of the distinguished forensic scientists at St Mary's, and A.Q. Silcock (1884), one UCH-trained physician, Sidney Phillips (1884), and two Guy's physicians, David Lees (1880) and Robert Maguire (1885). Anderson Critchett, later Sir Anderson, a London-trained man working at the Royal Free, was elected ophthalmic surgeon in 1881 and transformed a small, ill-equipped department into an internationally renowned clinic.[38] He raised the average daily attendance in the department from ten to fourteen to between seventy and eighty, and an assistant surgeon was added.[39] A retired Guy's man, Braxton Hicks, brought distinction to the obstetric department from 1887 to 1892, and in 1886 another gynaecologist, Montagu Handfield-Jones, son of Charles, was the only internal hiring of the period. Not all of the external hirings were impeccable: Robert Maguire was a drunk and in 1905 became the first junior not to be promoted to senior staff.[40] A brilliant young Mary's graduate, Horace Collier, named assistant surgeon in 1897, resigned in 1911 after his heroin addiction cost a patient's life.[41]

The teaching staff also decided that their thirty-year old buildings could not accommodate what they described as the "progress" of medicine. The medical school committee (MSC) borrowed several thousand pounds from the hospital to pay for the improvements, saddling itself with a crippling debt. The focus for this expansion was physiology, which across Britain was at the forefront of what historians describe as "the laboratory revolution in medicine."[42] In 1884 the royal colleges collaborated to design an integrated examination for the conjoint licence of MRCS, LRCP; for the first time, substantial histological knowledge was required of the students.[43] That same year the students at St Mary's revolted against the physiology teaching. Walter Pye, a surgeon who had replaced the inadequate Lawson a decade earlier, was now himself obsolete. The students complained that "Mr Pye's teaching is in many respects at variance with that of modern text-books."[44] The MSC decided that the school needed a separate physiology laboratory and "an expert in that Department, one who devoted his whole time to the subject, and who in return shall receive a higher and special salary" (£300). The "present state of Physiological Science," they concluded, required more than a surgeon if the department was to constitute "a chief feature in the Educational power of the School."

Salaried physiologists who were laboratory researchers rather than clinicians had already begun to appear in English universities, long after their appearance in continental universities; but in 1884 St Mary's became the first London teaching hospital to appoint a full-time physiologist.[45] The staff sought advice from the leading physiologists in Britain – Michael Foster in Cambridge and John Burdon Sanderson, now at UCL – who recommended Augustus Waller. The appointment proved a brilliant one for St Mary's, which acquired an active researcher who raised the profile of physiology in the University of London as a whole. Waller became known for work in anaesthetics and for his electrophysiology; within a few years of coming to St Mary's, he found a way to measure the electrical impulses of the heart, laying the foundation for the electrocardiograph. He brought prestige to St Mary's; and in 1889 the Physiology Society met there, its first meeting held in a hospital medical school.[46]

The students, however did not necessarily benefit from this new scientific atmosphere. In 1893 Mary's students complained they weren't learning aspects of histology preparation such as staining, hardening, and microtoming. Waller explained that he taught these skills only to a few pupils, but under pressure he agreed to make arrangements for the rank and file.[47]

These changes in the physiology department at St Mary's between the 1870s and the 1890s were obtained by students worried about failing examinations. This problem, essentially one of pedagogy, was resolved by bringing in a salaried researcher who had more in common with other physiologists than with physicians and surgeons. It has been said that Waller's electrocardiograph was not taken up by British medicine because British physiology was isolated from medical practice.[48] Waller did perform some research with the hospital electrotherapist, Armand de Watteville, appointed in 1881. But de Watteville, though editor of *Brain*,[49] was slightly marginal within St Mary's, refused membership on the MSC in February 1884. Waller also applied for university positions but failing to obtain one and having married into a wealthy family of biscuit manufacturers, he founded a physiology laboratory at South Kensington and left St Mary's.[50]

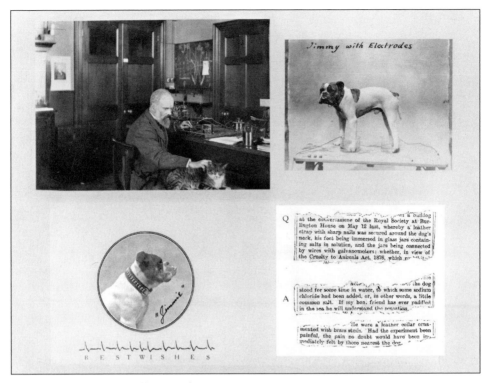

Augustus Waller. The Wellcome Library

He had been an outpost of laboratory science in a still very traditional medical school.

But by now the laboratory revolution had begun at St Mary's. A letter was sent out to the alumni announcing plans to fit up modern physiology laboratories, with the claim: "These Laboratories will place our Medical School at once, in a far better position, than it could otherwise attain for some years."[51] Science was thus seen as a short-cut to prestige. The revolution did not stop with physiology. The chemistry lecturer, Alder Wright, seeing the physiologist so well paid, demanded a raise, which he received in 1885. The following year, after chemistry requirements were reduced by the licensing bodies, the MSC decided that the chemistry teaching was too systematic, in a word, too *chemical* rather than medical, and voted to abolish the position. But Wright refused to be fired: he "asserted his belief that the School was in the position of a joint stock company and that the Board had no power to abolish a chair except on the ground of misconduct of its occupier. He believed that an action for damages by the Lecturer whose chair was abolished would hold good."[52] When the hospital's solicitors agreed

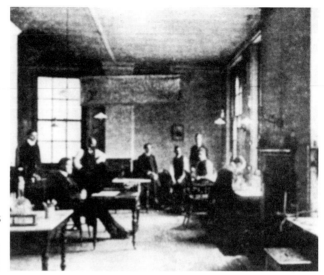

Old physiology
laboratory. St
Mary's Hospital NHS
Trust Archives and
the Royal College of
Surgeons of England

with him, Wright was kept on, but subsequent hirings were for fixed periods, subject to renewal.

The efforts to revamp the school paid off handsomely. The intake doubled almost overnight, rising from twenty-five in 1882 to fifty-two full time and twenty-nine part time students in 1885. Dean George Field urged still bolder expansion: the dissecting room was overcrowded, more benches were needed in the physiology lab, and the chemistry room was much too small. But it was now pathology that had the least and promised the most. Here, accommodation was "absurdly inadequate ... We certainly ought to have [a] proper pathology laboratory where men could be shown how to cut sections, & in fact could be taught the subject properly. This is really a want in London, for there is no such place in any School. I propose that we should take the lead in this matter, and show what ought to be done, for it would I believe have a splendid effect on our next entry."[53]

And so pathology was rebuilt, acquiring more lab space, raising salaries, and expanding the teaching from two to three hours a week. But pathology, unlike physiology, was becoming increasingly a medical department. New bacteriological and serological tests enabled it to encroach upon clinical diagnosis and even therapeutics during the 1880s and 1890s. Yet it retained enough of a laboratory focus to be organized around scientific concepts of research and experiment, as the clinical departments were not. Thus when St Mary's upgraded the pathology department, it ushered in powerful new forces for change. With the appointment of Sir Almroth Wright in 1902, St Mary's would move to the vanguard of the pathological revolution.

Field had other plans as well. In 1884 a conversazione organized by the consultants' wives attracted 3,000 visitors and, Field reflected, "did immense good by letting people know of our existence." He also revived the project of a residential college. Remarking that parents "were continually complaining to him of the impracticability of finding a satisfactory home for their sons,"[54] he rented a house nearby and installed junior staff as wardens.

Another area given attention was student culture. Ad hoc sports had appeared at St Mary's from the beginning: students played "singlestick" underneath the anatomy theatre, and they boxed.[55] Pick-up rugby games began during the early 1860s, and a rugby team was formed in 1866 under Owen's captaincy, though it had trouble getting a full team together, let alone a uniformed and drilled one. (The school colours were a ghastly blue and orange.) Some non-students often played for Mary's, such as William Teriss, the brother of a student, who was continually about the school; once, when no RMO could be found, he set a broken leg in casualty.[56]

When James Lane gave the inaugural school lecture in 1868, he urged students to join one of the clubs then in existence – rugby football, cricket, boating, or the united hospitals athletics club – with "a judicious combination of work and play."[57] When the rugby club fell into disorder in the early 1870s, Lane began himself to play for it. Not everyone enthused about sports: at the inaugural lecture of 1875, John Randall, lecturer in forensic medicine, "earnestly recommended [the students] not to enter into sports or games which would interfere with their attendance at lectures or more important instruction in the wards." His remarks were greeted with hisses.[58] Robert Farquharson was more popular the following year when he praised sports as making for a healthy body and an *esprit de corps*. Twenty years later, Farquharson, now an MP, was invited back to St Mary's to preside over a dinner held to celebrate sporting victories. He reaffirmed that sports produced men who "whether in cricket or in the battlefield, carry their side up to victory."[59]

An association football club was first sustained (though there had been earlier attempts) in the mid-1880s. A shooting club was formed in 1885. Cricket had its club, and cycling would get its club in 1895. Originally the lecturers' support was informal, but in 1883 the sports clubs were formally amalgamated and given £50 a year from the school kitty on the grounds that they were "integral & important parts of the School establishment, conducing largely to its prosperity, position, & success."[60] The school grounds were moved from Wormwood Scrubs to Castle Hill, and club teams now chose dark blue and white for their colours. After this, uniforms were regularly worn, though one footballer, B.W. Gonin, recalled that a player "had always to carry three lots of changes – one for his own use, one for somebody who hadn't any of his own, one for those whom we might pick up on the way to fill vacancies."[61] The rugby football club reached the cup finals for the first time in 1887 under the able captaincy of Frederick Ponsonby Hill, known as "the Bunter" for his habit of stopping men with a headbutt to the stomach. In 1888–89 Mary's supported first and second string rugby teams which played thirty-three fixtures. They were beaten by Bart's in the cup finals in a bloodthirsty game that left many players injured.

Colourful stories of club life during this period have survived, including one deathless account of a football match in 1900: "Sharples made two or three furious sprints after the ball: Gonin damaged his knee in what appeared to be a desperate attempt to foul an opponent: Cruise wrenched his leg in a frantic endeavour to kick the ball over his head, and retired to bandage it, with the aid of several ambulance men in khaki and readiness. There was no score."[62] In 1896 "Two Old Players" reminisced about their days with the football team: "We look upon our football days at St. Mary's, the teas in the dressing room at Wimbledon, the goodly fellowship upon the return journey, the comfortable tiredness which this exercise alone brings, with infinite regret at their departure forever."[63] There was much hilarity about the cycling club outings, with limping young men carrying battered bits of metal home on the train. At the annual school sports day

Rugby football Hospitals cup winners, 1900. St Mary's Hospital NHS Trust Archives and the Royal College of Surgeons of England

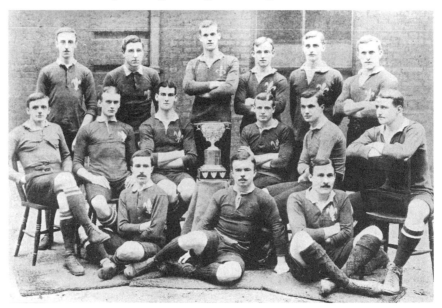

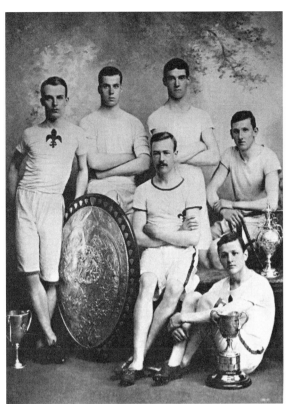

Athletics Hospitals
cup winners, 1900.
St Mary's Hospital
NHS Trust Archives

Winning teams of 1900. St Mary's Hospital NHS Trust Archives

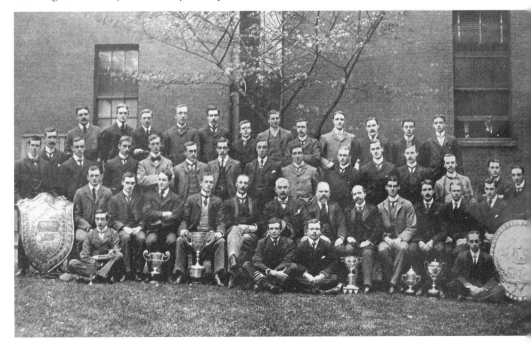

in 1895, the bicycles were just entering Kingston when a cat ran across the road "and in a second a confused heap lay in the road." Another highlight that year was the mile run in four minutes, forty-five seconds, by R.C. Leaning. Sports days were held at the Paddington recreation ground, with native Paddingtonians shouting hearty encouragement: "Buck up, long 'un! Go on, Curly!"[64]

There were other less sporty clubs such as the Musical Society, which held regular smoking concerts during the 1890s. Students doubled over with laughter to see men take women's parts in songs or perform in minstrel acts. The volunteers corps met weekly to practise drills, and had regular reviews at Netley or Aldershot. These were, of course, the activities that received the sanction and support of the teaching staff. Other forms of student sociability did not. The guest registers at the cheap hotels nearby where prostitutes took their clients were full of the names of the Mary's staff, inscribed by the more dissolute students.[65] The less dissolute formed Christian study classes.

The high-spirited games created a sporting attitude towards life. Graduates describing in the student newspaper their new lives in the colonies boasted of amputating limbs unaided. Alumni gone to the outreaches of empire claimed that "the sport was good." Innumerable tigers were bagged by those in the Indian Medical Service, and lions in the African service, while those who settled in the west country had to be content with stags, foxes and otters.

St Mary's offered an education beyond mere academic learning. Since 1866 there had been a medical society where seniors and students both gave papers or presented interesting cases, and that society continued to flourish. But the formation of professional identity by professional activities was not enough. From the beginning, school officers knew that a medical profession formed only by medical training would not have the cultural and political resources that it needed to make its way in genteel society. The poet T.S. Eliot once remarked that if culture is to be taught by the schools and not imbibed from other sources, then "elites will consist solely of individuals whose only common bond will be their professional interest: with no social cohesion, with no social continuity. They will be united only by a part, and that the most conscious part, of their personalities; they will meet like committees."[66] Whether or not the teachers of St Mary's could have formulated this notion as clearly, it was an abiding concern. Walter Coulson's replacement, A.T. Norton, made the case candidly in 1872 when he insisted that education was not enough. It might enable "shrewd and clever" minds in the East London slums to elevate themselves socially, but St Mary's would not want to recruit from this class: "They were yet unfit for professions. They were wanting in social and tender feelings, to be gained only by association."[67] The games and clubs were intended to foster these "social and tender feelings" and make students and the doctors that they would become meet as comrades rather than committee members.

The emphasis on sports was a dilution and a domestication of gentlemanly ideals of culture, a philistine adaptation of the high ideals of "sweetness and light" articulated by the poet Matthew Arnold in his influential *Culture and Anarchy*. Sports secularized the Christian ideals that had informed the hospital founders in 1850.[68] But it was easier to teach rugby than morality, or at least to teach rugby as morality. The earlier ideals of Christian morality and a good general education had aimed at elevating young men to something outside themselves. By the end of the century, however, the support of the faculty was directed towards the secular clubs, and the means had become the end. The bond of fellowship had itself become the ideal. Sports were more conducive to fellow-feeling than was religion, and more likely to create a loyalty to the profession.

Rugby provided a superb model for the profession as a whole: competition was kept within bounds and rules of fair play and was subordinated to camaraderie and collaboration. Rugby encouraged loyalty to the school and enhanced sociability among schools. To use the language of social science, sports are a "liminal" field where participants can explore bounded forms of carnival and competition, without these forces threatening to subvert professional stability and solidarity.[69] In the long run the camaraderie of the rugby players would be translated into professional solidarity. For example, the *Hospital Gazette* denounced those bounders who accepted a panel practice – that is to say, a salary from a friendly society. Their subservience threatened the independence of all private practitioners.[70] Without a legal ban on such lèse-profession, social pressures couched in the terms of "fair play" could exert some influence. Mary's men did not stop accepting group practices, for many were too poor to say no, but accounts of their activities disappeared from the *Gazette*.

The attempts to build up St Mary's Hospital Medical School succeeded. By the early 1890s St Mary's had the third-highest intake of London schools, below only St Bartholomew's and Guy's – more than seventy full-time students and dozens more doing special courses. These exceptionally high numbers must have strained school resources almost to breaking point. Profits rose to nearly £2,000, though most of this was reinvested in the school. By the end of the century the school had a number of distinguished alumni, several of whom had joined the staff. The staff achieved honours in their profession, in the royal colleges, in the University of London, and the medical societies and press. Students were scattered around

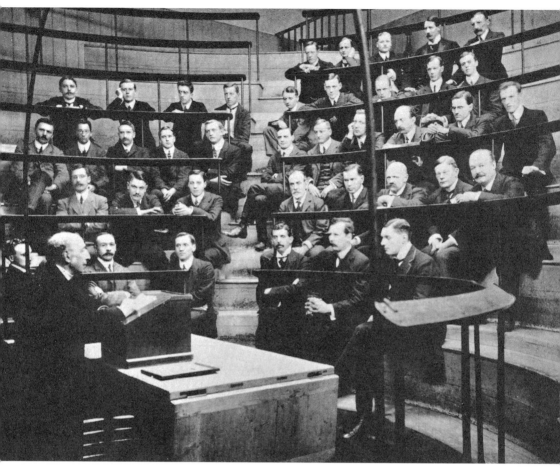

Cheadle's last lecture. St Mary's Hospital NHS Trust Archives and the Royal College of Surgeons of England

the world, carrying the Mary's banner. They had been taught the basics of medicine – they could ausculate a patient, make up histological slides, or do a spot serum diagnosis. They had probably attended and perhaps even spoken at a medical society, where the ideals of good diagnosis and the advancement of original research were put into practice. They had taken their knocks on the rugby field or sung carols around the stairwell at the Christmas concert. They had, in short, benefited from a well-established medical school. St Mary's had come of age.

FROM THE LATE VICTORIAN PERIOD
TO THE FIRST WORLD WAR

The Changing Hospital 1

ST MARY'S HOSPITAL changed a great deal in the late nineteenth and early twentieth centuries. For a start, it looked different, thanks to the addition of two new wings, Stanford and Clarence. Finally the governors had frontage on a major street; no longer would cab drivers look puzzled when directed to St Mary's Hospital. Randolph Churchill, MP for South Paddington, had advised the governors to become "more get-at-able," and at last they were. A spacious new casualty department was opened in 1912. Nurses wore uniforms. Governors were now elected to a closed board of management. Some of the changes were driven by an internal logic and local experiences, and some by wider changes taking place in London and throughout England. This chapter explores the sources of change, seeing them in the confrontation between professional and lay (financial and political) forms of authority. Lay interest in the rationalization of hospital services grew as the authority of the lay governors within the individual hospital diminished.

The Hospital in Its Setting: Local Culture, National Opinion

By the end of the century St Mary's Hospital had 281 beds, nearly twice as many as in 1853. But it could not keep pace with the rapid population growth in North Paddington. In 1877, when the new parish church of St Luke's, Kilburn, was consecrated, sheep still bleated at the church door during sermons; fifteen years later, houses splayed out in all directions.[1] Paddington's population grew to 75,000 by the 1870s, then doubled again

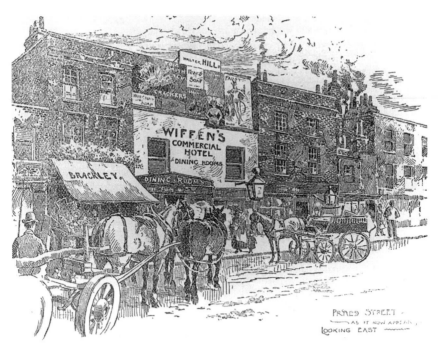

Praed Street before the Clarence Wing. St Mary's Hospital NHS Trust Archives

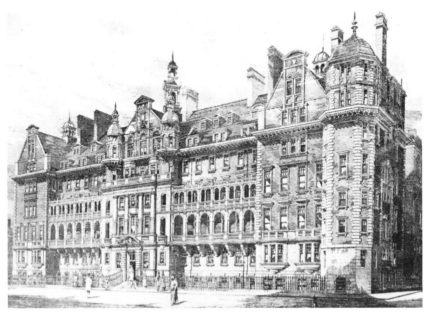

The Clarence Memorial Wing, 1896. St Mary's Hospital NHS Trust Archives

by the end of the century, surpassing Marylebone. The pauper population also grew: between 1888 and 1898 it hovered around a thousand, rising sharply to more than two thousand by 1905, though the rate of poverty remained half the metropolitan average. The census of 1901 found 618 souls in the workhouse, 210 in the infirmary, and 54 in the casual wards. Only about 5 per cent received out-patient relief. The average cost per patient was 8s. 3¾d. in the workhouse (usually the elderly infirm) and £1.3s. 4d. in the infirmary. In St Mary's, the average cost per patient was £6.10s. 5d.

Among the thirty registration districts comprising London in 1891, Paddington was the fifth wealthiest, a mere 21 per cent of its population living in poverty, according to Charles Booth.[2] It had only a few of the classes Booth called "semi-criminal" living around Tyburnia and along Harrow Road. The area around St. Mary's between Praed Street and Harrow Road was mostly inhabited by the labouring class, "not very poor, but rather rough, including dustmen, bricklayers, labourers, carmen and canal men." There were also decent shops and houses with artisans, postmen, clerks, railwaymen, and foremen. To the east and west of this neighbourhood were respectable middle-class neighbourhoods and beyond them, great wealth. Booth also identified pockets of great deprivation in northeast Marylebone and Kilburn. St Mary's Hospital admitted many patients

Building the Underground under Praed Street. London Transport Museum

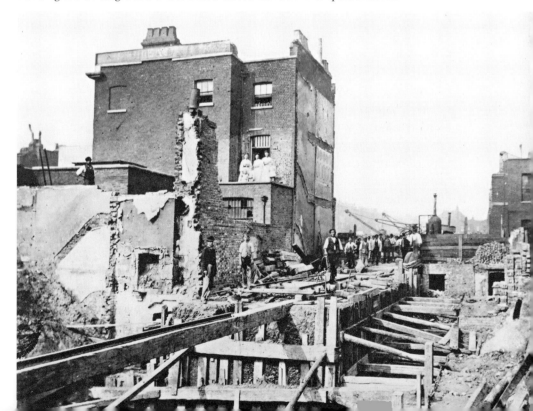

from these areas. According to the census of 1901, Paddington had 33,661 tenements, some frightfully overcrowded. Families of half a dozen or more might be crammed into three, two, or even single rooms. Overcrowding caused disease and burns and scalds, as Jerry White remarks of another London slum, "due to the sheer impossibility of living safely in crowded rooms while using coal fires to cook on and candles and oil lamps to light your way."[3]

Paddington drew builders and servants, neither of them lucrative occupations. Until well into the twentieth century, more than half of its working women and a third of its working men were servants. Manufactures were of the cheaper and dirtier sort.[4] Paddington was also a community of newcomers. In 1891 only a quarter of East-Enders were born in the country, whereas in the West End, the figure was 37 per cent and in one Paddington parish, St John's, more than 50 per cent. The Bishop of Marlborough, speaking on behalf of a congregation in Kensal Green (which was trying to move out of a potato shop into new premises) remarked, "Work in the new poor West parishes is extremely difficult. There are none of the ordinary elements of parochial work and life, and there is none of that *prestige of misery* which attaches to the East of London. People will not believe that such misery and poverty can exist in the West of London."[5]

Paddington became a more eclectic and less Anglican community, and so did St Mary's. The vestry was reformed in the mid-1850s with a return to a single-vote system, and church rates were swiftly cut. A synagogue opened in Bayswater in 1863 and another slightly east of Edgware Road in 1870.[6] Spiritualists held seances in Bayswater, and Freemasons met in Westbourne from the 1850s.[7] There was an Athaeneum for the middle classes and working-men's clubs providing libraries and evening classes. Physicians from St Mary's taught Sunday school and examined working men on their knowledge of sanitary science,[8] and St Mary's too had its own Freemason's Lodge, Sancta Maria, the better to cement professional solidarity.

Anglicanism was on the defensive in St Mary's, as rabbis and Catholic priests complained of proselytizing and obstruction. In a sermon preached in 1888, the chaplain, Reverend W. King Ormsby, denounced nonconformists and was censured. Two years later, when the governors vetoed his banishment of a lady visitor, Ormsby refused, Beckett-like, to submit to this lay meddling in matters spiritual and insisted the matter be referred to the bishop of London. He further embarrassed the governors by printing and circulating his complaints.[9] Ormsby never forgave the governors for the earlier censure, which had undermined his authority and left him unwelcome in the wards, confined to the vestry, a small, nasty, cold room that gave him rheumatics. Relations between chaplain and governors deteriorated beyond repair, and they were relieved to accept his resignation when he found a curacy in Chislehurst.

By the 1890s, religious fervour had declined. When it came time for the hospital to elect a new chaplain in July of 1894, the governors twice failed to draw a quorum of seventeen. This marked a change from the days when the election of a chaplain would bring out all the paid-up governors. Admittedly, there had been some unfortunate appointments in between. A chaplain elected in May 1867 promptly had a nervous breakdown, which his doctor blamed upon "an over amount of anxiety connected with his late contest for the Chaplaincy of your Hospital," though he added reassuringly, "His notions are still very large but not so large as when brought here."[10] In September 1874, the Reverend Thomas Dunn resigned after being caught cohabiting under an assumed name with a woman.[11]

Charitable activity flourished in Paddington, and by the 1870s the list of local charities spanned eighteen printed pages in the report of the Paddington Charity Organisation Society. The COS had been formed with national and local branches to coordinate all the various charities available and make philanthropy efficient and rational. The Paddington branch founded in 1869, was one of the earliest. Its first act was to demand plain-clothes detectives to disperse the vagrants in the parish, but soon afterwards it was dispensing money, bread, coal, and soup tickets, and arranging loans and finding work for applicants.[12] Member organizations included the Bayswater Female Bible Mission, which visited sick and poor families and encouraged uplift: "Our great object is to make the mothers feel that we really love them, and seek their good; and having gained an interest in their hearts, to induce them to have some feeling of self respect and some desire to rise out of the carelessness and neglect of their persons and of their homes, into which so many are pressed down by distress, and too often by ill-treatment."[13]

Crime continued to preoccupy Bayswater residents, well aware that their palatial houses drew thieves from across London. In a farce staged at the Adelphi Theatre in the 1850s called A Night at Notting Hill, all the characters were portrayed as living in constant fear of burglary. In 1860 seventy constables patrolled Paddington; by 1890 the number had risen to 430 for Paddington and Kensington. But the residents always wanted more. Often the thefts were connived by servants, as in October 1861 when a septuagenarian widow on Paddington Green "was alarmed by the sudden and stealthy entrance of two determined-looking men into the room" who "ferociously attacked her with life preservers."[14] (In the popular press, thieves always "looked determined," just as suicides always "walked determinedly" toward the Serpentine or the canal basin.) Paddington Green

("Paddington Brown") drew open-air preachers and "ruffians" who lobbed obscenities and occasionally stones at genteel passers-by. Caravans gathering for a fair in the field next to All Saints Church would, it was complained, "ensure the ruin of a considerable number of servant girls this year, as notoriously happened here from the same cause in the last two years."[15] According to the report of the MOH, Burdon Sanderson, the large number of servants led to high rates of illegitimate births and infanticide. In Paddington, infant deaths accounted for 12 per cent of total mortality in the late 1850s. Burdon Sanderson blamed the "fatal influences which the proximity of wealth and luxury exercises."[16] During the 1860s dead babies were found at the rate of two or three a week as Paddington and Hyde Park became a dumping ground for infanticides from across London.

Burdon Sanderson didn't exempt the canal basin from its share in the mortality: "Foul and pernicious gases are constantly bubbling up from the putrescent deposits with which the channel is covered and poisoning the neighbourhood."[17] Even so, the basin did not fester enough to prevent another parochial nuisance, "indecent bathing," with which the son of a Kilburn clergyman was charged in July 1861. Sanderson's successor was William Hardwicke, who was more concerned with private than public insalubrity. Hardwicke blamed overcrowding and lack of domestic hygiene for a scarlet fever epidemic of 1869–70 that killed 135 people in Paddington.[18] Occupancy on stricken streets was as high as twelve to thirteen people per house and two per room. "Many families are living happily on their limited means, paying 3s. 6d. or 4s. a-week rent for a kitchen in a clean and respectable house. It is a puzzle to me to know what to do with a family so circumstanced, and more so if the people are dirty in their habits, and if Scarlatina or Measles break out with one of the children. They cannot be treated as paupers." Yet many, Hardwicke reflected, were more poorly housed than criminals, paupers, and the insane. People working in dirty trades – "the dust women at the yards on the Canal basin, carmen, coal porters at the dust and coal wharves, horsekeepers from the numerous stables, blacksmiths, engineers, stokers, firemen from the railway" – often lacked running water, and there was no public laundry. Hardwicke closed his report on a wistful note: "Why should industrious, prosperous and wealthy communities see their people perish year after year at appalling rates, without trying some radical and effectual measures of reform?"

The public mood was changing. The medical officers of health produced monumental stacks of statistics registering death, disease, dirt, and dearth which, once known, became hard to ignore.[19] These malevolent forces threatened the middle classes. In 1890 genteel women living in Bayswater organized a Flower Girls' Guild that provided flower-storage facilities, to prevent the spread of infection, it was said, from the girls' homes.[20] Also in 1890, when four children died of diphtheria, a vestryman blamed bad drains and observed that although diphtheria was nothing new, now "the disease is spreading from the poorer parts of the parish to the more wealthy, with the effect that public opinion is at last being roused."[21]

Elected officials could not ignore public health. No longer a private matter, health had become a public good. In the late nineteenth century a new "idealist" school of British philosophers and Fabian socialists rejected the rampant individualism of the past and advanced a more organic view of society.[22] Democratization also raised interest in public health. Jose Harris identifies a new collectivism in politics and a new mass political culture, as the old limited polity was superseded by a more comprehensive and pluralist citizenry. What were intended as minor adjustments to the suffrage created a massive new constituency of lower middle-class and working-class voters from 1870. This newly enfranchised group demanded better working and living conditions.[23]

After the disastrous South African War of 1899–1902, when many recruits were found medically unfit for service, the state began to intervene more in the provision of health care. But even before the war, public interest in social questions was growing. A local example is provided in the reminiscences of John Clifford, who came to preach at the Praed Street Baptist Chapel in 1859 and spent his long life in the service of his church, his community, and liberal politics.[24] Shortly before his death in 1923, he reflected upon the changes he had seen among parishioners. In the early days, young people asked moral questions about resisting temptation; later "the social problem emerged," and the young people became "more inclined to throw the blame for personal failure on society and environment."[25] This attitude was very different from that of the 1830s which tried to reform society by threatening unfortunates with the workhouse.

From above and below, the result of changing middle-class sensibilities and rising working-class votes, there emerged a new collectivist tone in politics. It reflected the discovery of "the social" no longer as something that individuals constituted but now as something that constituted individuals, who were born into conditions beyond their power to alter. Still, the old Smilesian gospel of self-help died hard, and many still argued that voluntarism and self-discipline alone could solve social problems. This dispute famously divided the royal commission named to investigate the Poor Law early in the twentieth century. The Webbs, spokespersons for the collectivist view, were outvoted, but penned a minority report that proved in the long run the more influential.[26] Gradually the collectivist view won over British public opinion. Health served as a bridge towards this collectivist understanding of the relationship between the individual and society. The causes of illness – contaminated water, dirty trades, contagion – were beyond the scope of individuals to surmount. The female physician Elizabeth Garrett Anderson remarked of the Paddington and Marylebone District Nursing Association that its energies could not be misapplied, "seeing that the illnesses seen to were brought on by no wrong-doing of the people."[27]

The great question was how to promote health without promoting dependency. One solution was the Nursing Association, formed in 1877 to provide skilled nursing to the working classes and reduce their reliance on in-patient care. One supporter, the Reverend E.B. Ottley, believed that the well-to-do "could have no idea how the poor shrank from going into a hospital, for that often meant to them the breaking up of their homes; and it would be a great misfortune if the children were left to shift for themselves while their father was at work and their mother at a hospital." The association cooperated with hospital officers, some of whom served on its executive, including Cheadle, Broadbent, and Felce of St Mary's.

The District Nursing Association was just one of a number of mid- to late-Victorian organizations aimed at fine-tuning access to health care and especially to the hospitals. The early Victorians feared a Malthusian "brawny and many-breeding pauperism" that threatened to engulf the rest of society. The late Victorians were more worried about freeloading. The poor, while troublesome, no longer threatened social stability but only efficiency. For the late Victorians that was reason enough to interest themselves in hospital governance, which they began to scrutinize closely. The founding governors at St Mary's had been masters in their own house, spending their time soothing ruffled subscribers and dictating terms to the hospital staff. Their late-Victorian and Edwardian counterparts had to justify themselves to public opinion and especially to powerful voluntary organizations such as the Charity Organisation Society (COS).

Concern about hospital abuse centred on the use of the out-patient department (OPD) by people who could afford medical care. If they couldn't afford a private practitioner, they could at least subscribe to self-supporting provident dispensaries. Philanthropic busybodies campaigned to have OPDs abolished; physicians and surgeons tended to favour a means test. The debate, waged at such places as the COS and the Royal Medical-Chirurgical Society, intensified from 1870.[28] At St Mary's, OPD attendances rose from 4,000 to 5,000 in the 1850s to above 10,000 in 1870. The medical staff demanded a reform, but the governors opposed it. They did agree to let the COS investigate for abuse in 1872. Twenty-six of the "better class" of patient were investigated and the results were: five cases able to pay, twelve more suited to a dispensary, two false addresses ("in itself a suspicious circumstance"), seven suitable cases, and one irate governor who asked hotly "upon what ground or by what right have you questioned my veracity or discretion?"[29] The governors recoiled from further COS investigations as being "conducted in so searching a manner, including character as well as means, that they are likely to lead to annoyance and offence not only to the patients themselves but also to the supporters of the Hospital."[30] After that, very occasionally a flagrant case was rejected – the daughter of a furniture-maker in Portobello Road or the wife of a saddle-maker living in Lancaster Street. Attendances and tensions rose. During the early 1890s, under pressure, the House of Lords inquired into hospital administration. Nothing was done; vested interests were too strong.

Power and Money: Who Controls the Hospital?

As well as to the COS, hospital governors had to justify themselves to grant-giving agencies: the Sunday Fund from the 1860s, the Saturday Fund from the 1870s, and then the Prince of Wales' Fund at the end of the century. They tried to resist these encroachments on their autonomy, but growing financial dependency forced them to do business on the societies' terms. Above all, these organizations introduced the principle of public accountability, which paved the way for a much wider debate in the twentieth century. As with the District Nursing Association, there was much overlap in their membership. Edward Parker Young, an early graduate of St Mary's and a board member, oversaw the conversion of the Western General Dispensary into a provident dispensary, and he testified before the COS medical committee.[31] Sir Thomas Pycroft chaired board meetings at St Mary's Hospital and the Paddington branch of the COS.[32]

The Saturday and the Sunday funds collected money from the public and distributed it among the London hospitals. Traditionally many churches devoted sermon offerings, perhaps two or three a year, to their local hospital, with especially rich pickings at the harvest festival when flowers and fruit might also be sent. From the late 1860s the Sunday Fund was set up to organize this collectively, with an appointed day for sermons and a committee to distribute the funds according to the needs of the hospitals and the services provided. City guilds, which had traditionally donated directly to hospitals, began to channel donations through this fund. The Saturday Fund collected weekly sums from the working class and used them to subscribe to hospitals and receive letters of admission. The idea was to make the working class more self-dependent. In the event, on a "no taxation without representation" principle, the Saturday Fund became a voice to represent working-class interests, and it began after much opposition to name governors to hospital boards.[33] In 1899 these governors convinced the board at St Mary's to rewrite its form letter inquiring into patients' means, making it more tactful.

Voluntary organizations and hospital officials did agree that hospital accounts should be standardized. The Sunday Fund wanted to compare the cost incurred per bed in each hospital to ensure that funds were well spent. So did hospital officials: from the 1860s successive secretaries at St Mary's championed the development of standardized accounts.[34] They did not have much success until the Sunday Fund began to second the demand in the 1890s. Hospital administrators were as anxious as reformers to uncover extravagance. Without comparative figures, governors could only compare the consumption of spirits or bandages over time and make such weak resolutions as that of January 1887: "Resolved that the Physicians' attention be called to the great increase in the number of Chicken Diets ordered for their Patients with a suggestion that Rabbits might sometimes be substituted."[35] Only by comparing consumption across hospitals could governors prove that their medical staff were profligate. In 1890, after writing around to the other hospitals, the governors discovered that St Mary's patients guzzled mineral water and alcohol at a rate several times that of other hospitals' patients.[36] Subsequently, they had only to consult published figures, as in February 1894 when they found that dispensary costs per bed were higher at St Mary's than at any other London general hospital. The *Annual Report* for 1904 asserted that "The Board are giving their serious attention to the reduction of those items of expenditure in which St. Mary's Hospital exceeds other Hospitals, and to the maintenance of its relative position in regard to those items in which it compares favourably with other Institutions."

The figures didn't satisfy everybody. It was axiomatic that the more efficient hospitals were also the cheapest; yet while hospitals with a high turnover could treat more patients, they cost more per bed because acute care was more expensive to provide than convalescence. When St Mary's opened a convalescent home in the 1880s, hospital costs per bed rose because the turnover increased: the average length of stay fell from twenty-eight to twenty-three days. But it was easier to conform to the statistical norm than to engage in special pleading, so governors drove costs down to par (about £77 per bed in 1895).

In 1897 the King's Fund ushered in a new age. It began as the Prince of Wales' Hospital Fund, inaugurated to mark the Diamond Jubilee by creating a capital fund to channel money towards the London hospitals which were, for the most part, experiencing financial difficulties.[37] (St Mary's balanced its books only when somebody exceptionally rich and well disposed died.) From the beginning the King's Fund aggressively demanded conformity to abstract standards constructed by statistical averages. It sent inspectors around to all the hospitals and formed strong opinions on such matters as laundering. (The fund recommended that hospitals do their own washing, whereas St Mary's had been sending it out since it had discovered that staff were bringing in laundry for their friends and family.) Because the King's Fund quickly commanded immense funds, the hospitals had to dance to its tune. When St Mary's applied for a grant in 1898, fund inspectors spent two hours going over the hospital to ensure that everything was in order – that, for example, the lavatories didn't smell and the nurses looked healthy. They found that St Mary's was overcrowded, with obsolete wards and equipment, but also that "these deficiencies are not due to negligence or to ignorance & that given money & time, the Managers will place this Hospital in the position it deserves in the estimation of the public."[38] Most urgently, St Mary's needed a new OPD, at a cost of about £12,000. The existing one was so crowded that only one officer could work it, and throngs of above a hundred people waited in the hallway, sometimes until midnight, to be seen.

Power followed money, and money increasingly came from centralized organizations rather than individual subscribers. The parish still housed some of the grandest grandees of England, and the *Bayswater Chronicle* filled columns with the doings of local lords and ladies as they came and went for the season. But that was precisely the problem. Those with estates elsewhere preferred to spend their charitable money at their country houses; when playing Lady Bountiful, one got more bang for the buck in the

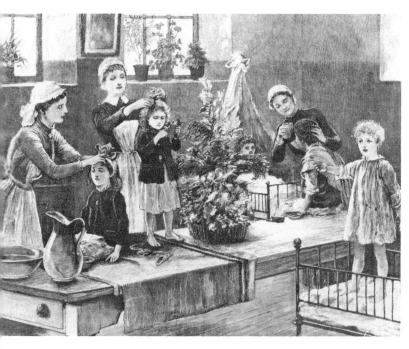

Preparing for
a royal visit.
St Mary's Hospital
NHS Trust Archives

countryside. The servant population was on the decline, and so fewer employers subscribed. By the end of the century the number of titled subscribers had been cut by more than half, and they tended to subscribe only a guinea or two. Legacies, tiny in the early years, grew to substantial sums, and occasionally they made for a "prosperous" year. But they were unreliable, and from the mid-1890s death duties cut into them.

More and more the hospitals relied on smaller donations from lowlier classes. Some were former patients who had made good, such as the carpenter treated in the OPD in 1870 who became a successful builder and a life governor.[39] One big-hearted benefactor was John Barrable, a humble rate-collector for the parish who died leaving an estate worth £6,276: £2,500 went to St Mary's and another £1,000 to the parish poor.[40] Thanksgiving offerings from grateful patients began to mount up to hundreds of pounds. Supporters were overwhelmingly from Paddington.[41] Subscriptions were inadequate, but there was no point in raising the price, because a letter was no longer required for admission.

Subscribers continued, nonetheless, to complain. One woman who had a fit in an underground station was brusquely told not to expect "the observances" of private practice in an institution for the sick poor.[42] Courtesy no longer mattered as it had done fifty years earlier, when the hospital could offer little else. Complaints about the standard of care received equally brusque treatment from a new standing committee. In 1908 the complaints of a patient were rejected after inquiry: she *had* been given morphine, she *had not* been made to drink out of a jamjar, there *were* enough bedpans and it *was not* proved she had cut her arm on a broken pan. On the other hand, the "remark attributed to Mr. Lees that 'beggars must not be choosers' was, as he admitted, actually used by him. Though we think the observation was an unfortunate one, we are satisfied that it was not intended offensively, and that it was made under great provocation." The woman, a former nurse, was "unusually exacting and self-opinionated" and renal disease made her subject to "mental derangement."[43]

Hospital officials who dismissed complaints summarily were probably responding to the greater aggression of newspaper reporters and lawyers. Patients as well as doctors were being empowered by all the new technology, and the doctors didn't like it. In 1899 Edmund Owen reflected upon the threat posed by the x-ray, which provided "inconvenient" illuminations of badly set fractures so that "our mistake is nailed upon the barn-door." He told of patients who consulted him, hoping to sue for a misdiagnosis, and who received scant sympathy from him.[44]

Complainants could still threaten to "go public." In 1903 a drunk woman was turned out of St Mary's and deposited almost naked on the footpath outside the door for the police to collect. She died a few days later of pneumonia consequent upon a spinal injury that the casualty physician had failed to diagnose.[45] The newspapers played up the story and a clipping was sent to the King's Fund inviting inquiry into the case. The coroner exonerated the hospital: the injury was difficult to spot, and the police surgeon had also missed it. Moreover, the casualty physician had recommended that the woman, Rose Askew, be taken to the infirmary; but the waiting policeman decided to take her to the police station to sober up. Different witnesses gave contradictory accounts as to how long she was naked (her skirt fell off as she was carried out) and how long she lay on the ground waiting for the police. St Mary's censured the porter and ruled that henceforth patients should not be brought out until the ambulance was ready for them.

There were other worrisome murmurings of dissatisfaction. Mrs Thomas Wright of Westbourne Terrace refused to renew her subscription in March 1899 on the grounds that "no poor person in want of medical or surgical assistance will accept an Out-Patients letter of recommendation to St. Mary's Hospital." Having had three letters rejected, she sent them all to the cleric of a poor district in Lisson Grove, only to have them returned, for the clergyman couldn't give them away either.[46] Two months later Mrs Rowcliffe of Regent's Park reported that "St. Mary's is *not* a popular Hospital. Patients have to wait often for hours before their turn is taken."[47] There were also waiting lists for surgery, and one house surgeon, finally able to admit a patient from the list, was told "Sir, I thank you for the bed and I have been to Charing Cross Hospital and come home again."[48]

Even graver stories were aired before the Lords' Enquiry into the Metropolitan Hospitals in 1891. One speaker told of "an absolute sale of in-patients' letters outside the door of the hospital." The Paddington COS reported that a man with fractured ribs had applied three days running for admission into the hospital, being told each time to return the next day; pneumonia was the result. A practitioner in St John's Wood, F.H. Corbyn, told the Lords he had sent a thirty-year-old woman to St Mary's with a bad cough. St Mary's referred her to the Brompton Chest Hospital, but the Brompton sent her home with some medicine. She died the following week, and the post-mortem revealed extensive disease throughout the lungs and viscera. Corbyn blamed the Brompton, but on questioning he admitted that St Mary's should have admitted the patient.[49] The hospital did not normally take consumptives, but it did admit those near death, whatever the disease, and so was censurable along with the Brompton.

Yet for all their complaints, the middle classes were beginning to demand admission to the teaching hospitals, and this suggested a solution to the financial problem. In May 1894 a local man offered to contribute towards a paying ward at St Mary's, saying "it would be a great boon to persons with limited means and be a source of revenue to the hospital. As you are aware, there are a great many families in Bayswater such as retired military officers, government officials and others with limited means who are obliged to live in apartments or boarding houses and have neither the means nor accommodation for proper attendance for their families. It would save them being sent to the public wards, which must be very trying, especially to ladies."[50] In January 1896 the Reverend Ridgeway moved for the introduction of paying wards. From the early 1880s St Thomas's and Guy's, their endowments hard-hit by agricultural depression, began taking private patients rather than close beds. But the governors at St Mary's refused, perhaps because they feared alienating local medical men.

The governors knew that already a "considerable" number of respectable patients were finding their way into the wards.[51] Increasingly, the medical and surgical staff began to admit patients who could afford a GP but not the expensive skills of a consultant surgeon. In February 1899 Anderson Critchett raised the case of a woman needing a cataract operation who could afford to pay twenty-five to thirty shillings a week for her care, but could not afford the fee of an experienced eye surgeon. The board admitted the case.[52] In November 1900 Sidney Phillips asked to admit a clergyman with a wife, five children, and £200 a year, for an operation; again the hospital approved.[53] In June 1899 when Edmund Owen was called in to explain why he admitted an alcoholic publican with a large hernia, explain he did in his usual forthright manner. The referring GP, an alumnus, had sent the patient because no wise man would have performed this operation in a private house; it took a great deal of skill and five assistants to effect the reduction. Owen sent the publican home with orders to abstain for two months and then return, at which point he was admitted for two more weeks of dieting and Epsom salts before the operation was performed: "I had to take away his testicle and a large amount of fat from the interior of the rupture; then we had him upside down and after great difficulty managed to stow the truant bowel back in his belly." He looked back on the case with extreme surgical interest and satisfaction.[54]

The governors were beaten, and they knew it. Henceforth the Mary's staff were free to admit whomever they liked, so long as they recorded all such special cases in a book. Former students were among the first to be admitted regularly for operations they wished to have performed on themselves by their old teachers. Thus, while the hospital still looked like an institution solely for the sick poor, an opening had been made for the middle classes. The persistence of charitable ideals, however, prevented the governors from capitalizing on the change.

For practical, political, and philosophic reasons, the English middle classes were growing interested in the provision of medical care. They wanted to be sure that their guineas were well spent. They read with horror and outrage the scandals trumpeted by the press. They also began to demand therapies that were available only at a hospital. A growing burden of expectation was being placed upon hospitals, and yet there was widespread distrust of hospital management. Some told the Lords' Select Committee in 1890 that the hospitals should be nationalized. In 1905, when a speech at the annual prize-giving at St Mary's praised Germany where "all the hospitals were under public authority, and maintained out of public funds," the students and their families applauded the remarks.[55] Students speculated in the *Hospital Gazette* that nationalization of the hospitals and state salaries for doctors were inevitable and even desirable: "The present generation, bred on a diet of Pathology and Bacteriology, have come to regard medicine as an exact science; the humbug which is part of the burden of practice is not to their taste, and they are prepared to swallow a reasonable remedy. They resent being dependent on the caprice and ignorance of patients, they look more each day to the public services for an independent position, where they would not be compelled to commit the humiliating concessions and the treacheries to science that are now forced on them as general practitioners."[56] Everywhere, pressures were beginning to mount in favour of state intervention in medicine.

Medicalizing the Hospital

Growing interest in the rational administration of hospitals at the macro or societal level reflected the waning lay control at the micro or institutional level. In one hospital after another, doctors seized greater control over administration, a process that the historian Charles Rosenberg has described as "medicalization."[57] Historians dispute the degree and the causes of this process. Medical men of the day argued that the growing efficacy of medicine enabled them to do more for their patients and that the concentration of medical technology and expertise in the hospital made it a particularly efficacious and therefore attractive locus for medical care. Sceptical historians have produced evidence to show that the medical profession gained power without any great advance in therapeutical efficacy. They argue that the impetus for transforming the hospital came from administrative rationality and that, if doctors did obtain power, it was a result of broader changes in political culture that saw "the retreat of private judgement" and a growing intellectual division of labour.[58]

A survey of changes in therapeutics, the growth of specialization, and hospital administration will help to assess the extent of medicalization at St Mary's. Regarding therapeutical efficacy, the evidence is mixed. Most people didn't benefit in any obvious way from improved treatments. In the OPD, for example, people queued up to get a quick look-over and a bottle of salts or minor surgery. The wards were hardly any better, according to Ida Mann, a student at St Mary's in the 1910s: "One made the diagnosis and put the patient to bed. He either died or got better."[59] Casualty had little in the way of special apparatus beyond heaps of bandages until the x-ray apparatus was introduced at the end of the century. Germ theory did enable physicians to explain disease more satisfactorily, and in a very few cases – diphtheria, tetanus, rabies – it provided specific remedies. The tone was set by Sir William Osler in his great textbook *Principles and Practice of Medicine*, published in 1892. Osler was more sceptical than most of his colleagues as to the efficacy of much that passed for therapy, but, as his became the textbook of choice around the world, his opinion prevailed.[60]

Yet it would be wrong to characterize the period as one of pessimism and stagnation. Chemistry laboratories were producing new drugs such as salicylic acid that were tried out with great enthusiasm. Heroin was first produced in the labs at St Mary's in the 1870s. New technologies were being developed, such as x-rays, which could treat cancer, diagnose fractures, or find swallowed pennies. In March 1896, the physics lecturer A.P. Laurie advised his colleagues that "the process known as photographing with the Röntgen rays may be of considerable importance from a clinical and diagnostic point of view if introduced into the Hospital and thus justify the expenditure of Hospital money in providing the necessary apparatus." The board agreed to spend twenty pounds on the purchase.[61] The next month Laurie asked if he could charge outsiders ten shillings for a session. (The answer was no.) When Silcock tried to have an x-ray done in October 1897, he was told that Laurie had taken the apparatus "to Scotland to lecture."[62]

Early twentieth-century writings convey palpable excitement at the dizzying array of new therapies. In 1890, soon after Koch announced a cure for tuberculosis – tuberculin – a consultant, Malcolm Morris, sent a young man to Berlin to experience the treatment. The Paddington press followed the case with great interest.[63] Tuberculin proved disappointing, but there seemed always to be something new just around the corner. Fourteen years later, Sir Malcolm Morris reflected ruefully on the changing treatment of *lupus vulgaris*:

During that period the researches of Koch have modified our conception of the disease, while the discovery of new methods of applying physical agencies has almost revolutionised its treatment ... I have given the principal new methods which have come before the profession with adequate scientific credentials the fullest and fairest trial. I have treated my cases in the spirit of Lord Strafford's principle of "thorough." I have scraped, scarified, burnt, applied caustics, injected tuberculin, used light and the x rays, given thyroid and urea, fed my patients on raw meat, &c., with a zeal born of the "wish to believe" which theologians tell us is the basis of faith. This, I venture to think, gives some value to my experience; for it enables me to say with some confidence that where failure has occurred it has at any rate not been due to half-heartedness in the application of the treatment.

And, he concluded, the newest treatment, Finsen rays, really did work, though he couldn't prove it statistically because in most cases he had mixed treatments.[64]

Changes in surgery were more dramatic. In 1909 A.J. Pepper, speaking at the Harveian Society of London, reflected on some of them.[65] Pepper had begun his surgical education with five years' apprenticeship in the Midlands before entering University College Hospital. He came to St Mary's in 1878 as museum curator and surgical tutor, and, making a good impression, was named supernumerary surgeon in 1880. In the 1870s, he recalled, "surgery of the cranium and its contents consisted of little more than the treatment of fractures, Pott's puffy tumour, and wounds of the middle meningeal artery." Pepper himself specialized in surgery of the head and its cavities. In 1898 he pushed forward the boundaries of the operable when he broached a large cirsoid aneurysm of the ear in a young woman. The case had been exhibited at the recent exams for the FRCS, and Pepper's house surgeon recollected, "any candidate who advised operation was severely criticised for recommending the impossible." When the case came under Pepper, recurrent bleeding threatened to kill the woman, so, before a crowd of students in the operating theatre and amidst torrents of blood ("every one of the Spencer Wells forceps in the theatre was used"), Pepper excised the aneurysm – hardly an operation for the kitchen table. The woman survived to bear many children.[66]

When Pepper joined the surgical staff, "intraperitoneal surgery was in its infancy." By the time he left it, he, like Edmund Owen, urged more frequent resort to intraperitoneal surgery in gallstones and appendicitis where medical treatment was merely a "simulacrum of treatment." In the old days, fractures were left to join together as best they might, and the treatment of fracture and dislocation of the neck of the humerus was particularly nasty: one drove the upper end of the lower fragment into the top so as to form a new joint "and let the head of the bone take care of itself." Now, the aseptic method enabled the surgeon to open the joint and fit the bones together. Varicose veins could now be excised. Arterial aneurysms could be ligated.

The growth of surgery followed the adoption of Listerian techniques, but exactly what constituted those techniques was never entirely fixed. In the early years, Pepper recalled, after carbolic spray had been liberally applied, "the surgeon, calm in the assurance that no floating germ could have survived the ordeal, wiped the stump with a soiled towel." By the turn of the century asepsis had replaced carbolic acid spray, and overalls had replaced the soiled old frock coat that hung at the back of the theatre. But there was still some leeway in the question of gloves, which Edmund Owen thought were overrated. (Another half century and gloves were routine – but not yet masks.) Surgeons now claimed for themselves diseases traditionally treated by physicians, such as appendicitis and gastric ulcer. Citing statistics comparing medical and surgical outcomes, Pepper argued for immediate operation in all cases of appendicitis on the grounds that a "person who has had an attack is like one walking near the brink of a precipice."

There were few authoritative guides to best practice. Statistics were as reliable as their author. One young medical student of 1909, trying to advise his parents on whether to undergo a gastreoenterostomy for a gastric ulcer, commented: "You can tell nothing from published results as results are unconsciously cooked by keen people."[67] He may have learned this from Edmund Owen, who thought that "no surgeon should be allowed to prepare his own statistics. It may be putting him to too severe a moral strain."[68] Textbooks, like Owen's *The Surgical Diseases of Children* (reviewed as "an accepted *résumé* of accepted knowledge on the subject written in a bright practical manner"), tended to eschew statistics. They did little to reduce eclecticism in practice. One example of therapeutic eclecticism which historians are fond of citing concerned a patient treated at St Mary's for double pneumonia by two consecutive physicians, the first departing on vacation. The patient found himself with hot poultices over one lung and cold packs over the other.

Specialization as a Factor in Medicalization

Specialization did most to end therapeutic eclecticism. The public flocked to the special hospitals that were sprouting like mushrooms across the metropolis. These hospitals might have a few charity beds, but they catered to fee-paying patients. While the general hospitals were contemplating bankruptcy, the specialist hospitals raked in profits. Specialists saw thousands of patients with similar conditions on which to practise their specialized surgical techniques and therapies, which were then disseminated into the general hospitals. Ovariotomy followed this course. Though the elite consultants of London denounced narrow knowledge, and though

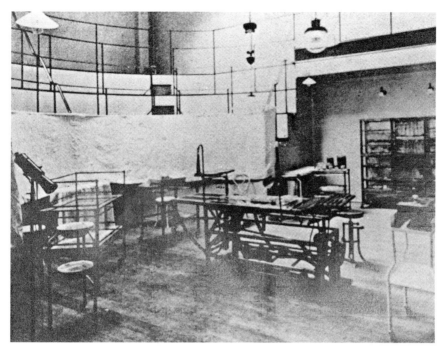

The operating theatre. St Mary's Hospital NHS Trust Archives

British medicine was slower to specialize than American or continental medicine, the process was irresistible.[69] St Mary's grew more specialized despite itself. The early specialist work was done by the general medical and surgical staff who had cross-appointments at specialist institutions catering to cases the general hospitals didn't generally admit – paediatrics, obstetrics, and venereology.

In 1867, as a way of reducing the threat from special hospitals,[70] St Mary's created skin and throat out-patient clinics. Handfield-Jones, assisted by Cheadle, ran the dermatology department, and when Cheadle advanced to the senior staff in 1882, Malcolm Morris took it over, obtaining the first new specialist appointment at St Mary's. A graduate of St Mary's, disappointed in provincial practice, Morris had visited Vienna to study in a specialist clinic and then set himself up in London as a specialist practitioner. As a paid-up governor of the hospital, he regularly attended board meetings and urged expansion of the hospital work into dermatology. In 1879 he was named joint lecturer with Cheadle on skin diseases; in 1880 he began to assist in the OPD clinic; in 1882, the year he published a popular *Manual of Diseases of the Skin*, he took charge of it. Morris's decision to specialize paid off handsomely, earning him wealth and a knighthood from a grateful monarch. (Morris advised a colleague, Arthur Conan Doyle, to follow his example of a short period of study in a Vienna clinic and then a specialized London practice; but Conan Doyle whiled away the idle hours in London by writing and decided to change professions.[71])

From 1867 to 1888 the throat department remained in the hands of generalists: first Sieveking – who was fascinated by the new laryngoscope – and then A.T. Norton, who ran it in a "perfunctory" way, using only a huge tongue depressor and some flawed mirrors. R.H. Scanes Spicer, a graduate of St Mary's working in an infirmary, saw his opportunity. After the obligatory stint in Vienna, he offered his services to Norton, who was glad to give up the work and persuaded the governors to place it in the hands of a "genuine expert."[72] A medical-school lectureship came three years later, in 1891. It was said that few were safe from Spicer's tonsil guillotine, least of all his family and friends. Wilfred Harris, another pioneer specialist, began work in the electricity department, founded in 1881 as a service to the general departments, and parlayed it into a neurology out-patients clinic in 1903. These new specialists aggressively pursued status and business. They founded specialist societies like the Laryngological Society and fought for special sections within the BMA and the Royal Society of Medicine.

The 1880s were the decisive decade for specialization. At their start St Mary's had only five special beds: two paediatric cots, two beds for eye patients, and one for "diseases of women." In 1887 George Field, who was dean of the medical school as well as aural surgeon, convinced his fellow governors to mark the Royal Jubilee by expanding the hospital onto Praed Street so that they might gain frontage and build special wards. Field observed that "it was notorious that Special Hospitals received almost as much in yearly subscriptions as the General Hospitals and that this would not be the case if the General Hospitals put their Special Departments on a proper footing as at Paris, Vienna & Berlin."[73] The governors agreed, and by the end of the decade St Mary's housed eight ophthalmic, four dermatological, four aural, and three dental beds. Thirty-four beds were set aside for paediatrics, though the lay governors continued to refuse the obstetricians' demand for in-patient beds for ordinary cases. In 1900 an advertisement in the local paper described St Mary's as "A GENERAL HOSPITAL and a combination of SPECIAL HOSPITALS." Specialization was propelled by the public and by ambitious medical men, and the hospital governors had to adapt to it, even though it further enhanced the intellectual and institutional authority of the consultants.

The evidence on medicalization at St Mary's suggests that an ethos of therapeutic progress reigned, and there did exist new technologies, techniques, and treatments that sustained and replenished that ethos. The mortality rate among the medical patients dropped by nearly a half between the 1870s and early 1880s when it hovered around 15 per cent, to single digits in the

1900s. The surgical death rate rose slightly, but this reflected the development of new operations, and it is certain that many more lives were saved.

At the same time a growing division of labour within medicine enhanced the perceived expertise of the medical professional. The lay governors at St Mary's had never seriously encroached on the clinical expertise of the hospital consultants; they had merely invoked administrative and financial rationality as a higher goal. Increasingly at the end of the nineteenth century, administrative and financial rationality was being generalized across the hospital scene, with central bodies setting new standards of knowledge and efficiency to which local hospital administrators now aspired. Nevertheless, when lay and medical authority clashed in regard to the individual clinical encounter, lay authority had to bow to medical expertise. The governors of St Mary's freely admitted the fact before the Select Committee of the House of Lords in 1890. When asked, "How would you manage to check extravagance in diet on the part of the medical officers; the committee could be no judge, could they, of whether the diet was necessary or not?" Colonel Stanley Bird admitted that the governors were powerless.[74] In 1891 when Robert Maguire was asked to sign for each special diet ordered, he refused outright. The board's tactics of governance – the special books requiring signatures for special diets, special admissions, or long attendances – were simply ignored by the consultants.

The governors were no longer governing but were now managing, and in 1891 they changed their title to the "Board of Management" to reflect this. A closed board was finally accomplished. Stanley Bird told the Lords that the change was effected so as to concentrate power among experienced governors at a time when there was "great difficulty in exciting the interest of the public to attend the board." The change also reflected and increased the power of the medical staff, who had pushed for it, according to Herbert Page.[75]

The consultants relegated the governors to the status of handmaids. They began to have more influence over policy and administration within the hospital and to change the character of social relations within it. Hospital behaviours became less ritualized and more directed to maximizing therapeutic impact. Surgery was no longer a weekly spectacle attended by the whole surgical staff and student body. Admission and discharge, previously done once a week before a meeting of the governing board, from the 1880s were quietly negotiated between doctor, patient, and registrar at all times of day and night. Lay supervision was entirely removed, and admission was solely on medical grounds. The old restrictions on admissions were dismantled, and none were turned away save those thought by the medical staff to pose a danger to other patients – lunatics and the contagious – for

whom state-funded hospitals existed elsewhere. The physicians and surgeons demanded more power within the hospital and were, finally, placed
on the all-powerful House and Finance Committee.[76]

The consultants' demands became more flagrant at the end of the nineteenth century. In 1894, for example, Edward Sieveking argued that out-
patients should only be accepted if they were interesting teaching material;
all the others should be sent elsewhere. Sieveking had taken this position
since the 1860s, but he now adopted a new, more aggressive tone. He admitted that the governors might be alienated if their subscribers' letters
were thus made worthless, but "it is to be hoped that, when they understand the importance of doing everything that is possible for the advancement of the most beneficial of all professions, and know the sacrifices made
by those who cultivate it, their objections may yield."[77] The justification
was not therapeutical efficacy nor even scientific prowess but the "devotion" and "sacrifices" of the profession – quite a remark coming from
someone who had garnered prestige, wealth, and a knighthood by his "sacrifices." The hospital governors met Sieveking halfway. In 1896 they created the post of casualty physician to perform triage by treating minor cases
himself while sending the best patients on to the OPD.[78] In this as in other
respects, the consultants commanded a new authority within the hospital,
a change they owed to a complex mix of administrative, therapeutic, and
wider social changes.

Medicalization beyond the Hospital

Similar changes were taking place even in the workhouse infirmaries. The
increase in professional competition raised standards and improved medical care. It could no longer be said, as the *Lancet* had in the 1860s, that
the workhouse infirmaries "are closed against observation" and "pay no
toll to science."[79] The physician to the Paddington Infirmary, Dr T.D. Savill, brought in such state-of-the-art therapies as Koch's tuberculin in 1891,
presented cases to medical societies, and showed colleagues around the
wards. The guardians, including some governors of St Mary's, notably
Felce, usually supported Savill's efforts. In the 1880s the infirmary was en-
larged, and from 1889 the creation of short-term clinical assistantships introduced a steady stream of keen young physicians and surgeons. Two
years later Felce and Savill convinced the guardians to permit clinical lectures in the infirmary, the first given in a Poor Law institution.

The career trajectory of the infirmary medical officer was changing. In
the early 1880s the guardians of Fulham Union erected a hospital to replace
the old workhouse infirmary. The infirmary work was performed by H.F.E.

Harrison, an old Mary's man whose "sporting tendencies" and large private practice kept him too busy to service the new hospital. He advised Scanes Spicer (not yet a throat specialist) to take over and coached him on how to woo the tradesmen on the board of guardians – namely, at the turf. Spicer made his appearance suitably horsed and dressed in plaid trousers, smart spats, melton coat, cravat, field glasses, and a black hat that had cost him a guinea on Jermyn Street. As well as winning back his expenses by judicious betting, he was duly elected medical superintendent at £500 a year, a position he held for four years.

For Harrison and Spicer, a Poor-Law appointment was a stepping-stone towards a more lucrative career. For A. Remington Hobbs, it was a worthy career in itself. Hobbs entered St Mary's in 1894 and distinguished himself in sports, music, and freemasonry. In 1905, after doing house jobs at St Mary's, he became a clinical assistant at the Paddington Infirmary. He went on to get his MD in 1908 and after private practice and war service became an infirmary medical superintendent, first in Bethnal Green, then in Kensington. Interested in puerperal sepsis and its treatment by glycerine irrigation, he published eleven articles and obtained his MRCP in 1930, two years before his death from illness.

Under the influence of this new breed of medical officer, the infirmaries came increasingly to resemble hospitals. In 1891 the Paddington Infirmary still had only nine nurses for 300 beds (compared to sixty-one nurses for 255 beds at St Mary's), but as its medical work expanded in the decade before World War I (admissions rose 30 per cent between 1910 and 1914) the guardians increased the staff, added beds, and expanded the surgical facilities. In 1910 Paddington Infirmary had by far the best ratio of medical staff to beds in London, one to 94.6, as compared to an average of one to 178.7 beds.[80] Therapeutic serum was purchased in 1904, from the Lister Institute. An x-ray machine was acquired in 1911, fifteen years behind St Mary's, and a pathology department was opened in 1914.

The process of medicalization was set well in motion, and it was led by the teaching hospitals. These developments in the infirmary revealed the growing political influence of the medical profession, and they presaged a closer relationship between infirmary and hospital and between governors and guardians.

Nursification

The shifting relationship between lay and medical parties within the hospital was complicated by the transformation of nursing. In 1851 nurses were laywomen, few in number and largely uneducated. By 1900 they were trained professionals. Doctors were often hostile to the Nightingale reforms that introduced new ward disciplines and challenged their authority. Across London one Nightingale matron after another fell into conflict with staff physicians and surgeons.[81]

The original nursing establishment at St Mary's consisted of the matron and eight nurses. By 1891 the hospital's twenty-three wards were nursed by the matron, ten sisters, thirty-seven day nurses, twelve night nurses, and one night-time superintendent. Twelve years later the nursing contingent was eighty-three. The increase accounted for much of the rise in hospital salaries, from £13. 5s. 4d. per week in 1851 to £100 per week by 1892. The founding of the school in the 1870s had helped to keep costs down: twenty-three of the thirty-seven day nurses in 1892 were probationers and virtually unpaid, while others actually paid to learn nursing. In the late 1880s and early 1890s the school was at its peak and covered about one-third of the annual nursing costs, about £500 of £1,500. The growth in nurses outpaced the growth of beds as standards and surgical work grew. A night theatre nurse was added in 1900.

As early as 1857 the governors had expressed a wish for a "more stringent mode" of appointing nurses. In 1859 and again in 1865, wages were raised in order to obtain "a better class of woman" and match the other hospitals' wage of about £30 per annum for a ward sister. Nurses were also given a uniform, it being thought that "an uniform helps to maintain discipline and order."[82] Nurses were divided into two classes, one exclusively devoted to nursing and the other to bring up patients' meals, clean the grates, and do other casual ward cleaning. Their diet was improved in 1863 to include more meat and again in 1873. Beginning in 1861 St Mary's took in a few women for some months' instruction in nursing. In 1867 the practice was put on a formal footing, when the hospital agreed to take six resident and six half-day probationers from a London training school; but following quarrels over disciplinary standards, the agreement ended in 1870.[83] Paying probationers were still accepted by St Mary's directly, and, as well, a few genteel women paid to acquire a "slight" knowledge of nursing, useful for missionary work or for visiting the poor.

In 1876, when Alicia Wright retired, St Mary's hired a Nightingale-trained matron, Rachel Williams.[84] Williams had entered the training school at St Thomas's in 1871 and worked there several years before serving as assistant matron to the Royal Infirmary at Edinburgh. She was a special favourite of Florence Nightingale, who took matters in hand from the start, seeing St Mary's as "a great opening for noble work in the good nursing cause." The hospital, she promised, would "not know itself in a year." A collection of 186 letters from Nightingale to Williams have survived,

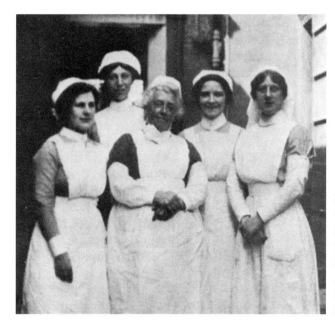

Nurses: Grannie
Colbeck in front,
Princess Alexandra
to the left. St Mary's
Hospital NHS Trust
Archives and the
Royal College of
Surgeons of England

fired off at the rate of three a day in times of crisis.[85] That razor-sharp mind
and administrative genius of Scutari was now directed towards the management of St Mary's, and no detail was too small to interest her, down to
the custody of the maternity linen bags.

Getting Williams in was the first concern. Nightingale arranged for letters, including one from her own cousin, Paddingtonian Henry Bonham
Carter, who described Miss Williams as "a lady by birth and education and
in manners," as well as well-trained, principled, conscientious, and tactful.[86] (Bonham Carter was too sanguine, for it was a lack of tact that finally brought Williams down. Nightingale herself would have known the
description to be untrue: her nicknames for Williams were "Goddess" for
her imperious moods and "Baby" for her self-pitying ones, and by frequent
and affectionate use of them, Nightingale would cajole Williams into
good humour.) Nightingale's own letter of recommendation emphasized
Williams's mastery of the technical and theoretical points of nursing, and
her ability to teach others. Nightingale complained that the physicians' recommendations "invariably omit the essential point, a thorough knowledge
of nursing: in order to be able to teach, 'superintend,' & train in it for a
'Superintendt.' of 'Nurses.' (What would they think of me if I were to recommend an 'amiable' lawyer for the post of Surgeon?) 'Amiability' is not
an international power, nor an Institutional Power: nor is it by any means
our characteristic."[87] The comments reveal just how novel her conception
of nursing was. As Susan Reverby has pointed out, nursing was not a job

one trained for but was, rather, the essential quality of being a woman.[88] Medical men recommending a good nurse would emphasize her caring personality. For Nightingale, on the other hand, nursing involved theoretical and technical knowledge that had to be formally mastered. Her goal was to translate nursing from tacit into formal knowledge.

St Mary's was notorious among the Nightingale School officials: back in 1867 the matron at St Thomas's had written to Bonham Carter of an applicant: "I was no more favourably impressed with her appearance than you were, very untidy, & too short & during the last five years as occasional nurse in St Mary's, has not of course been subject to regular or systematic control."[89] Williams expected the worst of her charges and remarked in a private letter, "I am told by the Drs. at St. Mary's, that the night nursing is even worse than the day, in the lawlessness of the nurses." She entered her new position at St. Mary's full of plans for improvement and within a few months of arriving had drawn up a new scheme for a nursing school. When the governors forced Williams to scale it down on grounds of cost, Nightingale commented pessimistically to her, "I should not like to be your Probationers, to begin with. They are so certain to be made drudges: & 5 at least of your Sisters to be incompetent to teach." Williams did manage to establish a small library and common room. Consultants gave lectures on medicine, surgery, and obstetrics, and there were occasional classes in cookery or from St John's Ambulance. Williams admitted sisters and even outsiders to the lectures on the grounds that this was "very good rivalry. Nurses see that Lectures are thought something of."[90]

Gradually Williams revamped the nursing staff. She brought three nurses down from Edinburgh and added others recommended by Nightingale and the matron at St Thomas's, Miss Wardroper. These additions were highly trained women: in 1883 her night superintendent was lured away to become matron of King's College Hospital. Williams also weeded out older nurses who refused to adapt to the new regime. In December 1876 she dismissed two women for insubordination and insolence. But her reforms stirred up animus among the medical and nursing staff which surfaced in 1877 in the matter of Sarah Saunders, Sister Victoria. When Saunders repudiated a complaint that she failed to dress a patient's sore leg, the matron dismissed her for telling lies. Saunders complained to the governors, and two of them, Broadbent and Thomas Chappé, took her part. They packed the next board meeting with forty-eight members – about forty more than usual – and rescinded the resolution that had supported Williams.[91] Sieveking, James Lane, Edmund Owen, and other supporters of Williams rallied their forces, and the next week the sixty-six governors present rescinded the rescission. Immediately, according to a previously negotiated compromise, Sarah Saunders resigned. Rachel Williams had won.

Nightingale, who had sustained Williams through this crisis with ex-hortations and hams, celebrated the victory, though she knew the war was far from won: "You know perhaps that I think the next two years will see us everywhere on our trial again: especially as to the trained Matron's authority we require, & justly. May we not be found wanting!" Rachel Williams lasted another eight years. In 1884, when she was offered a position elsewhere, the board offered her £250, an increase of £100 above her present salary, to stay at St Mary's. Hostile governors persuaded their fellows that she had exaggerated the offer and her salary should be reduced again. Against Nightingale's advice (Crimean battles were much relived in the letters), Williams resigned in January 1885 and set off for service in Egypt, taking with her a silver tea service subscribed by 198 supporters.[92]

Though this was defeat, it was not a rout, for the nursing school remained in place. William's successor, Matron Medill, increased the number of lectures from twenty to thirty in 1888 and raised the period of training from two to three years in 1893. She also doubled the nursing staff and obtained an entire floor of Clarence Wing as dorms for the nurses. Mary's nurses began to acquire a considerable reputation; they were called in to nurse royalty, and they distinguished themselves during the South African War. Between 1895 and 1905 at least eight became matrons at other institutions, including Cheltenham General Hospital, Mount Vernon Hospital for Consumption, the new St Mary's Infirmary in Highgate, and the British Lying-In Hospital on Endell Street. These were just a few of the nurses who flowed out of St Mary's Hospital into private and institutional situations, prompted by better pay. Investigation in 1897 and again in 1900 revealed that St Mary's nurses were the poorest paid in London. As they filled positions across England and Wales, it began to be said that St Thomas's trained the matrons, but St Mary's trained the nurses. Rachel Williams had left a considerable legacy.

In nursing as in medicine, St Mary's set a path far in advance of the infirmary but one which that institution eventually followed. In the mid-1860s a workhouse reform association staged an inquiry into nursing in Paddington after the first trained nurse to be appointed there complained of the conditions. The paupers who did most of the nursing were found to be incompetent, cruel, or too ill themselves to provide adequate care. One stole the soap from the lying-in wards so that mothers and babies were unwashed for days. Another removed the pillows from dying patients to make them "go" quicker. One pauper nurse, Mary Windsor, admitted to drinking but shrugged off accusations of neglect, saying "the paupers would always complain if she was not always 'paddling about for them.' They were like a nest of young birds; if she got out of bed to assist one, they all required something done." Windsor "didn't do anything for a patient she didn't think was required, and she was the judge of that." Reproached, the matron said placidly that it was very difficult to get good pauper nurses. Meanwhile, the medical officer and the master of the workhouse insisted that the patients had everything they needed – even oysters.[93]

Into the 1890s the infirmary had less than ten paid nurses, with paupers still providing much of the care. As late as 1906 the Local Government Board reprimanded the guardians for failing to appoint a superintendent nurse for the chronic beds in the workhouse, leading the journal *The Hospital* to exclaim, "This is Bumble in his worst form."[94] In 1890, when Savill asked the board for two guineas to buy a skeleton so he could instruct the nurses, a guardian, Mrs Charles, loudly opposed the purchase: "The duties of the nurses were to look after their patients and not to study anatomy. In time the nurses would be such swells that they would not do their duty." Within a decade, however, probationers on the wards were raising the standard of care. St Mary's staff served as examiners.[95]

The Patient's Perspective

The professionalization of medicine has been accused of silencing the patient, because doctors preferred objective symptoms to subjective complaints.[96] Ausculation, however hard to teach, seemed more useful than the patient's account of where it hurt. Temperatures, blood pressures, and other statistics recorded on standardized forms replaced the meandering narratives that once characterized case records. The physician's moral and intellectual authority was itself a powerful weapon in the healing arsenal and could be exercised untrammelled on the pauper patients. One student

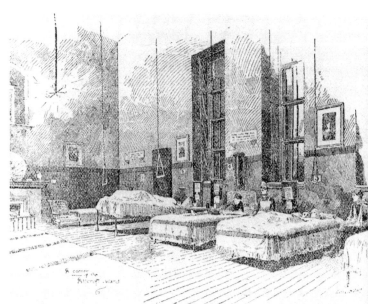

Hospital ward.
St Mary's Hospital
NHS Trust Archives

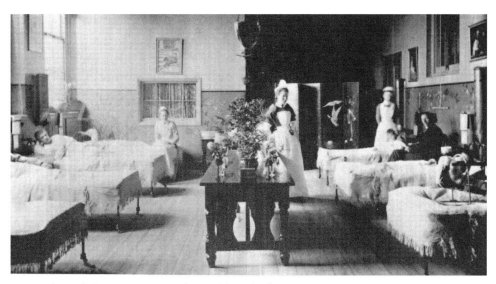

Hospital ward. St Mary's Hospital NHS Trust Archives

during the 1910s recalled the fierce therapeutics of Wilfred Harris, a man she described as "without fear or pity": "I have seen him pick up a girl with hysterical paralysis by the scruff of her neck like a kitten and set her on her feet saying 'Walk.' The girl folded into a flaccid heap on the floor a dozen times, but Harris's demonic will power won in the end, and at the last fierce, 'Damn you, girl, walk,' she stiffened up and staggered down the ward to escape him."[97]

Patients were not entirely helpless. Often they flouted medical advice. In 1895, an artist was diagnosed with sarcoma of the eye and advised to have it out but, according to the surgeon, "like many, he refused immediate admission and said he 'would go home and think over it.'"[98] Others who demanded admission were discouraged with something known mysteriously as "the towel treatment." One woman, "our Annie," undeterred by this tactic, regularly appeared feigning epilepsy and often took in a green house physician. In 1896 she presented with a broken back, having been knocked over by a cab. When she threatened the staff with her crutch (a trophy from another hospital), they took it from her, whereupon she sat up and complained. Hot strapping applied by the nurse and dresser ended that encounter. Six months later, she came in with a "broken knee cap" which she refused to let anyone examine: "'Slit your own blooming bags up,' was her chaste retort, and finally she was helped out by the night porter."[99]

Physicians and surgeons were not unaware of the dangers of treating the patient as a mere piece of flesh. In 1908, speaking to the student medical society on the "Patient's point of view," Maynard Smith, a hospital surgeon, explained how to interpret the stories that patients told. Patients often said a lump they'd had for some time was new because they were afraid to hear that it was cancer. They also had their own etiological theories: "To the average man or woman the conditions we meet with in surgical practice are due to one or two causes. Either there has been some injury – a blow or fall or strain – or else there is some constitutional defect in the patient, a defect which is a family defect, due to heredity and likely to be handed on to future generations. There is no more bitter blow to a patient than to feel that there is a suspicion cast on the constitutional well-being and strength of himself and his children." Smith advised a homely "cheerfulness" and a healthy respect for differences of opinion.

Paediatrician Reginald Miller also taught how to translate folk explanations into medicalese. "With a little experience the mothers' histories of their children's illnesses may be turned to great account and on occasions they are of the utmost importance. Nothing is more foolish than to disregard as a matter of course everything the mother tells you about her child." Coughs were "stomach coughs," "croupy" (which meant hoarseness rather than diphtheria), "chisicky," and "'acking." "Gone off his legs" could mean paralysis, rickets, or scurvy. The remark "'e ain't quite right in 'is pore li'l 'ead" was as likely to describe bad digestion as cerebral disturbance. Miller playfully translated everyday descriptions into scientific jargon: "An infant is not easily examined in its mother's arms, for at the first whine it is snatched from you and oscillated violently both horizontally and vertically."[100]

Doctors did listen to patients and did take their accounts seriously. Personal human qualities like fear and confidence, trust and suspicion, kindness and cruelty, playfulness and portentousness all continued to characterize the doctor-patient relationship – an obvious point but one worth repeating. Vast impersonal forces for change were ultimately translated into human acts of caring or uncaring and were shaped as much by the interplay of these personal qualities as by the conjunctions of power, knowledge, and money.

By the early twentieth century the forces that would lead to nationalization of the voluntary hospitals were already in place. Parliament, local authorities, and lay associations had begun to take an interest in the configuration of hospital management and distribution, for reasons of public health and financial efficiency. Doctors further urged the national importance of their work, justifying it by reference to their devotion to the public good and their increasing therapeutical efficacy. In the short term these claims helped the medical officers obtain greater power within the hospital. In the long term, they would subject them more closely to political authority.

Almroth Wright and Pathology

IN THE BEGINNING pathology was the humblest department at St Mary's. The work was salaried, always a sign of low status, usually done by a young man waiting for an opening on the consulting staff. His duties included mounting specimens for the museum, performing post-mortems, and giving practical instruction to the students. The department was chronically understaffed, and unmounted specimens often piled up.

By contrast, at the outbreak of World War I pathology was St Mary's most celebrated department. From the unprepossessing material available to him at one of the smallest teaching hospitals in London, Almroth Wright built up an important research institute. Among the first major medical research establishments in England, it helped to define the type. This chapter describes how pathology was transformed from an ugly duckling into a swan, as part of a broader change in the intellectual structures of medicine. The focus is on pathology and pathologists; the next chapter will look more closely at relations between the pathology laboratory and the clinic.

Pathology was powerfully invigorated from the 1860s by the spread of cellular pathology, germ theory, and bacteriology. With the discovery that animalcules were responsible for infectious diseases, and with Pasteur's development of vaccines for rabies, anthrax, and chicken cholera, the promise of therapeutical efficacy seemed unbounded. Germs provided much greater analytical purchase for laboratory investigation than had miasmata. As the tuberculous bacillus, the cholera vibrio, the syphilis spirochete, and other pathogens were identified, diagnosis was placed on a new footing. These discoveries excited prolific theorizing about the nature of the immune response. At the end of the century two hypotheses were advanced, each with an affinity for different constituents of the bloodstream. If blood is centrifuged, it will separate into three elements: red blood cells, white blood cells, and serum. The Paris school of bacteriology, under the influence of Eli Metchnikoff, emphasized phagocytosis, a process whereby some of the white blood cells (also known as phagocytes) "attacked" invading disease cells and ingested and destroyed them. Infection, according to this theory, occurred when the white cells were outnumbered or their power of activity was diminished. Paul Ehrlich and the German school of bacteriology emphasized the bactericidal power of the blood serum, where antitoxins were formed in reaction to toxins.[1] Ehrlich developed a complicated chemico-physical theory of immunity based on the relationships between toxins and antitoxins. More practically, Emile von Behring developed diphtheria antitoxin made from horse's blood serum, which could neutralize the disease.

The Development of Pathology at St Mary's

As pathology became a specialized discipline, teaching hospitals had to hire specialized pathologists and bacteriologists to perform routine analyses and to ensure that students passed examinations which were now set by bacteriologists and pathologists. Until the 1890s, physiology was the glamorous and high-tech side of St Mary's, with the only full-time paid lecturer. Pathology was by comparison a backwater, taught by a clinician. About two hundred autopsies were performed each year.[2] Students wandered through the small museum like "yokels at a village fair," exclaiming "Oh, I say, just look at this!"[3] The contents were miscellaneous and included a bad wax cast of a face eaten up by syphilis, prepared by the porter: "A friend of mine down at Woolwich. I went down and took him after he were dead."[4]

Within a few years all the medical schools erected new pathology labs, including large teaching labs with water, light, gas and microscopes, and separate research labs equipped with centrifuges and refrigerators for preparing cultures. Under Dean George Field, the school at St Mary's went into debt building new pathology labs during the 1880s and 1890s. Pathology clerkships were introduced, systematic teaching was increased from two to three hours a week, and practical bacteriology was taught from 1895, rather late by London standards. Practitioners learned how to do their own serum diagnosis of diphtheria using forceps, a probe, scalpel, test-tube, glass dish, spirit lamp for sterilizing, 1 per cent soda solution, cotton wool, and an egg.[5]

The growth created acute problems of staffing for the impoverished school. William Willcox, a former student who did the chemical analyses and practical teaching in pathological chemistry, performed thirty demonstrations or lectures and a growing number of analyses for the hospital, for the inadequate salary of £50. In 1901 he analysed thirty specimens; in 1906, ninety specimens; and in 1908, 282 specimens.[6] Some analyses were exhaustive. In 1902, for example, asked to examine a specimen of faeces, Willcox described its appearance (pale and creamy, the case being acholia), alkalinity, water content, and histological make-up, noting the presence of epithelial cells, phosphate crystals, and food debris. He dried a sample until there was only an oily cake, which he burnt, obtaining a smoky flame, and then estimated the fat content, comparing it with a normal control to show that it was unusually high. He repeated the analysis several times in the course of treatment.[7]

The school pressed the hospital to pay for the work and wrung £100 from it in 1897, which was raised to £200 in 1900. In 1905, when the hospital took over the pathology department, the work cost about £700 per year, plus £230 for the teaching. In 1896 the school hired H.G. Plimmer as a part-time bacteriology lecturer, and in 1899 Plimmer assumed the pathology teaching as well. Two former students, F.J. Poynton and Alexander Paine, were named as assistants. They did the routine pathological and bacteriological work, leaving Plimmer with time to perform research. In 1899 he proudly boasted, "We are in this Hospital very favourably situated with regard to investigation and research, for here clinical and experimental work, when necessary, go hand in hand. In some London hospitals scientific and experimental work is discredited and not allowed; but here, thanks to the large mindedness of our staff, every facility is placed in our hands for investigation and research, and I feel sure that this plasticity of mind with regard to the great problems at present before us will bear fruit."[8]

These were heady days in the pathology lab at St Mary's. Plimmer, Poynton, and Paine were making a name for the hospital with bold assertions in favour of the bacterial origins of diseases considered non-bacterial: cancer and rheumatic fever. Cross-appointed to the Cancer Hospital, Plimmer had performed microscopic examinations of 1,278 cancers by 1899.[9] In 1,130 cases he found parasitic bodies. He found he could generate new tumours by inoculating guinea pigs intraperitoneally with cancer cultures and by scarifying rabbit corneas. He thought that the disease was transmissible but had trouble observing this in animals because, as he said, "cancer in animals, in my experience, is a very rare disease." (In fact, transplantation of tumours in rats was just on the eve of becoming a big business in the laboratory.) Many were unconvinced by Plimmer's theory. Critics argued that cancer didn't resemble specific diseases: the body seemed to incubate it rather than blasting the foreign colonies with lymphocytes. One claimed to have seen identical bodies in the spermatocytes of guinea pigs, and there was nothing either cancerous or parasitical about them.[10] In 1902 German authorities instigated an inquiry into the question, under the direction of Paul Ehrlich, and invited Plimmer to join it. He did not hesitate. Informing the school authorities that "it is quite impossible to undertake to do even the minimum teaching work in pathology properly if one has any other work on hand,"[11] he resigned.

Plimmer had been doing more than his own research work; he had also assisted other staff with their own investigations. Because he had a Home Office licence to experiment on animals, other staff would ask him to in-oculate animals from time to time. When Robert Maguire, an assistant physician, wanted to inject bactericides into the veins of tubercular pa-tients, he first had Plimmer try the substances in rabbits' ears. And when Poynton and Paine tried to reproduce rheumatic fever in animals, they se-cured Plimmer's help.

Poynton and Paine both qualified at St Mary's in 1897 and took various odd jobs there and elsewhere: Paine at the Lister Institute and Poynton at Great Ormond Street Hospital. The two young and inexperienced men suddenly hit the medical headlines when in 1900 they announced that they had isolated a diplococcus that caused rheumatic fever. They had taken tis-sue from the joints, the bloodstream, and the organs of rheumatic patients and had Plimmer inject it into rabbits, whereupon four animals had devel-oped swollen or arthritic joints, pericarditis, valvulitis, and pleurisy.[12] Paine and Poynton took their work to most of the medical societies around Lon-don.[13] A number of leading physicians and surgeons, on hearing the evi-dence, pronounced themselves convinced. William Osler and Clifford Allbutt, in the new editions of their medical textbooks, declared rheumatic fever to be a bacterial disease. Several people wrote in to the medical jour-nals to stake their claim to priority, based on obscure papers given decades earlier. Things were proceeding as a proper scientific discovery should.

Doubts crept in before long. Poynton and Paine had to argue that swollen joints and pericarditis were essential signs rather than complica-tions of the disease, and that arthritis and rheumatism were identical to rheumatic fever. They had to inoculate enormous doses of the culture in order to get results, so that the stiff joints and pleuritic effusions could be seen as non-specific responses rather than rheumatic ones. At the British Medical Association in 1901, their theory took a beating. During a discus-sion of the Gram method of staining bacteria, Poynton and Paine dismissed the method as unreliable. Three pathologists replied that the method was absolutely reliable so long as "the technical details were carefully observed."[14] This was tantamount to accusing them of sloppiness.

Immediately afterwards, Poynton and Paine gave a paper on their work, and they faced difficult questions, such as why other talented pathologists hadn't been able to find the diplococcus. Another weakness of their theory was the way it kept growing to encompass more and more diseases. The two men reasoned by analogy between the symptoms produced in animals and diseases in humans. They also claimed to find the diplococcus in these associated human diseases. But as the number of diseases that they declared to be rheumatic and infectious grew, distinguished clinicians and pathologists (most from St Bartholomew's) objected. Chorea was credible; so was malignant endocarditis. But when Poynton told the Medical Society of London in 1905 that gout was probably infectious and dismissed "the narrow views of that disease founded upon the uric acid theory," Archibald Garrod defended the latter theory, which his father had propounded.[15] T.J. Horder and W. Bulloch both denied that the diploccocus existed even in rheumatic fever, and Horder accused Poynton and Paine of having misidentified *Streptococcus faecalis*.[16]

Discreditation came gradually. In 1902 Poynton and Paine were still enjoying considerable acclaim when they both applied to replace Plimmer at St Mary's. The Medical School Committee decided to separate bacteriology and pathology, so there were two positions available. Each would have been a strong candidate – but neither was appointed. Almroth Wright, professor of pathology at the Royal Army Medical College at Netley, applied for both the positions at a combined salary of £400. This was still £200 less than he received at Netley, but Wright was anxious to leave the college. St Mary's was equally anxious to hire him, so anxious that the hiring committee did not even bother to read Poynton's testimonials. The committee unanimously resolved that "it will be invaluable to the Hospital to obtain the services of so skilled a Pathologist, and to the best interests of the Medical School to add to its teaching staff so eminent a scientific investigator, and so able a teacher."[17] Poynton moved to University College in 1903, while Paine followed Plimmer to the Cancer Hospital.

Poynton, Paine, and Plimmer failed in their attempts at bacteriological discoveries. Almroth Wright would be more successful. Both his typhoid vaccine and his theory of opsonization still survive. It should be noted that success or failure is no necessary proof of the wrongness or rightness of any of these men or their theories. The viral transmission of cancer was proved soon after Plimmer left St Mary's. Recent cancer trials suggest that auto-inoculations can improve outcomes.[18] A century later it is pointless to try to make a final verdict. A more fruitful endeavour is to understand what made

Almroth Wright more successful than Paine, Poynton, and Plimmer, by the standards of evidence of the day. Wright brought modern scientific investigation into St Mary's. He also exerted a considerable fascination over students, pathologists, and statesmen of the day.

Almroth Wright before St Mary's

By 1902, when he applied for the position at St Mary's, Almroth Wright had already made a name for himself. Qualifying in Ireland, he spent a year in Leipzig on a scholarship, working alongside another Briton, L.C. Woodridge, studying coagulation.[19] At the end of the year Wright came to London and studied law and then joined the civil service. He spent his leisure time doing independent research at the Brown Institution, again with Woodridge. This was shortly after John Burdon Sanderson had left there, but Wright was nonetheless influenced by Burdon Sanderson's work on inflammation. Wright then became demonstrator of pathology at Cambridge, also working in the physiological labs. Another scholarship, this one from the Grocer's Company, enabled him to return to Germany; he then briefly held a position in Australia. Returning to London in 1891, he began to do research on clotting at the laboratory erected by the Royal Colleges of Physicians and Surgeons on the Embankment so that medical men without access to laboratories elsewhere could perform investigations.

The following year, 1892, Wright was named professor of pathology at Netley in Hampshire. He had a minimum of teaching to do and pursued pathological research at the college's hospital. He continued his work on coagulation, but as he taught bacteriology, he became ever more interested in that subject. His first serious achievement was to find a diagnostic test for Malta fever, modelled on Widal's agglutination test for typhoid. Widal found that the blood serum of men who had had typhoid, when exposed to a culture of typhoid bacilli, caused the microbes to clump together. Therefore, the test could be used to diagnose typhoid. Working with Surgeon-Captain F. Smith, Wright found that Malta fever could also be diagnosed by agglutination. He then tried to find a vaccine that would provide protection, and when he thought he had accomplished this, injected himself with the vaccine and the disease. Recovering from the resulting bout of Malta fever, he decided he had had enough of that and turned his attention to typhoid fever, developing a killed vaccine. In a killed vaccine, bacteria were exposed to the atmosphere or heat or an antiseptic and then injected into a subject. Pasteur and Roux had found that a killed vaccine protected against chicken cholera. Wright killed his by exposure to heat and lysol.

It was one thing to produce a vaccine in the laboratory, another to test it

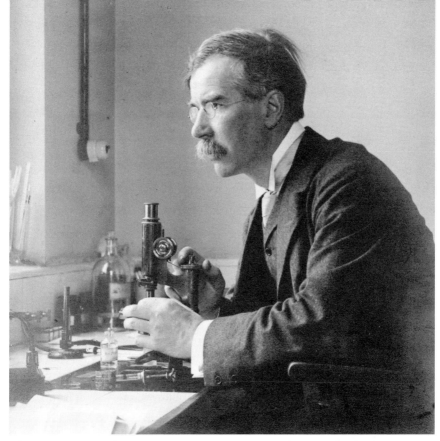

Almroth Wright at the microscope. St Mary's Hospital NHS Trust Archives

on humans, and still another to gather statistical evidence of its efficacy. An outbreak of typhoid in an insane asylum in Maidstone in 1897 provided the first chance to test the vaccine. Staff who volunteered to be inoculated remained healthier than uninoculated staff and patients. The next year Wright went on a commission to India to study the plague there. Indian authorities applied for a trial of his typhoid vaccine, but army authorities refused to spend money on a scientific experiment, although they agreed to permit private testing among volunteers.[20] The India trial was far from satisfactory because very little control could be exerted over the troops, who scattered during the hot season and had different levels of exposure. Nor was there much information about their susceptibility, which was known to vary tremendously depending on the length of sojourn. Because the inoculation of the troops was done on sufferance of their commanders and medical officers, Wright could only get informal and irregular reports.

A new opportunity to test the vaccine presented itself in the form of the Boer War. The British government was still loath to waste men or money on a medical experiment, but the vaccine was offered to volunteers, and thousands agreed to try it. Once again the lack of any formal control or

Right: Taking a blood
sample. The Wellcome
Library and Heinemann's
Publishers

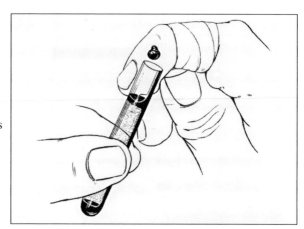

Below: Opsonisation
equipment. The
Wellcome Library and
Heinemann's Publishers

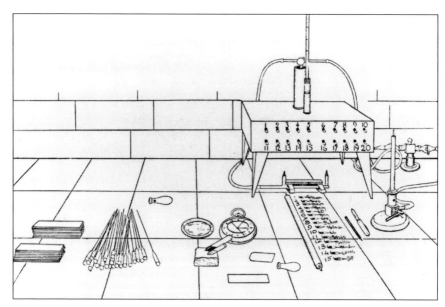

surveillance meant that many of the results were unreliable. The incubation period was not properly tallied in all cases. Some ignorant medical officers conflated illness and inoculation. That the vaccine could cause a nasty fever for a few days did nothing to enhance its popularity among the troops.[21] In some cases, the inoculation actually seemed to lower resistance to the disease. Wright investigated and found that a large dose of the vaccine caused a "negative phase" whereby the bactericidal qualities of the blood, as tested in vitro, fell for a few days, though they then rose above what they had been originally, thus conferring immunity. Wright drew an analogy with money-lending and repayment with usury. The negative phase could be averted if, rather than one big jab, two small ones were given.

Even then, the immunity conferred was not absolute but only an improvement on natural resistance, and it wore off in a few months.

Wright was unable to produce the sort of dramatic results that Pasteur had demonstrated at Pouilly le Fort with his anthrax vaccine.[22] You could not shoot men full of typhoid as you could livestock with anthrax bacilli. Moreover, Wright had to rely upon the agency of other men to perform the inoculation and register the results, and these men were not sufficiently disciplined to produce reliable results. To make matters worse, he made enemies in the army hierarchy who distrusted his work and went out of their way to discredit it. In 1902 an army board that advised the War Office on questions of science, acting on the suggestion of David Bruce (whom Wright had beaten to the chair in pathology at Netley), recommended that the inoculation be suspended.

Wright's vaccine was subsequently vindicated, but that lay years in the future. In 1902 Wright was a very frustrated man. He was surrounded by enemies and, as a pathologist, he lacked access to clinical material either to confirm his previous laboratory work or to pursue his new research interests. The problem with preventive inoculation was that it couldn't be proved in a laboratory or at the bedside but required a program of mass action. Wright did not have enough power in the larger world to coordinate that program. He returned to the lab to find a more direct measurement of efficacy, in the test-tube.

Wright firmly believed that measurement was the basis of science and should be applied to investigation of the blood. In the spring of 1900, during discussion at the Pathological Society of London on the changes that blood underwent during disease, he called for more thorough measurements of blood constituents. A clinician in the audience took exception to his remarks and dismissed as uninteresting mere quantitative changes in the blood.[23] Wright was not the sort of man to be discouraged by such a response; to the contrary. Within a few months he had written up an article on "a method of measuring the bactericidal power of the blood for clinical and experimental uses," which asserted the importance of quantitative measures. It described, in fairly idiot-proof terms, how to get a sample of blood serum, grow a bacterial culture, and then measure bactericidal activity, both before and after exposure to typhoid or the typhoid vaccine.[24] Wright found that if the blood and cultures were diluted according to a definite gradation, one could assign a "definite arithmetical expression for the bactericidal power which is exerted by a given blood upon a given bactericidal culture."[25] He distinguished between anti-bacterial properties in the blood (whereby the growth of bacteria was inhibited) and actual bactericide (whereby the bacteria were killed off).

Wright was now turning from prophylactic to therapeutic inoculations – that is, inoculations to combat an already existing infection. Therapeutic inoculations provided a more direct and immediate form of bacteriological warfare and a more precise calculus of victory. He would not need a statistical infrastructure to get results. Moreover, it was easier and more usual to experiment with sick people than with healthy ones. March of 1901 was a busy month for Wright as he presented his theories and findings at the Royal Medical-Chirurgical Society on 12 March, the Clinical Society of London on 8 March and 22 March, and the Pathological Society of London on 19 March. At the Med-Chi, Plimmer applauded Wright's work. At the Pathological Society, Wright announced some positive results that he and William Leishman, a military pathologist, were beginning to obtain with therapeutic vaccines, directed against such simple staphylococcus infections as chronic boils.[26] The theory was that in local infections (not, he emphasized, general ones), the inoculation of killed staphylococci would stimulate the body's powers of resistance. Other of Wright's papers, meanwhile, described improvements in laboratory technique such as a new cultivation tube that was easier to keep sterile, and more precise instructions for diluting cultures.[27]

In the physical manipulation of the laboratory equipment, Wright was one of the most skilled and inventive workers of his day. He worked out many techniques that later became standard. As Leonard Colebrook, one of his students, remarked, "the smooth-working modern syringe did not exist in those days. Its predecessor, with the plunger made water-tight by winding thread round it, was a very crude instrument. The taking of a sample of blood from a vein was almost unknown."[28] Wright developed techniques for drawing blood and making cultures in capillary glass tubes and for estimating bactericidal properties, and these methods had to be described alongside the results of his experiments. Thus every paper had a lesson in basic or advanced laboratory techniques – how to make the glassware and how to manipulate it – lessons that were later systematized in his books *Principles of Microscopy* (1906) and *Handbook of the Technique of the Teat and Capillary Glass Tube* (1912). Of the *Handbook*, W. D'Este Emery, the chief pathologist at King's College, conceded that one could quibble with some of Wright's techniques. (He, for one, preferred Henry Dale's methods to estimate coagulation time.) Even admitting all this,

we still think that the publication of the book marks an epoch in the study of bacteriology, and that anyone who wishes to make quantitative researches in this field in future must practise Sir Almroth's methods, even if he ultimately finds that others are more convenient for his own purposes, for they have great advantages: they will do the work for which they are designed, requiring only the simplest apparatus, nearly all of which is prepared by the experimenter himself, so that he is independent of the vagaries of the instrument-maker, and will do it with the smallest possible expenditure of material. The introduction of these methods has brought the clinical investigation of the reactions of immunity within the reach of practical politics.[29]

Quantification enabled Wright to make two claims: that his science was more rigorous than most medical knowledge, and that he was in the vanguard of medical science. It was hard to deny, as William Bulloch, bacteriologist at the London, told the Pathological Society, that Wright's methods were considerably more sensitive than older coarser methods of testing the bactericidal power of blood. To adopt his techniques meant, more or less inevitably, to confirm his findings, for to arrive at any other findings meant that one had not adopted his techniques. There was a circularity between method and outcome. In subsequent years the weak link would become these laboratory methods which, some critics claimed, created non-existent entities. But in 1902 Almroth Wright had established himself as a master of laboratory technique. Almost the only possible objection was that made by Dr John Washbourn at the Medical Society of London, who "did not consider that the immunity of an individual could be estimated by the bactericidal capacity of his blood."[30] This was an ontological claim rather than a technical one, a clinician's argument rather than a pathologist's. (Washbourn was the bacteriologist at Guy's, but he was also a clinician and served as a consulting physician in South Africa, where he developed a deep scepticism as to the value of the typhoid vaccine.) Clinicians regularly criticized pathologists and bacteriologists for their reductionism, but for the pathologists the goal was precisely that: to make the microcosm of the test-tube blood effectively represent the whole person. Wright accomplished this manoeuvre beautifully and was for that reason a pathologist's pathologist.

Wright was a better pathologist than Poynton or Paine. Whereas they had difficulty performing such common techniques as Gram staining, Wright was setting the standard for many kinds of laboratory manipulations. But this was only part of his appeal. In 1902 Wright was an older man, already established. His typhoid vaccine, if effective (as many were beginning to think it was), was a significant scientific accomplishment, one that would greatly reduce suffering and death around the world, and it put the discovery of the rheumatic diplococcus in the shade. Typhoid hampered imperial strategies by striking the troops.[31] It also broke out epidemically and, like all epidemic diseases, could disturb social relations, whereas rheumatic fever struck children sporadically and by the end of the nineteenth century

was rarely fatal. Finally, even in 1902, Wright was already the personifica-
tion of "The Pathologist." He was intensely, almost fanatically devoted to
science. It was widely believed that serious science could only be done by a
man possessing near-genius qualities who could infuse the entire laboratory staff with his rigorous standards and enthusiasm for knowledge. Almroth Wright had these masterful qualities in abundance. St Mary's Hospital
Medical School was lucky to get him. Plimmer, who worked with him, may
have advised him that at St Mary's he could freely perform clinical experiments without requiring bureaucratic approval as at Netley. Despite the
pitiful salary and minimal laboratory equipment, St Mary's offered Wright
the independence and scope he required.

Almroth Wright at St Mary's

At the turn of the century, pathology passed from being a low-status activity done by junior would-be clinicians to high-status work done by a star
player. The shift to professional, full-time research pathologists occurred
about the same time in the other London teaching hospitals. Wright's appointment was a throwback in that it lumped bacteriology and pathology
together, but he soon introduced a division of labour into the department
by delegating much of the work. The routine specimen analysis was placed
under assistant pathologists and then reorganized as a department of clinical pathology. J.H. Broadbent (son of Sir William) served as assistant
pathologist until 1905 when he became physician to out-patients. He was
the last clinician cum pathologist at St Mary's. The next two assistants,
though they trained in medicine at St Mary's, became pathologists. After
assisting from 1905 to 1907, Bernard Spilsbury was made clinical pathologist and lecturer in morbid anatomy at the medical school. E.H. Kettle replaced him as assistant pathologist and lectured in cellular pathology.
When Spilsbury left in 1919, Kettle was made senior clinical pathologist.
The two men became prominent pathologists in their own right, Spilsbury
in forensic science and Kettle as a specialist in cancer.

St Mary's had to make some adjustments when it brought in Almroth
Wright. The pathology facilities were rebuilt so that four tiny rooms became one spacious laboratory. The lab was equipped according to Wright's
specifications, including centrifuges, autoclaves, incubators and sterilisers,
microtomes, and white tiles everywhere.[32] But the MSC refused his demand
for a supply of electricity after hours, so that he had to work by the light
of bunsen burners. Not until July 1905 did the impoverished school agree
to supply the pathology and physiology labs with unlimited use of electrical current.[33]

Together with Major S.R. Douglas, who came with him to St Mary's and collaborated on the work, Wright developed a new theory of bactericidal action in the blood performed by a new laboratory entity: the opsonin. (Like Paul Ehrlich,[34] he sometimes invented new laboratory entities to explain experimental facts.) Hitherto, Wright had analysed the process of bactericide (or phagocytosis) by a reduction of scale. He diluted his bacterial cultures and lymphocyte solutions until he had almost reduced a bactericidal war to one-on-one combat, Horatii-style. Now he began to analyse the role played by the different constituents of the blood. There was, as has been noted, a debate raging between the French school, which attributed bactericidal action to the leucocytes, and the German school, which emphasized the role of blood serum. Wright performed experiments that resolved the matter.

Using a centrifuge to separate out the components of blood, he showed that while blood serum could produce antitoxins, it had no bactericidal action on staphylococcus or the plague. Leucocytes did exert bactericidal action by ingesting these bacilli. This suggested that in bacterial rather than toxin diseases, the body's defence system rested on the leucocytes. But Wright suspected that the immune system (as it has since come to be called) was more complicated than this simple experiment suggested. Performing further experiments, he found that when he replaced blood serum with a saline solution or separated it out, heated it up, and then re-combined it with the leucocytes, the leucocytes killed fewer bacteria. So the serum played an auxiliary or facilitator role alongside the leucocytes, he concluded, and this is when he gave the function a name: "we may speak of this as an '*opsônic*' effect (opsôno – *I cater for; I prepare victuals for*), and we may employ the term 'opsônins' to designate the elements in the blood fluids which produce this effect."[35]

The discovery of opsonins helped to reconcile the cellular and humoral theories of immunity. It also gave Wright something to measure in the laboratory: the "opsonic index." He was quite clear that, whatever he was measuring, it wasn't simple phagocytosis. He did an experiment to see whether it was the leucocytes or the blood serum that his vaccines were effecting changes in: he separated the serum and leucocytes of one immunized person and one control, and then swapped them around. Phagocytosis was stronger in the mix containing the control's leucocytes with the immunized serum, while the mix containing immunized leucocytes and normal serum showed "smaller phagocytic action."[36] So his vaccines were acting upon serum rather than leucocytes, and, he thought, opsonins acted directly on the bacteria, attacking them, perhaps weakening them, rather than by stimulating the leucocytes.

A steady barrage of papers now proceeded from St Mary's pathology department regaling clinicians with lab techniques, results of analyses, case histories, and bold statements about the implications for the future of medicine. Wright's first opsonin papers were given to the Royal Society, and then re-enacted for the students at St Mary's, with disrespectful asides aimed at traditional medicine.[37] He published ten papers in 1904 alone, and a small book on the typhoid vaccine, which gathered together the evidence from the Boer War.

By that time typhoid was back in the public eye. Two years earlier, when Wright had protested against the suspension of vaccination, the government consulted the Royal College of Surgeons, which refused to express an opinion, and the Royal College of Physicians, which praised the vaccine. So did another army committee, which in 1904 recommended trials on troops in foreign service. But Wright wanted more than small trials. He and William Bulloch resigned from the board, fed up with the slowness of army procedures. Relations were further strained when an article appeared in *The Times* maligning the scientific competence of the clinicians remaining on the army board. The subsequent trials performed by William Leishman, who had replaced Wright at Netley, confirmed the favourable verdict on the vaccine. Still the British army was slow to introduce routine vaccination, lagging behind Germany and the United States.

Having won the battle of the army board, Wright confronted a new barrage of criticism from Karl Pearson, a professor at University College London and the leading statistician of his day, who wrote an article for the BMJ condemning Wright's statistics. The groups inoculated were too small, the numbers too variable, and the variations not explained.[38] Wright wrote back hotly defending his vaccine and explaining some of the variations: one man reported inoculated wasn't, another had really died on the battlefield, and so forth. Pearson responded, and the debate was on.

The exchange did not descend to statistical minutiae but was largely waged at the level of principle. Pearson saw in the typhoid vaccine a chance to put forward a larger argument, that medical men should learn statistics and should recognize the authority of the statisticians: "Any inoculation process must ultimately come before the calm tribunal of a statistical inquiry." Wright retorted that this was like saying that a man who calculated about ships knew more about them than a practical seaman. Pearson's standards of knowledge were too impossibly high to be applied to clinical medicine, and the lower, realistic standards were good enough for those who understood medicine, especially in a matter so clear-cut as this. Even Pearson's supporters chastized him for underestimating the difficulties of laboratory experimentation.[39]

Despite these contraries, Wright's body of work was forcefully established in the years after his arrival at St Mary's. Papers continued to appear, describing new findings and reinterpreting old ones. He rehabilitated tuberculin which, he found, given in low doses, acted like a therapeutic inoculation. He also found that the opsonic index varied according to whether the patient had been at rest or in motion, and he concluded that movement acted like a vaccine by circulating the bacteria, and leucocytes, through the system. Motion was named "auto-inoculation" and became part of the therapeutical regime. Wright also assimilated opsonization with new work on internal secretions when he told the Chelsea Clinical Society in 1904 that antitoxins and all "protective substances" were really internal secretions, and if a man got acne, he "was defective in a certain internal secretion."[40] Wright collected a band of supporters and enlisted them in the great project of opsonizing medical theory. In 1907 forty-six clinicians and pathologists came from around the world to learn his techniques.[41] They then carried the gospel of opsonins into their own hospitals, schools, and labs. In effect, Almroth Wright created a research school, the first such school to be established within a voluntary hospital. In order to accomplish it, he transformed relations within the hospital.

When Kettle or Plimmer or Spilsbury did research, they could sit quietly in their labs cutting up specimens and putting them under microscopes. To perform his therapeutic inoculations, Wright needed patients. His early cases had been army men invalided back to Netley. At St Mary's he had to rely upon carbuncled medical students or referrals from medical men, usually of hopeless cases.[42] But Wright was too independent to rely upon the vagaries of clinicians for long. In 1905, the year that he was knighted for his typhoid work, he convinced the hospital to establish a Department for Therapeutic Inoculation. Patients could be transferred from within St Mary's, or they could enter it directly. Thus, unlike most pathologists, Wright now had access to patients. Moreover, the managing board let him levy charges on those able to pay,[43] even though no such charges were levied anywhere else in the hospital. The agreement was a lucrative one all round. The hospital had recently erected the Clarence Wing but could not afford to open it up to patients. In 1907 Wright rented five rooms in the wing for his inoculation patients, fitting up two laboratories for routine work and another for teaching. Dipping into his salary, he hired two assistants, Captain Douglas and a medical student, John Freeman.[44]

To run his department, Wright needed considerable sums of money, far more than the medical school or hospital could provide. Counting opsonic indexes was time-consuming. In 1906 alone some 16,000 were estimated, about 450 a week, each taking half an hour.[45] Two assistants were not enough; Michael Worboys estimates that this would have required four full-time workers.[46] There was also the clinical work: between 1 April 1906 and the end of the year, 314 patients were treated with over 3,000 attendances (in keeping with Wright's principle of frequent and low-level doses of vaccine). In 1907, 550 patients attended 3,889 times and 16,399 opsonic indexes were calculated. That year the staff consisted of Wright, three permanent assistants, and four student assistants. The next year three more professional assistants were taken on at £2.2s. a week. Patients' fees and donations paid for much of the expansion. They amounted to £694 in 1906, while tuition fees paid directly to Wright provided another £391; the students also helped out with the routine work. Another source of income beginning in 1906 was the commercial production of vaccines. In 1908 Wright secured a contract with Parke Davis, long an important source of income for the research institute, and this permitted him to hire yet more workers and researchers. Finally, he channelled proceeds from his private medical practice to the Inoculation Department.

Wright's Influence

By 1910 Wright's vaccine therapy had become respectable, if not orthodox. A lengthy discussion at the Royal Society of Medicine yielded little substantial criticism, and his supporters dominated the podium. Pathologist-historians have argued that his vaccine therapy was the making of British pathology.[47] St Thomas's Hospital opened an out-patient clinic for vaccine therapy in 1907, Guy's created a vaccine department in 1908, the Westminster's Department of Bacteri-Therapeutics appeared in 1909, and Manchester Infirmary and Liverpool Royal Southern Hospital also created vaccine departments, while several other hospitals added an opsonizer to their staff. However, Michael Worboys tempers this picture by suggesting that vaccine therapy was only a marginal part of pathological lab work, which had begun to expand enormously before Wright developed his vaccine therapy.[48] Indeed, St Mary's' decision to expand its pathology and bacteriology in 1902 followed the opening of new pathology labs in the previous two years, in Oxford, Cambridge, King's College, the Westminster, and the London. As well, the Jenner or the Lister Institute opened in 1902 as a place for bacteriological investigation and anti-toxin production. Wright benefited from rather than initiated the rise of the pathology lab.

Nonetheless, his vaccine therapy and his opsonic theory did shape Edwardian medicine. He created a European-style teaching and research laboratory – still something of a novelty in England, especially in the medical field. Michael Foster and John Burdon Sanderson had succeeded in estab-

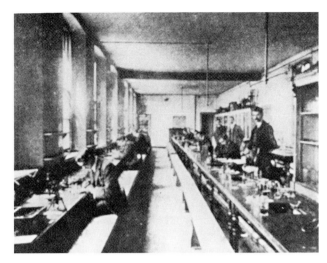

The Opsonic Department.
St Mary's Hospital NHS
Trust Archives and the
Royal College of Surgeons
of England

Inoculation Department tea party showing Freeman, Wright, Douglas, and Fleming in the foreground. The Wellcome Library

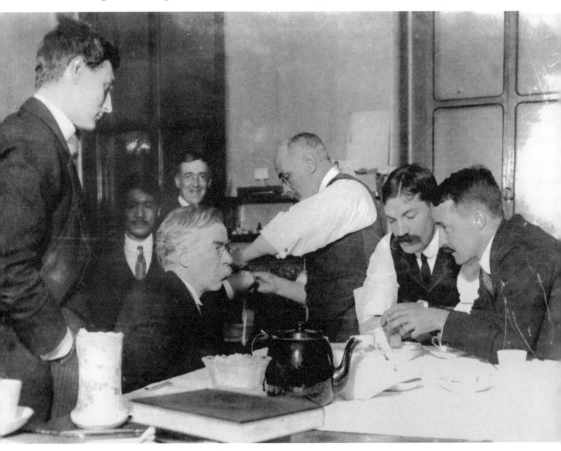

lishing physiological teaching laboratories, but Wright's was unlike theirs in having an overwhelmingly clinical orientation. There were other clinical research laboratories, funded by the sales of therapeutics, but none that so closely resembled the European model of a teaching and research laboratory which would come to predominate in university departments by the late twentieth century. Henry Wellcome, the pharmaceutical manufacturer, established the Wellcome research laboratories in 1894, but though some highly distinguished research was performed at these laboratories, they were not used for training students.[49] The Lister Institute in London and the Liverpool Institute of Comparative Pathology tried to build up research teams by selling bacteriological products, but neither was very successful, according to Steven Sturdy. The Liverpool Institute dissolved in 1911, while the Lister only made a profit by intense commercialization during the war; both had only tenuous links to medical education.[50] The Embankment laboratory owned by the Royal Colleges, where Wright did his early work on citration, ran out of money, and all research there stopped in 1902. (Outside England, on the other hand, the Royal College of Physicians of Edinburgh established a flourishing laboratory that accommodated thirty-five investigators in 1901.[51])

Wright's influence was twofold. First, the clinical applications of his work helped to make pathology more interesting and useful to hospital consultants and GPs. Secondly, he created a set of hypotheses and research problems that other pathologists could analyse and dispute. He created a research paradigm. Pathologists across the country began to hunt opsonins. Peter Keating has surveyed much of the early research on opsonins performed in the United Kingdom. In 1906 R. Muir and W.B.M. Martin added "amboceptors" or "immune bodies" to normal serum and argued that opsonins were a category of Ehrlich's complement. In 1908 Q.S. Shattock and L.S. Dudgeon studied phagocytosis using melanin rather than bacteria and found greater variation in outcomes if they swapped the leucocytes rather than the serum of healthy or sick people, something that Wright later conceded. In 1908 W. Watson Cheyne argued that opsonic readings did not register the well-known immunity of newborn infants.[52] There were many more such papers. Clinicians also carried the research into the wards and out-patient clinics where they tallied successes and failures. Keating counts sixty-one clinical papers published in Britain on vaccine therapy between 1906 and 1914, and twice that number in the United States.[53]

A discussion at the Royal Society of Medicine in 1910 illustrates some confusion as to what counted as evidence. Even some advocates of vaccine therapy distrusted the measure of its success, the opsonic index, and argued that taking the patient's temperature was a better guide. Others wondered

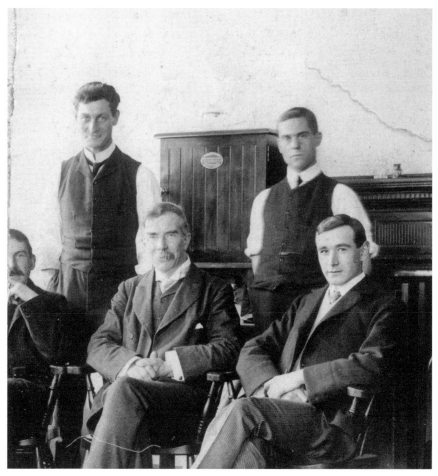

Douglas, Freeman, Wright, Colebrook, Noon. The Wellcome Library

what they were measuring. H.W. Bayley, assistant bacteriologist at St George's, couldn't get consistent results from parturient women. He echoed the objection Markham had levelled against Edward Smith half a century earlier, that "surely a method of examination of serum that is beyond the power of any careful laboratory worker ceases to be a practical test, although still remaining an interesting laboratory phenomenon."[54]

Wright, of course, would hardly be satisfied with creating "interesting laboratory phenomena." It was a strength of his methods as well as a source of vulnerability that he encroached upon the clinic. William Bulloch attributed much of the criticism of vaccine therapy to "a certain degree of resentment on the part of many of those who practise medicine among their fellow-creatures that others should enter the domain which, rightly or wrongly, they consider to be their perquisite, and should enter it especially in a spirit of commercial competition."[55]

Other criticisms concerned the difficulties of interpreting clinical signs. Diagnoses were loose, prognoses even looser, for even so-called hopeless cases sometimes cleared up by themselves. John Freeman tried to overcome these difficulties in what amounted to an early double-blind trial of a whooping cough vaccine. He divided a group of children so that half were given the vaccine and half treated as controls and given sterile salt solution. Unable to measure opsonic indices, he classified the "rambling remarks of parents" under the headings "much better," "better," "no change," "worse," and "much worse." But he found he couldn't trust his own impartiality: if a mother reported that the child was whooping more severely but less frequently, he registered this as "better" in a vaccinated case and "worse" in a control case. So he decided to keep himself in ignorance of the child's treatment until he had tabulated all the results. Vaccination, he found, cut the average length of illness by almost half.

Freeman thought that large-scale trials were impractical, leaving only the "quasi-statistical" test of experience with patients. But this method "only convinces the observer, and when he tells us of his conclusions we are left speculating on his status in our profession and on his capacity for judgement."[56] The reliability of the fact rested on the reliability of the speaker, to be judged by qualities extraneous to the dispute at hand: where he worked, who he worked with, perhaps what clubs he attended. One pathologist reviewing Wright's *Handbook* agreed that in cases of dramatic improvement, a prominent consultant's opinion was valuable, while that of his house physician "would not have been of the slightest value."[57]

It was difficult to follow clinical outcomes. Patients' accounts of their health were not to be trusted. At the Inoculation Department, when patients first came in to have blood samples taken (so that a vaccine could be made), the staff injected them with saline so as to let them think treatment had begun. On average, 20 per cent of patients reported no effect, 40 per cent claimed they got better, and 40 per cent claimed they got worse. Freeman remarked, "one does not want vaccine-therapy to be built up on nonspecific evidence of this sort."[58] Only half of the tuberculous patients seen at a surgical clinic in the Inoculation Department returned, even after the surgeon, Maynard Smith, wrote to them.[59] The OPD remained as treacherous as it had been for Broadbent. This problem plagued Almroth Wright's experiments from the beginning. His first paper on vaccine therapy, given in 1904, described four patients. The first, who had boils, remained perfectly free of them "for a period of weeks after the inoculation, when the patient passed out of observation." The second improved but "was lost sight of" within a week. The third "relapsed after free indulgence in alcohol." The fourth "relapsed, but did not come up for further observation."[60]

To conduct his research, Almroth Wright needed beds. St Mary's, which couldn't afford to fill its beds, offered him wards in the Clarence Wing if he could find £800 per annum to pay for them.[61] The proposal would have been prohibitively expensive for anyone but Wright, who had a knack for attracting the interest of prominent businessmen and politicians. His theories appealed to science-minded philanthropists because they promised to harness science to the body's own mechanisms of defence. Arthur Balfour, former prime minister, was subject to feverish colds and felt great benefit from vaccine therapy.[62] In April 1908 he called a gathering of friends and supporters at his chambers in the House of Commons to form an "Inoculation Department Committee." Present were some of the wealthiest businessmen of the land, including Henry Harben of Prudential Assurance (president of the hospital), banker Max Bonn, brewer and Tory MP Rupert Guinness (later Viscount Iveagh), and Lord Justice Fletcher Moulton.[63] Others belonged to the "smart set" that surrounded the Prince of Wales. Within a few months more than £21,700 had been promised, one-third of it contributed by another banker, Sir Ernest Cassell.[64] An agreement was drawn up between Moulton and Harben for the occupation of thirty-one beds in the Clarence Wing. Wright would have the right to admit and discharge patients, and the hospital would charge him for nursing and maintenance costs. Although he also applied to the King's Fund for money, it turned down the irregular enterprise.[65]

In 1907 Balfour and Moulton had used their private wealth and influence to sponsor medical research. Four years later they led the move to state sponsorship. When the National Insurance Act was passed in 1911, a subsidiary clause provided for the development of medical research on tuberculosis. This led to the creation of the Medical Research Committee, later named the Medical Research Council (MRC)[66]; its mandate quickly expanded to encompass research into other diseases. In the House of Commons Balfour defended the bill to create the council while Fletcher Moulton became the first head of the MRC committee. Wright was the obvious choice as scientific head of the new research establishment. It seems likely that his work, which promised a laboratory-driven therapeutical revolution in medicine, had convinced these leading public men that medical research should be state business.[67]

Surviving records of the negotiations between Wright and MRC officials illustrate what medical research was thought to involve. Because he had almost the only European-style, large-scale clinical teaching and research laboratory in the country, he was to some extent educating the members of the MRC on the requirements of such an institution.[68] Several of his key demands were rejected, including the five assistants that he asked for, though he was allowed Major Douglas. Wright was to be paid £1900, but would have to relinquish his private practice. He demanded an expression of support for his (commercial) vaccine department, but the MRC refused to commit itself on this point. He was more successful in arguing that serious medical research required research beds, and in August 1914 the MRC took over funding of his beds in the Clarence Wing. Another point Wright raised was that rather than having the research units entirely run by MRC staff, outside researchers should be able to "come up for study & practice" and then return to their own institutions, as happened with his own institute.

He also had fixed ideas about the research agenda. He argued that there should be a special investigations committee composed of MRC members and outworkers, to decide what research should be performed and how it should be done:

The duty of that Committee would be to read up and sift all information which is available on the subject and to see whether there was really a problem which could be investigated; if so, to formulate that problem in precise terms; and to determine whether there is at any disposal any experimental method for obtaining the desired information. Where there is no experimental method available it would be well to report whether there is any prospect of such a method being worked out. And where such is available and has already been employed it would be the duty of the Committee to report whether trustworthy, or untrustworthy and conflicting results had been obtained. In the latter case the Committee would have to report whether the method [that] had given these was worth pursuing, and if worth pursuing, how many experiments would be required to give a result which might be regarded as conclusive.

According to Wright's scheme, the MRC would publish these referees' reports, dismissing some projects as vague and impractical and others as impossible of resolution in the "present condition of knowledge."

This was a very top-down approach to research. Experts with special credentials would dictate terms to everyone else. The guarantee of expertise was experimental and methodological prowess. Researchers in the MRC must, Wright argued, have initiated research themselves ("an achievement which is not given to everybody") and must prove themselves useful on the research committee. He dictated details as well as principles, identifying promising lines of research and how to resolve them. Question 1, for example, asked: "Are protective (i.e., antigeni-tripic) substances elaborated at the seat of inoculation; or in the blood stream; or in the tissues after the antigen has been conveyed into these transudation from the blood?" The researcher was told to inoculate vaccines and toxalbumens lending themselves to in vitro measurement; to compare blood and lymph from different parts of the body; subject them to opsonic, culture, and agglutination tests, and so forth. Other questions invited investigation into tuberculin; opsonic or phagocytic powers in newborn animals and infants; the incubation of infectious disease; and the experimental production of scurvy.

By 1914 Wright had constructed himself as an exemplar of medical research and organization. He carried this persona into the army. Here he found his experiences of the Boer War both reversed and perpetuated – reversed, because in the dry African climate, bullet wounds were remarkably aseptic and the great burden of military medicine was combating and preventing typhoid. In the trenches in France, by contrast, typhoid was effectively controlled by Wright's vaccine, but nearly all wounds became horribly infected with faecal bacteria or gas gangrene as well as ordinary streptococcus. His vaccines worked, he showed, against streptococcus, but they were useless against the other pathogens infecting wounds.

More controversially, Wright argued that pouring antiseptics onto the wounds was no better. Assisted by Alexander Fleming and William Parry Morgan, he showed that standard disinfectants like carbolic acid did more damage to the tissue of the wound than to the pathogens. Fleming had already, in 1912, observed that infected wounds seen at the St Mary's casualty department tended to be made worse by the concoctions applied to them before admission.[69] In France he constructed an artificial wound, a test-tube that had been twisted and distorted to form the sort of uneven surface one found in wounds, and he showed that antiseptics did not reach all the nooks and crannies. Better, the team argued, to bring the mountain to Mohammed: to encourage the flow of lymph or leucocytes – which *could* kill the infecting bacteria – into all parts of the wound by irrigation with a hypertonic saline solution. This was the so-called "physiological treatment of wounds." Surgeons took offence at this assault upon their hero, Lord Lister, and upon their methods. Battle was joined in the pages of the medical press, even in the *St Mary's Hospital Gazette* where Fleming and the surgeon Zachary Cope crossed swords, or rather, lancets.[70]

In 1915, as in 1902, Wright had a plan to improve medical practice which he believed would save lives. In 1902 he had been unable to have his typhoid vaccine properly tested because the inoculation was done in informal fashion, often by ill-trained medical officers. By 1915 the typhoid vaccine was getting good results because, as he told the *BMJ*, it was practised "under direct instructions" from experts on high.[71] Now, however, he met all the old obstacles when he tried to reform the treatment of wounds.

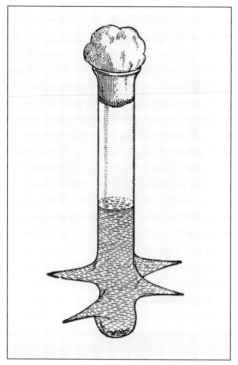

Fleming's distorted test tube.
The Wellcome Library and
Heinemann's Publishers.

Front-line surgical care was performed by civilians acting as military medical officers without laboratory training.[72] One had to know how bacteria, leucocytes, and serum behaved to follow their behaviour in the wound. As in 1902, a dispute about the efficacy of competing wound treatments – antisepsis versus saline solution – became a dispute about experience and authority. Surgeons argued that hypertonic saline solution was a nice laboratory theory but useless in practice. Wright replied that his theories were not properly tested because medical officers lacked the skills or directions to apply them. The surgeons replied with their own accusations of unskilfulness: "Antiseptics will always be 'disappointing' unless the details are carefully attended to," said one correspondent in the BMJ.[73]

The controversy, and a conviction that his discoveries were not given a fair trial, drove Wright to demand a reform of army medicine.[74] The war and the discipline that it required of medical officers provided a marvellous opportunity to smash all the old inefficiencies of civilian medicine. Wright announced that "it is a question of conflict between our cherished professional tradition that every medical man must be completely unfettered in his choice of treatment and the very foundation or principle of the army that every man shall work not as he individually thinks best but as part and parcel of a great machine." He called for an elite advisory committee, heavy on laboratory expertise, that would "plan and then carry out such investigations as would be calculated to bring into clear light the effect of rival procedures. That accomplished, there would be very little dispute possible and substantial agreement at least would be arrived at."[75] The MRC could provide assistance in organizing it.

Wright put his ideas into articles which he published in the lay medical press and in a memo to the minister of War. He observed that the Royal Army Medical Corps (RAMC) had an admirably efficient administration and system of evacuation, but there was no *medical* assessment of treatment, no way to collect records as to what worked and what didn't. The RAMC couldn't even prove that their policy of immediate evacuation was any better than treatment at the front. Army medics listened to this slur on their organization and values with rising indignation. Wright had not consulted his immediate superior, Arthur Sloggett, who took the affair as a personal insult and, puffing himself up in Colonel Blimp style, demanded Wright's resignation. More moderately, Director General Sir Alfred Keogh (who had done some post-qualification work at St Mary's) called together an advisory body of leading army consultants and asked for their verdict on Wright's memo and whether, in principle, the RAMC had "taken steps to fortify ourselves in all directions with the resources of modern science." One or two of these consultants agreed with Wright that evacuation was performed too quickly in such cases as compound fracture of the thigh. However, with one voice they all rebuffed the "insult" to the RAMC and insisted that scientists were on hand to aid treatment and investigation. Above all they rejected Wright's doctrine of standardization, which would, they insisted, arrest all progress, for progress sprang from diversity of opinion and friendly rivalry among surgeons. Sir Bernard Moynihan, a professor of surgery at Leeds who was not unsympathetic to Wright, insisted that "no one ever decided upon the right way of treating wounds. The whole progress of surgery has depended upon the different interpretation that different men have given to the different methods of solving the same problem."[76] Elite consultants commanded greater influence with the army hierarchy, and this was their opportunity to repay Wright for all the insults he had heaped upon clinicians over the years. Wright's plans for reform came to naught.

Nor was his program of research implemented by the MRC. By the end of the war Wright had evidently had enough of serving the state, and he chose not to take up the MRC position. No doubt the MRC (which vigorously denied having any connection with Wright's schemes for army reform) collectively breathed a sigh of relief. Probably the RAMC memo and its aftermath harmed him in official circles: Leishman, for example, was on both the MRC and the army medical advisory board. Moreover, Wright was fifty-eight by the end of the war and, Colebrook suggests, disinclined to spend his remaining years building up a new lab, though he did accept a grant from the MRC to sponsor his research at St Mary's. Instead Captain Douglas took up the position of chief bacteriologist, and enjoyed a successful career, becoming FRS in 1922 and deputy director of the MRC Institute at Hampstead in 1930. Back at St Mary's, John Freeman and Alexander Fleming vied to become Wright's right-hand man.

By 1918 Douglas was leaving a leaky, if not a sinking ship. Vaccine therapy was declining in public favour. A second debate in the Royal Society of Medicine, held in 1913, had already raised far more substantial criticisms than were aired in 1910. The stream of international students into the Inoculation Department fell off. If vaccine therapy had been a crutch for pathologists, it was one they no longer needed. The heyday of the St Mary's Inoculation Department was over, and its postwar existence would be rather different.

The School, 1900–1920
Coping with Science

BY THE 1890s the school's future seemed assured. Its student intake exceeded all but the endowed schools and even University College and King's College. Yet within a decade it was facing its most serious troubles to date and for the first (but not the last) time, had to contemplate the possibility of extinction. Student intake and income declined both absolutely and relative to expenditure. As the ancillary disciplines – anatomy, physiology, pathology, and pathological chemistry – became increasingly laboratory based, they caused a crisis in medicine. The costs of salaried workers and laboratories became prohibitive for the smaller medical schools. Moreover, clinicians found that their claims to possess special knowledge about health and illness were undermined by these ancillary scientists. Scientific researchers initiated a critique of the existing structures of medical knowledge that politicians then took up. Over the next two decades St Mary's weathered the crisis.

The School at the Brink

The move towards laboratories and salaried teachers at the end of the nineteenth century gathered pace in the twentieth. At St Mary's, anatomy was still taught by a clinician until 1911, but professional scientists ran the other premedical departments. In the physiology department, Augustus Waller left St Mary's in 1903 (exhausting attempts to keep his name on the books as long as possible) and a succession of his students replaced him. The first was Nathaniel Henry Alcock, a specialist in the properties of nerves, who worked with Waller on anaesthetics. Physiology remained the most expensive department in the school at £499 per year, but biology, chemistry, physics, and anatomy were creeping up behind. In 1900, salaries amounted to £2,500, half the total running costs of the school. Most of the money, the MSC observed, went towards the laboratory departments, which were "the very departments upon the efficiency of which St. Mary's' chance of coming well through the ordeal of reconstruction, on a University basis, depends."[1]

The laboratories were necessary but they pushed the cost of medical education beyond what tuition fees could support. The bigger, endowed schools with hundreds of students could afford to sustain a good premedical department, perhaps with an FRS as lecturer. University College and King's College, which became incorporated colleges within the University of London in 1905, also flourished. Both had close links with university science departments, and both were subsidized by the University of London. Student fees met less than half their running costs. The small, independent schools were driven to the wall. Their meagre income from student fees could not pay to build, equip, and staff preclinical laboratories capable of teaching to a university standard. At St Mary's by 1897 most of the teachers were spending their share of the profits on teaching costs. By 1900 there were no more profits: all the income went directly to the salaried staff and equipment. In order to keep the school operating that year, lecturers actually paid over £1,471 of their own money.[2] The situation was aggravated by the rise of provincial medical schools. In 1880 about 40 per cent of English medical students had trained in London, but by 1910 the figure was only about 25 per cent.[3]

The schools cast around for other sources of income. Two potential sources were the parent hospital and the state. Most hospitals subsidized their schools. One witness told the Lords in 1891, "Before the hospitals were utilised as medical schools they had no reputation as hospitals; it was only by becoming centres of learning and instruction that they established a reputation."[4] Because the hospitals needed their schools, they diverted money towards them. In 1899 when the lecturers at St Mary's asked for a reduced rent, the board met them part way by offering to pay for the routine pathology work and remit interest on the school's debt.[5] In 1901 the lecturers banged on the governors' door again, to ask for a loan of £3,000 on easy terms, following upon £11,000 already borrowed and still owing. This was the wrong thing to ask of hospital governors who, qua governors, saw it as their *raison d'être* to force clinicians to live within their income. They found the school guilty of financial mismanagement. The residential college, for example, had been running at a loss of about £600 a year for fifteen years. The school had also been taking compounded fees (whereby students received a discount if they paid the five years' fees at the start) and spending them as annual fees. Until 1899 it had actually been dividing these fees annually among the lecturers.

Lay governors with financial experience were straightaway named to oversee the school's finances. The governors also refused to make the loan, which they knew would become a grant, though they did increase the subsidy paid for pathological work and remitted the rent. The debt was paid for the school by Henry Harben, who, like his more famous father, was director of the Prudential Insurance Company and a generous benefactor of London hospitals. Henry Harben Jr was for many years the hospital's biggest supporter: he served as governor, then president, until his death in 1910.

Other governors also affirmed their support for the school: "Without such assistance as we have suggested, the Medical School must cease to exist; without the Medical School, St. Mary's Hospital must sink at once to the level of a second class Hospital." After 1905, when the King's Fund prohibited hospitals from subsidizing schools, the managing board simply annexed the pathology department and charged the school a small sum for teaching services. The governors tried to be as generous as possible, and after 1905 the accounts seem designed as much to disguise as to reveal the financial relations between school and hospital. Nonetheless, as things continued to worsen, the schools could no longer turn to the hospitals for help.

The hospital governors believed that the school could be run at a profit. They were wrong. Strict economies kept the budget below £5,000 for more than a decade but posed a serious threat to the school's academic standing. The number of medical students matriculating at the University of London remained stable during the decade before World War I, around 1,050 to 1,100. But fewer and fewer went to St Mary's: from 106 in 1904–05, numbers would drop gradually to 69 (around half the total student body) on the eve of the war.

A subcommittee named in December 1906 to suggest economies in the preclinical departments was at a loss and could only advise cutting back on research. It commented that "while recognising that the ideal is to encourage research in conjunction with efficient teaching, the Sub-Committee are of opinion that the present state of Medical School Finances renders it imperative that departmental expenses in connexion with research should be curtailed as far as possible."[6] This was a risky proposition, for university-standard teaching could only be done by men prosecuting original research.

The sub-committee also recommended an appeal to the state for funding. If the public, politicians, and civil servants could be persuaded that medical education was a public service, then money would follow. Already in the

1890s some witnesses at the enquiry into the metropolitan hospitals had demanded the nationalization of medical education, on the grounds that the public had an interest in being well doctored. Yet so long as medicine and medical education were remunerative, doctors resisted state intervention in their provision. Students entering St Mary's in 1900 were told: "The fact that medical education in this kingdom is independent of state aid is one of the bulwarks of the dignity of the profession of medicine."[7] However, as doctors felt squeezed by economic forces beyond their control, they changed their tune.

Thus the medical schools turned to the state, with St Mary's leading the way. St Mary's was neither so big that it could do without state funds nor so small that the situation was hopeless. It teetered on the brink of viability. Only small sums were needed to nudge it towards viability, and the staff determined to find those sums. The solution was to convince the Board of Education that St Mary's Hospital Medical School was a technical institute and deserving of funding earmarked for technical institutes.

Initially, in March 1907, the Board of Education turned down the application. The situation at St Mary's continued to deteriorate and by May 1908 had reached such a pitch that the medical staff undertook to pay an annual subsidy of £500 per year for three years so as to maintain the complete curriculum.[8] They also focused their drive for economies on the most expensive department: physiology. Alcock, the man with the most to lose by the threatened economies, continued negotiating with the Board of Education, and in October 1909 he announced that the board had agreed to pay an annual grant to St Mary's, set at £1,037. The following year the grant dropped to £857 to penalize the school for what the board saw as examples of inefficiency, including excessively high scholarships and excessively low salaries. The school quickly introduced the necessary reforms, allowing for salaries in clinical fields when funds permitted (a utopian prospect).[9] That the medical school was indeed brought to a new level of efficiency is suggested by a memo sent round to all the lecturers in December 1909 reminding them that in view of "the right of the Board's Inspector to visit the School, it is most important that all lectures shall be delivered regularly."[10] There were other demands: in 1911, the Board of Education forced the school to hire a full-time anatomist.

St Mary's, like the other hospital schools, grew to depend on the Board of Education's grant (later distributed by the University Grants Committee through the University of London). While fees grew mathematically, grants grew exponentially. In 1920 the board grant amounted to £3,000, half the sum obtained from student fees. By the end of the decade it brought in twice as much as fees (£10,000 and £5,000 respectively). By the late 1950s student fees amounted to approximately one-tenth of the grant (£25,205 and £225,491). In 1976 fees stood at £81,591, while the grant had soared to £1.8 million and, finally, in 1986-7, the year St Mary's became a branch of Imperial College, student fees produced £663,000, and the treasury grant stood at £4,778,000. Alcock's patient and prolonged negotiation had a profound effect on English medical education (though it did little for Alcock himself, who took up a chair at McGill University in Canada in 1911). Once they were on the state's payroll, the schools had to follow state policy. The Board of Education began to scrutinize their spending. Schools used scholarships to attract candidates from rival schools, but the Board of Education, caring little how the pool of London candidates was divided up, forced the London schools to reduce the sums paid.

Another area of change was in reducing duplication in premedical science teaching. Each teaching hospital had to have its own clinical teachers (who were unsalaried anyway), but it seemed feasible to centralize the costly premedical subjects – chemistry, physics, biology, possibly anatomy and physiology – that were beyond what the smaller schools could afford to teach well. As far back as 1885 the smaller schools had discussed joint classes for the preliminary scientific examinations.[11] St Mary's, which had just hired Augustus Waller, decided against collaboration, and nothing was done.

By the early twentieth century St George's and the Westminster had to farm out their premedical training to the two university colleges. These grew in size (their student numbers rising by one-third) and in power when, as internal colleges, they began to influence University of London policies. In 1905, worried that the royal colleges might steal a march, the university senate applied to its landlords, the 1851 Commissioners, for space to build an Institute of Medical Science "at which may be concentrated the teaching of Preliminary and Intermediate subjects of Medical study (viz., Chemistry, Physics, Biology, Anatomy and Physiology), now carried on in the Medical Schools attached to the various Hospitals of the Metropolis."[12] Already, South Kensington housed a University of London Physiology Laboratory, established by Waller in 1901. The laboratory provided central research labs, while leaving the actual teaching under control of the medical schools, which supported Waller's grand plan. The schools did not support this new plan to centralize both teaching and research.

But the university's plan was forgotten after the Royal Commission on the University of London, the Haldane Commission, reporting in 1913, argued against the erection of separate institutes for advanced science. The chairman, Lord Haldane, had studied philosophy in Germany, and he tried to import German research practices back to England. He was also influenced by the 1910 report by Abraham Flexner to the Carnegie Foundation on medical education that criticized the lack of academic influences on the British teaching hospitals. Haldane believed that undergraduate and post-graduate education should occur side by side, so that even undergraduate education would be suffused with the research ideal, and that clinical and academic sciences should cooperate closely with one another. Rather than funding outcroppings of academe scattered about the medical schools, Haldane wanted to make medical education as a whole more academic.[13]

The Haldane Commission urged the reconstruction of the University of London as a great imperial and metropolitan university. So long as the university consisted of a federation of eclectic institutions – including technical schools, proprietary schools, and incorporated colleges – with the university powerless to improve standards of administration and teaching and only able to insist on the standard of exams, would a London education be devalued. The Haldane Commission argued that these independent and quasi-proprietary medical schools stood between the university and greatness. There were too many schools anyway, more than the market could support. The university should instead concentrate resources to provide a high-quality academic medical education in three medical schools: UCL, King's College, and an unspecified third school. The state would pay £12,000 to each of the three centres to provide salaries for clinical professors.

The great endowed schools like St Bartholomew's might hold out against these sorts of pressures, but St Mary's could not. The Board of Education would not long agree to subsidize unnecessary competition against other state-funded colleges. St Mary's would be dismembered, compelled to cede its premedical scientists. The anatomist at St Mary's, J. Ernest Frazer, was living proof of the danger. Forced out of St George's when its premedical departments closed, Frazer took up a position with St Mary's in 1911 and immediately, according to Cope, turned the Anatomy Department into a great teaching centre and a place of research. Meanwhile, St George's only matriculated two students in 1911, as students gravitated to the schools with the most complete curriculum. But now St Mary's was threatened with the same rationalization that had devastated St George's.

The Haldane report marked a sea change in public thinking about the medical schools. Before 1913 many people expressed regret that there was so much competition and wastage in the London schools. But the system was venerable and was thought to produce the best practical doctors in the world. European and American students perhaps had a more scientific outlook but, defenders of the British system insisted, they had far less practical clinical experience and they viewed patients coldly as experimental subjects. The English preference for practice and experience over theory also militated against administrative reforms undertaken in the name of abstract ideals of efficiency. Sir Wilmot Herringham expressed a widespread view when he told Haldane that, if he were building up London medical education *de novo*, he would not establish so many medical schools; but now that they were there, he would not reduce their number.[15] The commissioners took the abstract and theoretical outlook. Again and again Haldane questioned witnesses how they would build up medical education *de novo*. A growing concern with national efficiency, with economic organization and scientific output, required just such drastic measures.

The meeting between the commissioners and the witnesses for St Mary's (clinicians Sir John Broadbent, William Willcox, and Ernest Graham Little, and hospital chairman W. Austen Leigh) was short and stormy.[16] Haldane did not scruple to call the independent medical schools "the adversary." Other interviews were cordial, as big schools might expect to gain from the rationalization, while small schools couldn't hope to stand out. Only St Mary's tried to defend its small, cheap premedical departments. When Willcox said he had taught chemistry, the commissioners insinuated that as a clinician he was incompetent to teach it at a university standard. The admission that their physics lecturer also taught at a polytechnic prompted Haldane to exclaim, "You see there it is; at once you get outside the atmosphere of university teaching with your teaching." When St Mary's pointed out that their biologist and chemist were first-rate, whole-time men and recommended for university readerships, Haldane denigrated even this standard: "There again, you may get gentlemen who are qualified to be Readers of the University, but it is not the same thing, is it, as coming under a great professor of Physiology with the stimulus that comes from his personality and the inspiration which he puts into his assistants." For the commissioners, all education was either university education directed by the best scientists in the land or it was a technical affair of rote memorization that narrowed the mind rather than broadening it. In vain did St Mary's protest that they didn't want to make scientists but doctors, and that they did not want a "big" scientist who would leave the teaching to assistants no better than the current lecturers. Haldane was unmoved. As far as he was concerned, independent scientific schools were dinosaurs, ripe for extinction.

The rest of the interview was no happier. Only St Mary's defended the practice of examining and licensing students trained elsewhere. Only St Mary's made no suggestions for reforming the Faculty of Medicine. The school apparently wanted to pursue its own business and leave the university to do the same. But for educational reformers like Haldane, the very existence of the school at St Mary's was an obstacle to reform. It was no better than a vested interest and must be sacrificed to national efficiency.

Nonetheless, Austen Leigh was able to make an unanswerable point in closing: namely, that whether or not the University of London needed St Mary's Hospital Medical School, the whole northwest region of London needed St Mary's Hospital, and that fact alone should render St Mary's eligible as a site for concentration.

St Mary's and the University of London fell out over academic standards on other occasions. From 1912 the university began to confer the title of "professor" or "reader" on teachers in the independent medical schools. To obtain recognition, the school had to prove that the teacher had sufficient salary, time, and laboratory facilities to perform research and teach to a university standard. St Mary's did not pay a single teacher enough to merit a university title. Its best teachers were entrepreneurial, supplementing their teaching salaries with other sources of income. In the case of Almroth Wright, it was private practice and vaccine therapy; for William Willcox, it was analytic work done for the Home Office; for the premedical teachers, it was private lecturing. The principal of the university wrote to the dean at St Mary's offering to recognize the chemist, George Senter, and the biologist, W.G. Ridewood, as readers, so long as St Mary's raised their salaries to £300 (which it did). William Willcox might have been a reader in pathological chemistry "but for the fact that so large an amount of time is taken up by duties outside those connected with his teaching post." As for Almroth Wright, he was ineligible for a chair for the reason that he received no salary (his was paid to workers in the department) and "engaged in professional practice and that his appointment cannot therefore be considered as a whole-time appointment" as university positions had to be. Still, one could hardly *not* recognize Sir Almroth Wright, so an exception was made.[17] The University of London did not have everything its own way.

Haldane did not live to see his scheme of concentration realized. The First World War intervened, and by the end of the war, numbers of medical students rose, so that even the small schools began to prosper once again. St Mary's played a part in warding off the scheme for centralization. Leading the battle was Ernest (later Sir Ernest) Graham Little, a dermatologist and political activist. Hired the same day as Almroth Wright, he played perhaps an equally important part in keeping the school alive. Nowadays he is forgotten, but he was one of the most prominent physicians of his generation, a senator of the university from 1904 until his death in 1950 and MP for the university from 1924, when he ousted William Beveridge, until 1950 when the seat was abolished. Graham Little gave St Mary's and the conservative outlook of the traditional London teaching hospitals generally a powerful voice in university affairs and in public life. He lost many battles, the final one against the NHS, but he secured many concessions.

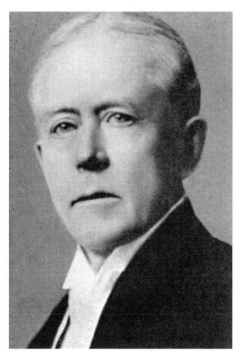

Ernest Graham Little. Heinemann and
St Mary's Hospital NHS Trust Archives

Born in Bengal and educated in South Africa, followed by St George's
and Guy's, Graham Little held various posts and scholarships before coming to St Mary's in 1902 to replace Malcolm Morris as the hospital dermatologist. His name is attached to a benign superficial epitheliomatosis,
which he was the first to see. He wrote scores of letters to the medical and
lay press in favour of health and political reforms, championing, among
other things, whole-wheat bread and the medical education of women.[18]
But his greatest efforts were directed towards the University of London,
where he exerted a weighty Marian influence that would be sadly lacking
after his death.

In March of 1913 Graham Little gave a paper to the medical society on
the centralization scheme.[19] He argued that the proposed Institute of Medical Science would cost more than the existing services and the teaching
would be performed in very large classes by underpaid and nameless
demonstrators. Who knew but that this unsatisfactory practice might be
extended to advanced medical courses? There were also plans to strip the
independent schools of their representation on the university faculty of
medicine, handing this over to the colleges. It was all very Germanic, he remarked, using what was in 1913 a telling phrase.[20]

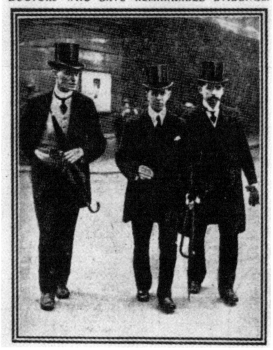

Crippen Again at Bow-street

DOCTORS WHO GAVE REMARKABLE EVIDENCE.

The Crippen-Catchers:
Bernard Spilsbury, Travers
Humphreys, and Willliam
Willcox. *Daily Mirror*,
17 September 1910,
by permission

The ensuing discussion foreshadowed later controversies. Speakers defended small classes, intimacy, and personal contact, with Spilsbury (soon
to leave Mary's for Bart's) insisting that smaller schools had better results
than the large ones. Aleck Bourne, a future socialist, asked if Mary's could
dispense with the government grant and go its own way. Impossible, the
youthful Charles Pannett replied, to go back to those days of make-do, for
modern facilities were needed. He recommended modern methods to sustain them, namely, advertising: "Modern buildings were necessary, and
great were the virtues of advertisement. St. Mary's might use the work of
the Inoculation Department to give her a world-wide fame." Graham Little agreed that St Mary's "did not set out her wares as advantageously as
she might – there were many chances of fame in the possession of men like
Sir Almroth Wright, Dr. Willcox and Dr. Spilsbury, the nature of whose
work made their names household words for the lay public; St. Mary's
ought to exploit these names for the good of the School."

All three men whom Graham Little invoked were laboratory men
(though Willcox and Wright also had patients at St Mary's). The senior
physicians and surgeons were nowhere in this plan to raise the school's
public profile. There may be several reasons for this. Consultants, qua con-

sultants, were supposed to shun any publicity more glaring than a discreet brass plaque on the door. Among the aristocratic social circles that elite physicians and surgeons cultivated, tacit knowledge was preferred to publicity, and the ideal was the stately royal physician to whom *le tout London* deferred respectfully. However, the nature of the public to which medicine was appealing was changing. The rise of the penny press had created a broader-based public opinion that did rest on publicity. Much of the penny press concerned itself with crime, and so it played up the forensic scientists who brought criminals like Crippen to book: Willcox and Spilsbury. When Doctor Crippen poisoned his wife, dumped the body in acid, and then buried it in his cellar, Spilsbury identified the bit of abdominal skin that was dug up as Mrs Crippen's by means of her ovariotomy scar, while Willcox detected traces of hyoscine in it. This extraordinary bit of medical detection quite rightly made the headlines.[21]

At the end of the war, when the different medical schools were canvassed by the Board of Education on their plans for reconstruction, St Mary's pointed to pathology, especially forensic pathology, as a possible basis for rebuilding the school: "Great developments would also be possible in the direction of Medical Jurisprudence, as St. Mary's has on her staff, at the present time, two of the leading Medico-Legal Experts." The school suggested that with separate forensic laboratory and museum facilities, it could fill a want in London medicine.[22] Forensic medicine could be sold to the state and the public as an exciting new laboratory science, but one organized around what were essentially diagnostic problems, just like clinical medicine. It neither required nor fostered a team-research approach, especially at St Mary's, where prominence was secured through a close relationship with the Home Office. After Willcox and Spilsbury retired, G. Roche Lynch took over the department and the Home Office work, serving as senior analyst from 1928. He published little, mostly a few articles on poison, and St Mary's was left behind in the developing clinical science of chemical pathology. Flexner criticized the lack of research in that department at St Mary's.[23] Forensic science at St Mary's was a domesticated science. In 1918 it provided a way to build up the school's scientific and popular prestige without threatening traditional clinical paradigms.

There were two other ways of building a scientific profile, but both posed a threat to traditional clinical authority. One was the research laboratory, the other the academic clinical unit advocated by the Haldane Commission. The development of scientific laboratories and academic units created a crisis of identity for the medical profession in the early twentieth century. The crisis was particularly intense at St Mary's. The dean of St Mary's from 1910–20, Sir John Broadbent, fought what he saw as the encroachments of both the Haldane units and of Almroth Wright (whose "opsonic process," he warned, "if applied too freely to the mental pabulum, is liable to debilitate the mental digestion"[24]). At St Mary's the epistemological crisis in medicine led to dramatic face-to-face confrontations, at committee meetings, on the wards, in the laboratories, and in the hospital medical society, as well as the wider medical press. The staff fought over the souls of the students, who revelled in the spectacle.

The Clinic versus the Laboratory

Almroth Wright was a controversialist. Soon after arriving at St Mary's, he launched a sweeping attack on traditional clinical medicine, on two grounds: it was impotent in the face of bacterial disease, and it did not advance knowledge of these diseases. In 1905 he argued this point at forums as diverse as the inaugural address at St Mary's and the *Liverpool Daily Press*. "The thoughtful and conscientious physician has absolutely no illusions," insisted Wright. "Confronted with an acute bacterial invasion, he does not conceal from himself, or from others, that he is quite in the dark, and that he cannot foresee or determine the issue of the conflict which is in progress in the organism. That conflict will culminate, as the case may be, in the recovery or death of the patient." Physicians were too concerned with money-making to undertake serious research, and consequently, he said "the medical profession is not an agency for medical research, nor are our hospitals instituted or administered for the purpose of solving the problems of medicine."[25] Progress depended on pathology, and the "physician of the future will be an immunisator."

Another lecture given by Wright in 1907 to the medical society was wittily summarized in the *Gazette*: "The Professor held forth, in his favorite rôle of Superclinician ... His confession of faith is something like this: Life is the relation of man to experimental science; Happiness is stated in terms of the opsonic index of man to immanent micro-organisms; the Laboratory is the source of a wise man's knowledge; the good man's morals are made in the Laboratory; the Clinician is a mere mechanical person, or the Hibernian equivalent thereof. This thesis he sustained delightfully in an hour's discourse that was pure joy to listen to, and at the end of it certain serious-minded persons left with an impression that the pathologist did them something less than justice."[26] Some of those serious-minded persons stormed angrily out of the meeting. Wright loved the cut and thrust of intellectual debate, which, he argued, gave a "vivifying personal interest" to dry intellectual matters. He believed that "all controversy is a warfare from which the one or the other of the parties has got to emerge discredited"[27] and humiliated his opponents ruthlessly, making many enemies. His colleagues at St Mary's tended to be for or against him. The surgeons were more favourably disposed than the physicians who bore the brunt of his attack on clinical medicine.

Before Wright's arrival, there had been much good-natured cooperation between clinicians and pathologists. For example, the physician D.B. Lees together with F.J. Poynton investigated the incidence of cardiac dilation in acute rheumatism, using post-mortem records.[28] Similarly, the St Mary's physician Robert Maguire worked out a theory that antiseptics injected into the veins might kill the tuberculous bacillus in the lungs. Since James E. Lane seemed to be having success by injecting a 2 per cent solution of cyanide of mercury into the veins of syphilitics, Maguire decided to try that and injected 30 minims in a 2 per cent solution into two patients at the Brompton. Thinking that this solution was too weak, he went to Plimmer and asked him to try injecting 5 per cent into a rabbit's ear. The rabbit was dead before the injection was completed. "I immediately hurried, as you may readily understand, to see what had been the effect of the weaker injection upon my tuberculous patients and found that both of them had become very collapsed."[29] He tried some other substances, getting Plimmer to inject them into rabbits first and then injecting himself. Maguire wasn't actually testing the drugs as therapies, because he didn't know how to give the animals tuberculosis. So he tested the drugs for safety on animals and for therapeutic efficacy on humans. He began to have some success, so he thought, with formic aldehyde.

There was some jealousy between clinicians and pathologists, to be sure. Pathologists joked that scar tissue grew over Edmund Owen's ward lectures, so the students could remember none of their earlier lessons.[30] But Owen, speaking in Canada in 1900, complained that when students came onto the wards, they thought they were merely putting the "finishing touches on their professional education." They had adopted a "bacteriological faith," and would demand surgical excision of any bodily parts tainted by tuberculous bacilli, whereas a surgeon would counsel restraint.[31] This was said with a wry humour quite different from the earnest tone Owen later adopted to criticize excessive faith in vaccinations. In 1909 he complained to the *Lancet* that vaccinists ignored clinical signs. He told of a woman with glandular swelling treated with tuberculin for what he diagnosed as chronic abscess of the tooth. "The time surely has not yet arrived that the vaccine-therapist can rise superior to those methods of investigation which are taught as the ABC to students as soon as they begin clinical work. It is far more important in such a case to examine the teeth than the blood."[32]

D.B. Lees too moved from a position of cordial collaboration to overt opposition. By 1907 he was determined to give no quarter to the bacteriologists, especially Wright, in regard to scientific methods or therapeutic efficacy. Lees claimed to be able to detect tuberculosis clinically, before bacteriologists or radiologists could find any trace of it, and he claimed that his treatment of pneumonia – ice packs – was far superior to vaccine therapy because lowered temperatures decreased microbial activity. "I claim, therefore, that the employment of ice in acute visceral inflammation is strictly a *scientific method* – as genuinely scientific as, for instance, the attempt to lessen the vitality of microbes and to stimulate the appetite of the leucocytes by the subcutaneous injection of substances of unknown composition: – equally scientific, and much safer for the patient." A case of pneumococcal pleurisy and pneumococcal pericarditis in Prince's Ward had seemed hopeless, so he had tried heroic remedies, including leeches and ice bags over the heart and lungs. He also applied lotions and sprays and an inhaler to stop micro-organisms coming in the mouth and nose. Hypodermic injections of strychnine completed the prescription. Still he feared that the case was hopeless. Then, he told students,

remembering the brilliant introductory lecture to which we all listened with so much interest two years ago, in which stress was laid on the powerlessness of the physician to deal with microbic infections, and on the superiority of the method of therapeutic inoculation as the only real hope in such conditions, I determined to seek the assistance of this latest development of science. With his usual courtesy and kindness, Sir Almroth Wright at once consented to give me his help, and himself took a specimen of the patient's blood. On attempting a cultivation, he found it to be sterile. In this case, then, of severe microbic invasion, the most advanced science found itself powerless. But I am glad to be able to add that the efforts of the physician, aided by the splendid nursing that the patient received from Sister Prince's, were crowned with success. It is the first case of the kind which I have seen recover.[33]

Opsonisers and radiologists did not let Lees's subtle attack pass, and critical exchange continued in the *Gazette* up until 1912.[34]

Lees's confidence in the superiority of clinical medicine was seconded by the greatest clinician of the age, Oxford regius professor Sir William Osler, who visited the school and warned students, "Stop your ears with the wise man's wax against the wiles of that Celtic siren, Sir Almroth, who would abolish Harley Street and all that it represents." This view was seconded as well by John Poynton (who, like John Broadbent, had competed for Wright's position in 1902). In 1909 Poynton insisted that only clinical judgment could tell if a vaccine worked or not: "Because a so-called vaccine alters an index which is, after all, to a great extent an artificial conception, it does not follow that we have unlocked the mystery of the healing process-

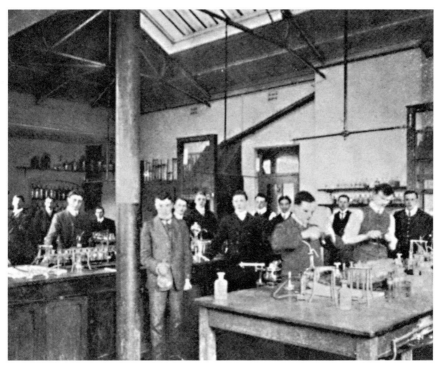

Students in the laboratory. St Mary's Hospital NHS Trust Archives

es even in the infective diseases: because a serum is of value in diphtheria, it does not follow, as we know only too well, that sera will cure all infective processes. It is clinical observation which will eventually sift out the degree of truth in these matters; and in no form of disease is clinical observation more needful, I think, than in the study of unexpected recoveries."[35]

The younger generation of Mary's physicians and surgeons responded more enthusiastically to vaccine therapy. Leucocyte and opsonic indexes challenged clinical judgment with increasing success.[36] For Edwin Ash, who entered as a student in 1898 and became a neurologist, leucocyte counts provided a more reliable measure of the gravity of patients' conditions than clinical symptoms.[37] Compelling evidence was provided by John Herbert Wells, a student who crossed over to the Inoculation Department. He accidentally inoculated himself with the glanders bacillus and, long before clinicians could diagnose the disease, Wells charted his terminal decline with opsonic indices. He died in 1909, aged only thirty.[38]

Two men who joined the staff at St Mary's the same time as Wright adopted his ideas. Leslie Paton qualified at Mary's in 1900 and was appointed assistant ophthalmic surgeon in 1903. In 1905 the *Gazette* observed:

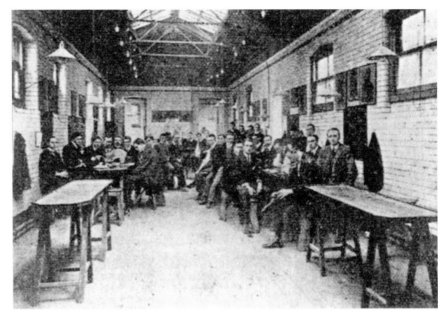

The dead room. St Mary's Hospital NHS Trust Archives

"Mr. Paton has been preaching the gospel of Opsonins in a paper read before the Ophthalmological Society, on November 9th, on 'Phlyctenular Conjunctivitis and its relation to the Opsonic Index.'"[39] Ernest Graham Little, the dermatologist hired in 1902, was another early enthusiast for Wright's therapies which were, indeed, largely directed at skin disorders.[40] Another convert was Sir William Willcox, who was Lees's house physician and became assistant physician to St Mary's in 1907, by which point he was already using leucocyte counts and opsonic indices to diagnose patients.[41] In later years "Swillie" became a proponent of focal sepsis, which he grafted upon his understanding of Wright's theories. In obstinate cases of low fever or arthritis or even diabetes, he pulled teeth and had Almroth Wright make up vaccines.[42] The students mercilessly mocked his theories. In 1932 a parody appeared in the *Gazette*, written in the manner of A.A. Milne. Willcox asks Wright for a vaccine, but Wright refuses, and the nurse suggests instead some emetine thickly spread:

Sir William said "Bother," and then he said "O deary me," and went to bed,
"I only want some sepsis in the patient in that bed."

Happiness is eventually restored when Wright agrees to make up a vaccine, sending Willcox joyfully sliding down the banisters.[43]

Students passing through the school responded variously to Almroth Wright. In the year of his appointment the number of incoming students rose, and some wended their way to the Inoculation Department. Alexander Fleming was the most famous, but there were others, including John Wells, Leonard Colebrook, and John Freeman, as well as William Parry Morgan, of whom the *Gazette* remarked, "Like so many of our best men, he has been gathered into Sir Almroth Wright's net."[44] The complaint was made that science was becoming more popular than rugby at St Mary's and the result was a "low opsonic content in sports."[45]

The *Gazette* was ambivalent about the Inoculation Department, its tone varying depending on the editor. Some admired Wright,[46] but most were irreverent. J.B. Rous, a talented writer (who died while working at the *Lancet* in 1910), remorselessly sent up the opsonists, as when he described them as "Modern Mrs. Beetons who have concocted the new cookery book entitled 'Opsonins or Dainty Dishes for the Million.'"[47] This reflected a wider student culture that playfully satirized all aspects of school life. (The preceding paragraph joked: "About 6 P.M. the most placid of physicians is liable to become without patience with Out-Patients.") But Wright and his opsonins were especially targeted.[48] The preceding issue of the *Gazette* had summarized a paper given by Wright to the medical society on "The Physiology of Belief" which classified fallacies as "hyperekeigonogenetic presentations," "hypereikonokinetic responsiveness," and so forth, all of which was a gift to the *Gazette* wits. An anonymous piece on "The Differential Diagnosis of Folly and Genius" mocked "the Eikonikinetic-Kinemeturgical" standpoint and other nonsense jargon: "Centrally the katabolic tendencies obtain their objective, whilst peripherally the anabolic endeavours are crowned with success."[49] Laughter, for the students, was a weapon against pretentiousness. It replaced disorderly conduct in the classroom as the informal policing mechanism against anything that breached student sensibilities. The students learned this from teachers like Edmund Owen, who mercilessly ridiculed and humiliated unprepared students. The *Gazette* provided the bacteriologists with a forum to convey new techniques and ideas, but it could equally be a conservative force, mocking these techniques and ideas.

In short, St Mary's Hospital Medical School had an ambivalent relationship with Almroth Wright. The extent to which he benefited the school is debatable. A student described him as a "fierce, hoary lion of a man who never spoke to a woman, who hated students of any sort and who refused to teach except for the few statutory lectures he had to give."[50] Wright tried to resign from the pathology lecturing entirely and, when the Medical School Committee refused, quietly handed the teaching over to his employees.

In 1911, just before classes began, Wright wrote to the dean from on board a ship to South Africa, where he was about to perform pneumonia trials: "With regard to the bacteriology I want you please to let me resign the lectureship. I have not done the work for the last year, and have been handing on the cheques to Freeman who as Assistant Lecturer has been doing the work."[51] That fall the *Gazette* lamented: "In spite of the fact that the pathological laboratory has never been served with greater skill or devotion than now, it must be admitted that the existing arrangements do not admit of all the work of the department being entirely carried through. Our students receive no training in practical clinical pathology, nor is there anyone at present with the time to teach them. This must handicap them in seeking residential posts in other institutions and in their practice."[52] Wright had his way: Douglas was named lecturer and John Freeman assistant lecturer in bacteriology. Practical teaching still failed to satisfy, and in 1912, the dean asked Wright to arrange for some instruction in "serum diagnosis and immunisation." Wright deputized the work to Alexander Fleming. As well, E.H. Kettle was made assistant lecturer in pathology.

Developing the Academic Units

For Almroth Wright, science occurred in the lab, not the clinic. One possible response to this argument was the academic clinical unit. Sir William Osler warmly advocated academic units to the Haldane Commission, and to the Northumberland and Durham Medical Society in 1911, where he observed that Wright's "funeral oration" for clinical medicine was premature, given that "the medical and surgical staff at St. Mary's are still on duty!"

A clinical or Haldane unit consisted of a salaried professor of medicine or surgery chosen from among the medical men capable of serious scientific research (whom some thought to be plentiful, others almost non-existent), with beds, a laboratory, and a few young assistants. Some thought the professor should be forbidden to engage in private practice, while others maintained that he should be permitted a few hours each week to keep his hand in. To be salaried, some argued, was to be a creature of the government and to be deprived of the bracing stimulus of economic competition. Moreover, a really good clinician could expect to make a fortune in private practice and, as witnesses before the Haldane Commission testified, would be unlikely to relinquish private practice for less than a small fortune. Haldane replied that they wanted men with a bent for research rather than a passion for money.[53] In other words, if it was the complaints of scientists that they were overworked and underpaid that prompted the attack on the traditional medical schools, the very fact that scientists came so much more cheaply than consultants provided Haldane with the solution.

The larger and collegiate medical schools told Haldane they would entertain the prospect of academic units, but Sir John Broadbent remained hostile. At the annual school dinner in 1913 he argued that surgeons with emergency practices could not set aside definite hours for private work. Moreover, the proposals would lower morale: they would relegate patients to the category of mere teaching material and would erode local patriotism.[54] As late as 1918, when asked by the Board of Education how it would like to reconstruct the school, given enough money, the MSC made no reference to academic units.[55] Within three years, however, the school had done an abrupt turnaround. Broadbent stepped down, and the new dean, Charles McMoran Wilson, persuaded his colleagues that they must institute academic units of medicine and surgery. The reversal was prompted by the Board of Education which in 1919–20 established units in medicine and surgery at four London teaching hospitals (St Bartholomew's, UCL, St Thomas's and the London), and another in obstetrics and gynaecology at the Royal Free.

Wilson saw in the appointments a death knell for the old system of medical education and the beginning of "a race for existence among the remaining London Schools."[56] This was not paranoia: officials in the Board of Education had been won round to Haldane's view, and they anticipated that "Schools that do not become Unit Schools are going to die a natural death."[57] Wilson was determined that St Mary's would survive and was well qualified to direct the effort.[58] A former Mary's student and a former captain of the rugby team, he was, despite his slight build, a force on the field by reason of his speed and determination. He believed that in life, as in warfare and rugby, the fittest would prevail.

St Mary's needed business methods and efficiency, Wilson proclaimed in the *Gazette*, which he edited from 1919. Without them, the school would fail: "We are passing into a highly-competitive world, in which institutions which are not run like a business must presently perish according to the laws of this business world … This is our little war for existence, and if we want to win it, we must be as thorough. There is no place for compromise. We are late in the field; we have given a start to rivals who have the assistance of tradition; we must make up leeway by an unceasing quest for efficiency." Two months later, in March 1920, Wilson repeated his warning that it was "a question of the survival of the fittest" among the non-unit schools. Already the Middlesex had raised £20,000 from wealthy patrons, while Guy's could fall back on a tradition of clinical research dating back to the days of Bright and Hodgkins. Wilson insisted: "We cannot have a first-class school with a third-class waiting room masquerading as a laboratory, *and if we cannot have a first-class school we cannot have a school at all*. It has come to that."[59] The rugby player handicapped by his small

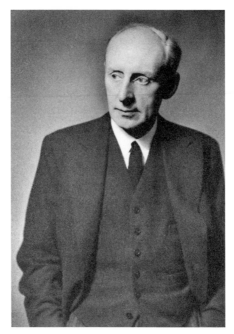

Charles Wilson.
St Mary's Hospital NHS Trust Archives

size became the spokesman for a school handicapped by its small size, still convinced he could overturn the bruisers by sheer force of will.

Wilson had been elected to the staff of St Mary's Hospital in 1919 largely on the strength of his solutions to the crisis. His appointment, which he described minutely in a series of letters to his fiancée, illustrates how one became a consultant at that time.[60] He had not been particularly promising as a student, spending too much time on the sports field. Still, in a school where rugby was taken seriously, this and his evident brains were enough to secure him a post as medical registrar (beating out the more scholarly Charles Singer for the position). However, he tired of school politics and set off to see something of the world; but a stint in Egypt was enough. He returned to London and, by extraordinary exertion, obtained a gold medal in the University of London MD exam. A staff appointment was now a very real possibility, as one of the lecturers, Wilfred Harris, informed him. Already Wilson knew his rival: Alfred Hope Gosse, who was "handsome, self-confident and debonair. He had the assurance that physical strength (he had rowed at Cambridge), good looks, easy manners and the innate knowledge of his own ability give to any man when he is young." Wilson, by contrast, was less attractive physically, with a crooked slant to his face, and his personality lacked Gosse's sunnyness. But as Wilson told

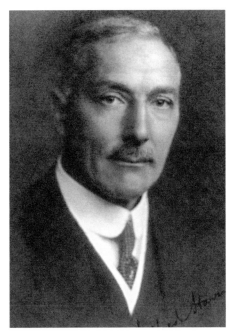

Wilfred Harris.
St Mary's Hospital NHS Trust Archives

his parents in 1913, "Gosse is very popular and I hold trumps as far as work is concerned." He had imagination and craftiness where Gosse had not.

After the First World War, finally in 1919 a junior post became available, with Gosse and Wilson the two strongest candidates. Gosse had already published articles, while Wilson had not, though he was trying to write one up. Still, Wilson remarked, "There won't be 'any damned nonsense about merit.'" The matter was decided entirely on the basis of partisan politics. Three men dominated school policy: Harris, who supported Wilson, and Willcox and Broadbent, who supported Gosse. The other staff members all had to be canvassed, by tradition. Gosse invited them all to his club, while Wilson tried to persuade them that the school would fail unless he were appointed and given a free hand to establish academic units. Broadbent and Willcox pooh-poohed the threat, but gradually, with the help of Harris and Charles Pannett, Wilson persuaded the staff that his appointment was indispensable. All parties were placated when the governors were persuaded to appoint a supernumerary physician, with Gosse taking that post. Neither man would make any great contributions to medical science.

Once elected to the staff, Wilson turned to the matter of the clinical units. St Mary's was not, in fact, terribly late in the field. Negotiations between the Board of Education and the four chosen schools were proceeding slowly, as the existing consultants demanded that the professor be named from among them, while the university wanted to bring in new men appointed in open competition. Wilson did not become dean until 1921, but he assumed direction of academic policy immediately after his appointment and persuaded the consultants and governors to sanction the appointment of salaried clinical professors.

Late in 1919 the hospital Medical Committee reported to the board that clinical units were necessary to both the school and the hospital. Modern medicine required researching clinicians: "If the type of man seeking election to the staff of the hospital in the future is to be maintained at the present level, facilities for research must be provided during the years of waiting and the ability to carry out original work should play a larger part in selection." Moreover, the Board of Education had determined to weed out the weaker schools: "Survival means acceptance of their terms. The Grant is to be employed as a weapon in enforcing policy and incidentally of automatically bringing about that reduction in the number of schools which the Board and all the Royal Commissions have advocated. This cutting down, indeed, is an inevitable part of their policy as it is clearly impossible to subsidise all on the scale the Board deems essential for efficiency."[61] The hospital was suitably alarmed and voted to sanction the units. In the spring of 1920 the MSC asked the University of London to recognize two senior consultants, Wilfred Harris and W.H. Clayton Greene, as directors of clinical units. The Board of Education had intimated that it would allocate one more academic unit to the school that submitted the best scheme.

At that point, Wilson ran into a roadblock. In July the University of London refused the MSC's request on the ground that neither Harris nor Green was a full-time teacher, and neither had been hired in an open competition. (The hospital appointments were filled on open competition as were premedical lectureships, but clinical lectureships were filled by those already in post at the hospital.) Wilson then paid a visit to George Newman and Sir Wilmot Herringham of the Board of Education, and both advised him that Mary's should give up teaching undergraduates and devote itself to graduate medical education. Herringham's idea of a suitable professor was a David Ferrier, an outstanding scientific researcher, rather than a glorified traditional clinician.[62]

Wilson refused to give up. He persuaded his colleagues to give the units a one-year trial. This took some persuading. The staff agreed to relinquish some beds to the units, and the hospital board agreed to guarantee £5,000 of the £7,000 salaries, the rest to be met by the medical school. At the end of the year, it was hoped, the Board of Education would reward the experiment by picking up the tab. The positions were duly advertised, but "it was seen that no responsible Physician or Surgeon could be expected for one year to give up his private practice."[63] As a compromise, the directors of the unit, who had to be men of some professional standing, were permitted to do some private practice, and the unit assistants, who were keen young men, would be salaried, whole-time workers. Harris and Clayton Greene agreed to the terms, and the units were formally instituted. In April 1921 the Board of Education did indeed agree to pick up the tab and pay three-fourths of the unit salaries, as at the other four schools. St Mary's was saved.

Then disaster struck again. King's Fund officials served notice that, according to the regulations of 1905, any hospital subsidy to the school would disqualify the hospital for King's Fund funds, which had amounted to £7,000 the previous year. The governors tried to argue that patients would benefit from the more systematic investigations that the clinical professors could undertake. The King's Fund rebuffed this slur against the methods in use elsewhere, but did agree that the costs of the extra tests and x-rays might reasonably be considered hospital charges.[64] When the governors told the school that it must find the money for the salaries, Wilson replied predictably with warnings of economic catastrophe; but in the end he had to find the money.

The clinical units were in place, but not quite as Haldane had envisioned them. Those at St Mary's, as elsewhere, were a triumph of reality over idealism.[65] Clayton Greene and Harris soon made way for Charles Pannett and Frederick Langmead, the most junior members of the hospital staff (excepting only Gosse and Wilson). They were too young to have lucrative private practices, and they were more open to experiment than the stately senior staff. Both were good clinicians and good practical teachers, but neither was a clinical scientist. Their appointments ensured that the consultants would dominate St Mary's Hospital Medical School for another two decades.

The clinical units were only one of Wilson's schemes for the school. The lack of beds had long been a problem: there were only 124 general surgical beds in the hospital, and regulations required that a unit have sixty beds. The other surgeons would not have accepted such an ignominious, second-best position. Wilson formed an agreement with the Paddington Guardians to permit teaching rounds in the infirmary, and by this stroke added six hundred new beds. As he triumphantly pointed out, this also ensured that students would see clinical material not ordinarily admitted to a teaching hospital but the bread-and-butter of general practice: fractures, tuberculous hips, late-stage cancer, pulmonary tuberculosis, and other chronic diseases. For Wilson, collaboration with the Poor Law hospitals was not mere expediency but part of a long-term strategy to preserve both institutions. In 1920 he told the Harveian Society that to meet growing demand for hospital treatment, "the infirmaries must be converted into modern hospitals," and the best way to accomplish that was to introduce students.[66] But this implied that two modern hospital systems, voluntary and state run, would compete directly with one another. Voluntary hospitals couldn't hope to compete against municipal hospitals commanding state resources. Survival lay in collaboration. Wilson's scheme was widely greeted as an important innovation and a beacon for the future of medical services and education. At the same time, he arranged for teaching rounds at Paddington Green Children's Hospital, led by Reginald Miller, who had paediatric appointments at both hospitals.

Wilson had many other plans for building up St Mary's. The committee that recommended academic units in 1919 also recommended reorganizing the pathology department. It quoted the Haldane Commission's observation that "University and hospital authorities would do well to make provision in every medical school for the establishment of a pathological institute, or arrangements equivalent to it."[67] Wright would no longer to be left to reign unchallenged in the Inoculation Department. After 1920 it and the medical school – pathology and medicine – began to inch their way back together, propelled by developments in science and politics.

The Interwar Period

Colour Plates

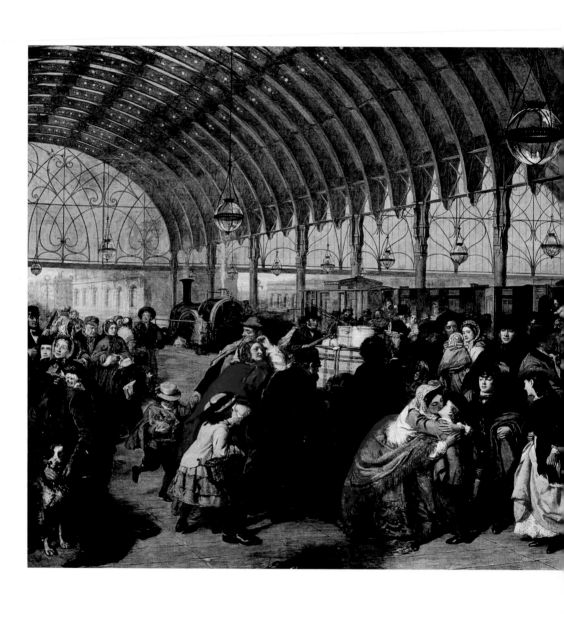

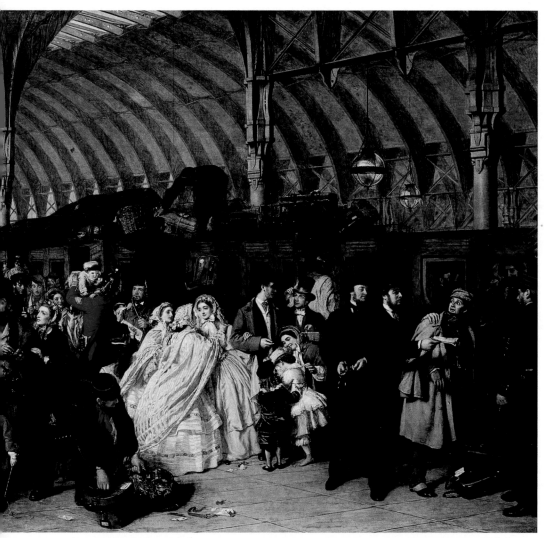
William Powell Frith, "The Railway Station" (1862), showing Paddington
Station. Royal Holloway, University of London

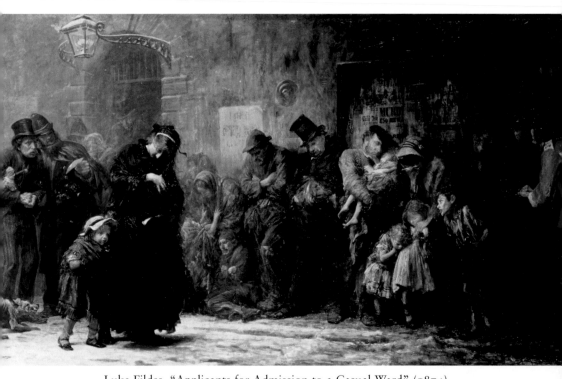

Luke Fildes, "Applicants for Admission to a Casual Ward" (1874).
Royal Holloway, University of London

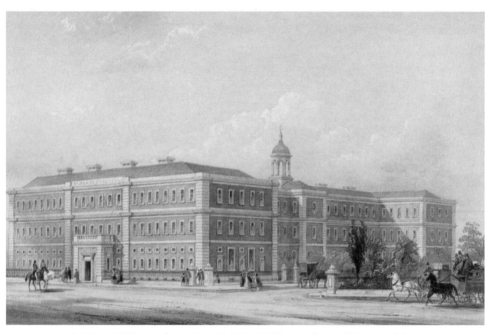

St Mary's Hospital in 1852. St Mary's Hospital NHS Trust Archives

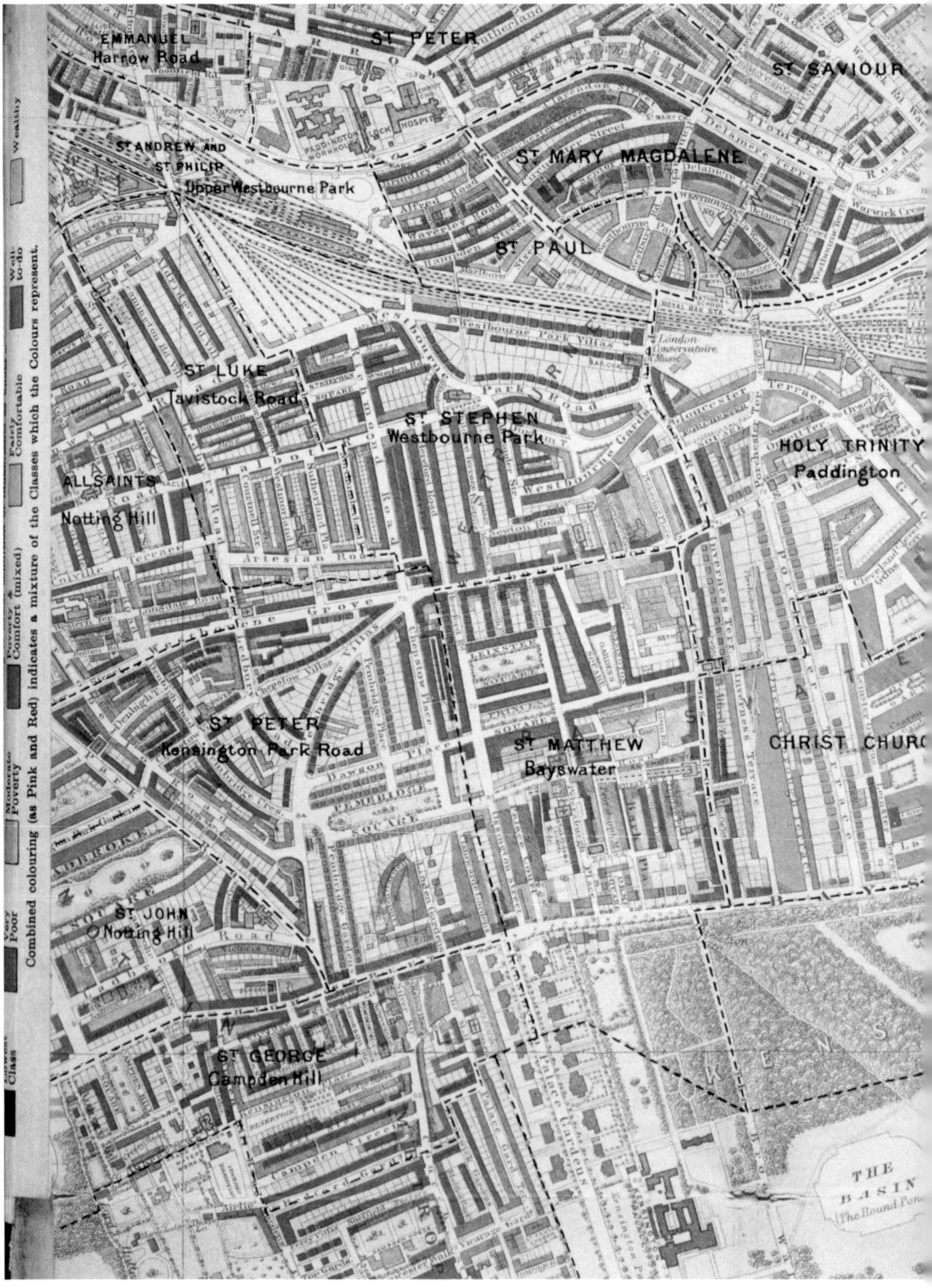

Combined colouring (as Pink and Red) indicates a mixture of the Classes which the Colours represent.
Very Poor
Moderate Poverty
Poverty & Comfort (mixed)
Fairly Comfortable
Well-to-do
Wealthy
EMMANUEL
Harrow Road
ST PETER
ST SAVIOUR
ST ANDREW AND ST PHILIP
Upper Westbourne Park
ST MARY MAGDALENE
ST PAUL
ST LUKE
Tavistock Road
ST STEPHEN
Westbourne Park
HOLY TRINITY
Paddington
ALL SAINTS
Notting Hill
ST PETER
Kensington Park Road
ST MATTHEW
Bayswater
CHRIST CHURC
ST JOHN
Notting Hill
ST GEORGE
Campden Hill
THE BASIN
(The Round Pon
Westbourne Park Villas
London Conservatoire of Music
Royal Oak Sta.
Arlesian Road
Chepstow Villas
Pembridge Square
Leinster Square
Princes Square
Campden Street
Palace Gardens

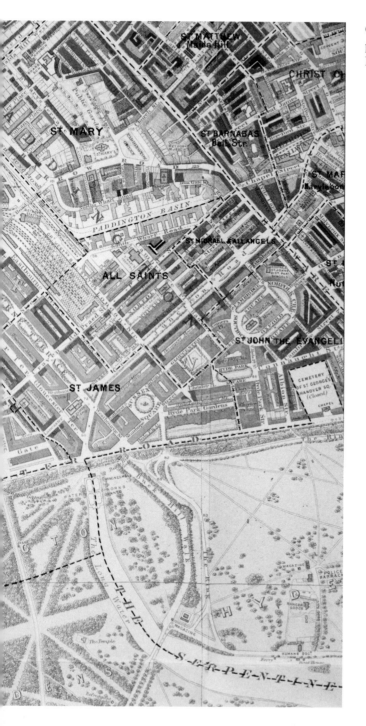

Charles Booth's map of
poverty in London, 1889.
British Library

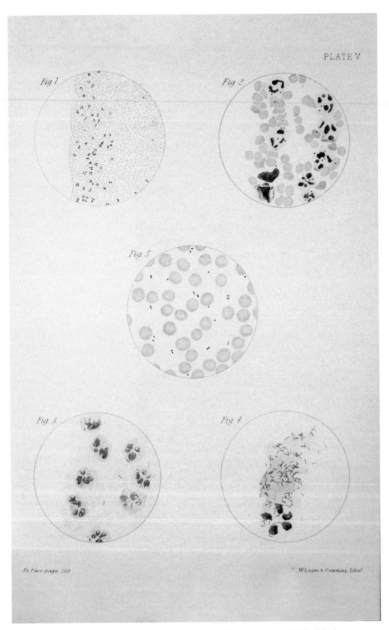

PLATE V

Fig 1.

Fig 2.

Fig 5.

Fig 3.

Fig 4.

McLagan & Cumming, Edin.

Opsonization. Wellcome Library and Heinemann's Publishers

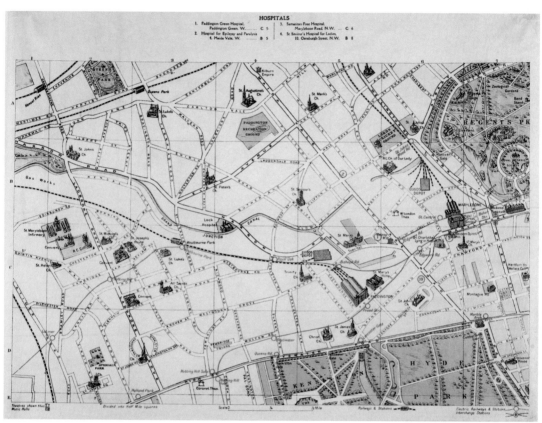

Map of Paddington in 1913 showing sites of medical interest (done for the International Congress of Medicine). St Mary's is shown, as are the Western Ophthalmic Hospital and the Lock Hospital, but not the Paddington Workhouse and Infirmary next to the Lock. The Wellcome Library

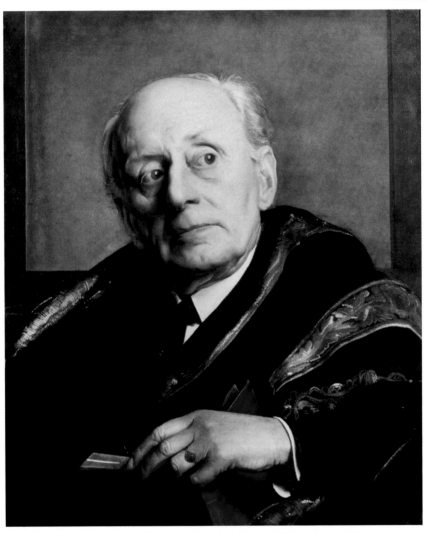

Annigoni's portrait of Moran. Royal College of Physicians of London

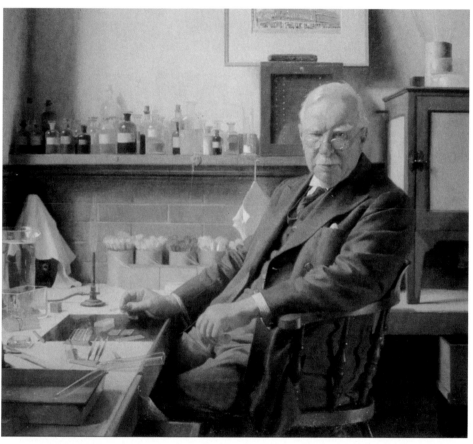

Gerald Kelly's portrait of Sir Almroth Wright. St Mary's Hospital NHS Trust Archives

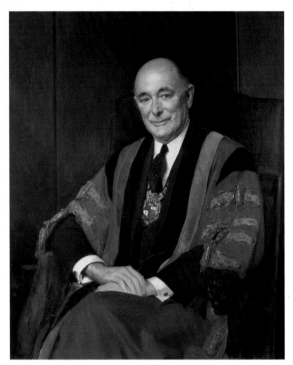

Arthur, Lord Porritt of Wanganui.
Royal College of Surgeons of England

The Changing Hospital 2

DURING THE FIRST half of the twentieth century the London voluntary hospitals lurched from crisis to crisis. From the early 1890s they were
so short of funds that there was serious thought of a bailout by the state.
At St Mary's, sixty beds stood vacant in the new Clarence Wing for want
of funds to administer them. War, then depression continued to threaten the
voluntary system. Subscriptions and donations formed an ever-diminishing
proportion of hospital revenues, requiring hospitals to cast about for other
sources of income.[1]

At St Mary's in 1900 subscriptions and donations made up 35 per cent
of the hospital's income (nearly £8,000 of a total income of £22,000), and
legacies accounted for another 35 per cent. Central funds – the Saturday
Fund, the Sunday Fund, and the King's Fund – made up 16 per cent, divi-
dends on investments 9½ per cent, and the rest was made up in various
ways, including a mere £2 from the local churches. The income was about
£8,000 less than was needed to run the hospital. St Mary's ran up annual
deficits each year, usually ranging between £2,000 and £10,000, depending on how many rich benefactors had died that year.

There were some outstanding benefactions. In 1901 a city merchant
named S.R. Zunz left £100,000 to charity, and the executors offered
£25,000 to St Mary's on condition that the hospital raise a like sum –
which it managed to do, thanks to a last-minute donation from Rothschilds. In 1912 the hospital was left an Australian estate worth more than
£46,000 by Frederick Griffen, which it sold piecemeal. The governors allowed the old custom of annual dinners to lapse and instead staged regular

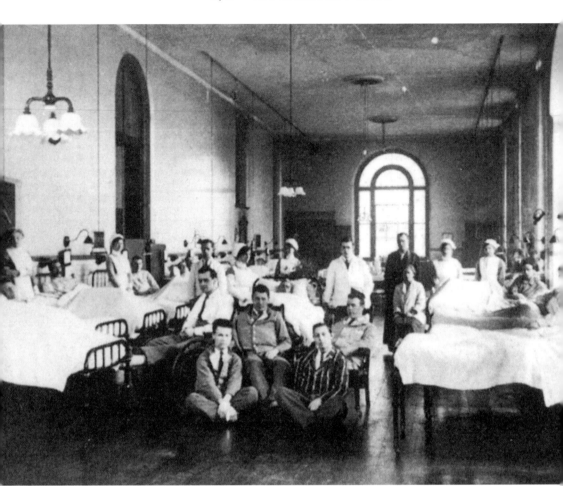

Soldiers on the ward during World War I. St Mary's Hospital NHS Trust Archives

bazaars, with different neighbourhoods of Paddington competing against one another. The first such, held in 1899, generated more than £21,000. During World War I the charitable income declined considerably, but government payments for the treatment of soldiers made up the difference.

After the war, subscriptions and donations failed to pick up again. By October 1920 St Mary's had accumulated a running deficit of £16,000. Bankruptcy loomed. As a last resort the hospital board drew up a voluntary payment scheme for patients. In 1921 patients' payments raised more than £9,000, and this went a long way towards meeting the costs, though a large operating deficit remained. The following year patient contributions accounted for 17 per cent of the hospital's income, almost as much as subscriptions and donations at 20 per cent. Total charitable income was at 60 per cent and slipping downwards at about 1 per cent per year. Payments from local authorities amounted to 10 per cent of the hospital's income. The hospital was still, barely, a charitable enterprise.

Fifteen years later, this was no longer true: most of its income came from payment for services, from local authorities (20 per cent) or patients (42 per cent). The central charitable funds provided for 6 per cent of expenditure, while subscriptions, donations, and legacies came to 20 per cent. Even so, the hospital could not make ends meet, and that year it had an overdraft of £70,000. By the end of the Second World War it had become obvious that the voluntary hospital system was unsustainable, and that something else would have to replace it. (See tables 1–4.)

This chapter outlines the causes, nature, and consequences of these changing patterns of hospital finance. The first half describes events at St Mary's itself: the admission of well-to-do paying patients and the establishment of clinics financed by local authorities. The second half turns to the larger picture and the introduction of a national health service. The lobby for nationalization developed at both the local and the national level, among the public and the medical profession, arguing from both the successes and the failures of medicine. St Mary's helped to shape the national debate.

The Triumphs of Medicine

During the first half of the twentieth century, vaccine therapy was one of many new treatments that came into public demand. Others included antitoxins for tetanus and diphtheria, both available at St Mary's from the 1890s, insulin for diabetes, liver extracts for pernicious anaemia, vitamin treatments for other deficiency diseases, arsenicals for syphilis, and light and radium therapies for cancer. Hormone therapy came into fashion: in 1921 a seventy-four-year-old Paddington man went to Paris to have monkey glands grafted onto his body in hopes of rejuvenation.[2] And then there were the mounting triumphs of surgery, facilitated by the development of saline injections,[3] followed by blood transfusion. By the early 1920s collapsed obstetric patients were being transfused by Aleck Bourne.

By trumpeting these medical triumphs, the daily press fuelled public demand for medicine. In 1906, for example, an article in the *Standard* bearing the headline "The Surgeon Twixt Man and Death" described a surgeon being called onto Albert Ward: "Within twenty minutes he has explored the patient's interior mechanism, found a something that clogged it, removed that something, cleansed the machinery, and sewn up the incision."[4] The public took their semi-enlightenment to whomever would cater to it, as evinced by the epidemic of green urine seen among patients in 1912 after a

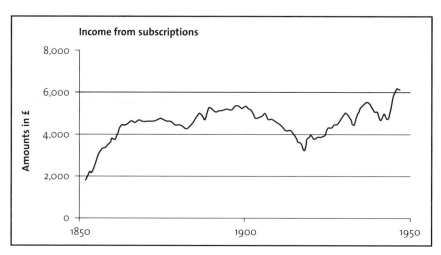

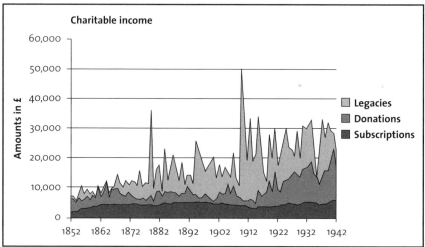

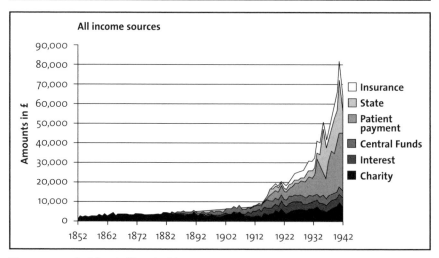

Figures 1–3: St Mary's Hospital income

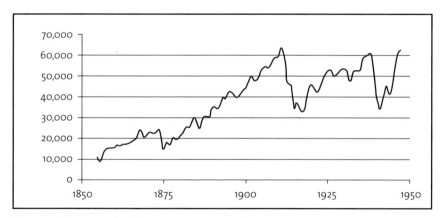
Figure 4: Patients admissions

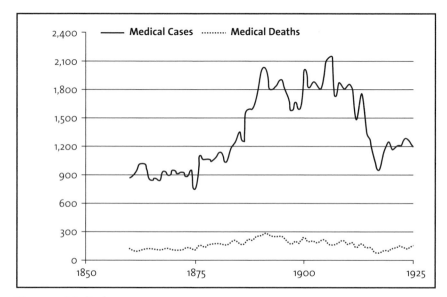
Figure 5: Medical cases

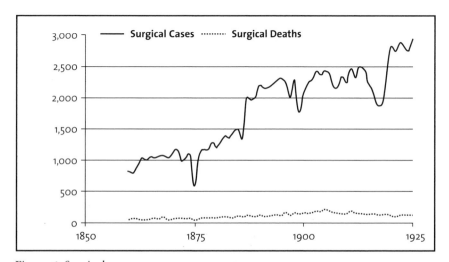
Figure 6: Surgical cases

salesman peddling "De Witt's Kidney and Bladder Pills" passed through Paddington.[5] One would-be patient wrote to Sir John Broadbent asking for a typhoid inoculation to cure his dyspepsia.[6]

People were everywhere demanding more medical care and greater access to hospitals. Increasingly, they were being born and dying in hospitals. The Medical Officer of Health tallied the figures: in 1914 only 13 per cent of births among Paddington residents took place in institutions (and .4 per cent in St Mary's); by 1923 the figure was 27.8 per cent and St Mary's, having opened an obstetrical ward for ordinary cases, accounted for a third of these.[7] During the 1930s the hospital competed for the patronage of parturient women: Bourne suggested wooing them with chloroform capsule anaesthesia, free milk for ten days, and a visit by himself "in a big car every Friday morning after the round to a few of the homes. This always creates an impression."[8]

Paddingtonians also began to die in public institutions in greater numbers: 22 per cent of them in 1901, 32 per cent just five years later, and 45 per cent by 1923. In the poorer districts the figure was over 50 per cent, and even in the wealthier ones it was near or above 30 per cent. By this time St Mary's accounted for only about 9–10 per cent of deaths among Paddington residents, and 15 per cent of the total deaths in the parish. During the 1890s, for every 100 patients who died at St Mary's, 61 had died in the infirmary and workhouse. By the early 1920s, the proportions had been reversed. In round numbers, roughly 612 died in the infirmary and workhouse to 425 at St Mary's (as compared to 207 and 336 respectively during the 1890s). Elsewhere in the parish, roughly a dozen people died at the Lock each year, several dozen at Paddington Green Children's Hospital, and 100 to 200 died in St Luke's Hospital for the Dying.

St Mary's could not meet the demands upon its beds and turned away patients, some of whom went to the infirmary. The hospital tended to reject chronic respiratory diseases like pulmonary tuberculosis or bronchitis but to admit tuberculosis lending itself to surgical treatment. From 1901 to 1905, pneumonia cases tended to go to St Mary's; from 1906 to 1910, the two institutions were almost on a par; by 1914–1918, pneumonia was more likely to wind up in the infirmary. Cancer might be admitted to either. Old age killed hundreds each year at the infirmary, but it didn't appear on a single death certificate from St Mary's during these years. Its twin, heart disease, was only gradually distinguished from old age; it too led to the infirmary. St Mary's preferred to admit people in need of heroic intervention: accidents, attempted suicide or other violent trauma, as well as acute abdominal disorders such as appendicitis. (See figures 7–9.)

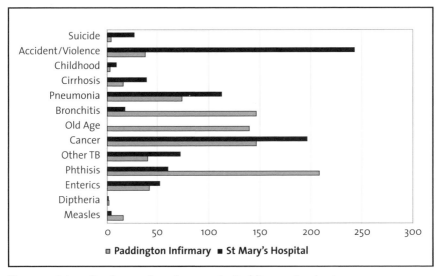

Figure 7: Mortality from selected causes in Paddington Institutions, 1901–05

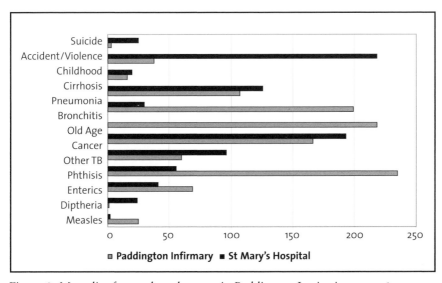

Figure 8: Mortality from selected causes in Paddington Institutions, 1906–10

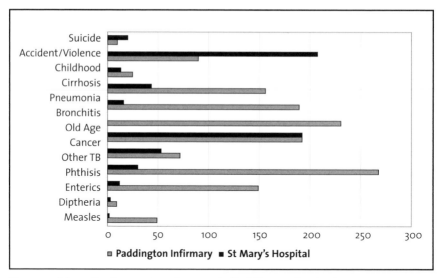

Figure 9: Mortality from selected causes in Paddington Institutions, 1914–18

As therapeutical efficacy increased, it came to seem unreasonable to deny admission to people who might afford some sort of medical care outside the hospital but who, everyone knew, would be better served inside the hospital where the latest technology and skilled nursing were on offer. Ernest Graham Little remarked to the St Mary's medical society in 1927, "It has always been something of an anomaly that the best medical attention in this country under present conditions can be obtained only by two classes, the rich and the poor, and both classes are attended by practically the same medical advisors." Not surprisingly, therefore, the middle class was "clamouring for treatment in voluntary hospitals."[9]

When the St Mary's Hospital board drew up its payment scheme in 1920, it effectively invited the middle classes to enter the wards. Nonetheless, the hospital was still seen to be primarily an institution run by the middle classes for the working classes. In 1920 the South Paddington District League of Mercy met to discuss the problem of voluntary hospitals. One woman argued, "People had not yet grasped the need to come forward and help these institutions, and it was chiefly to the class of people who used the hospitals that they must make their appeal," namely, the working classes. The Dowager Lady Dimsdale, president of the St Mary's Hospital Ladies' Association, agreed, as did the Reverend Charles Knight, who asserted that the "working-classes would give if they were only approached properly."[10] At St Mary's, patients were asked to contribute not towards

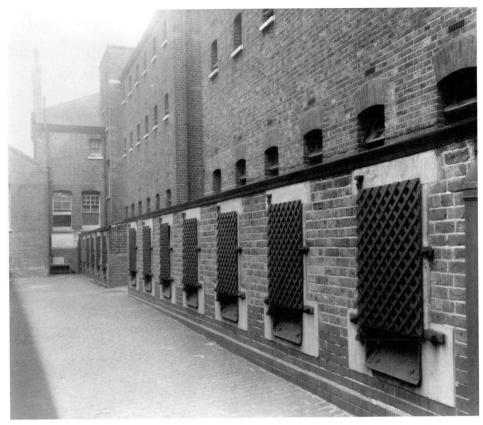

Paddington Workhouse Casual Ward cells in 1938. National Monuments Record, English Heritage

the medical treatment, which was free (else the governors would have to indemnify the honorary staff), but towards maintenance costs. Food alone cost 21 shillings per week and, with other necessaries, the cost of a bed amounted to £3.11.1 per week.[11] In 1926 a survey showed that half of patients paid nothing, while 30 per cent paid ten shillings or more.[12]

There were two reasons for the hospital's financial troubles during the 1920s. On the one hand, new therapies, technologies, and trained nursing staff drove up costs. Between 1914 and 1921, domestic and salary costs more than doubled. Spiralling postwar inflation exacerbated the problem. Bad as the hospitals' problems were, however, those of the general population were worse. The local press regularly reported on people driven to desperate measures. One woman living in Campbell Street, Paddington, was summoned for stealing clothing from a vicar. Her husband was laid up in the infirmary with rheumatism and her son by an accident. The policeman who went to arrest her found the family in such dire straits that he gave them food.[13] During the 1920s people entered the hospital in a starving condition. This could be shocking to the medical students, many of them raised in comparative affluence. One young Canadian, tall, athletic, and well nourished, was all for an immediate laparotomy when confronted with an acute abdomen case during the late 1920s; his senior, who had seen such things before, counselled waiting, and after a few hours it was discovered that aggravated hunger had produced the symptoms.[14]

On the other hand, the bitter class hostility of the period meant a complete absence of the benevolent good will upon which voluntary hospitals relied. The capitalist classes expected that society would return to its prewar state, and the Russian Revolution horrified them. They blamed bolshevism and industrial unrest for the economic problems and fretted at the spectacle of unemployed men – more than two thousand of them registered in Paddington in 1920 – marching down Westbourne Grove, waving banners and passing around collection boxes. A patently inadequate local labour bureau was their response. The *Bayswater Chronicle* commented: "We breathe an atmosphere of openly expressed dissatisfaction; few seem contented with their lot, things – to quote people's own words – were 'never so bad as they are at present,' and grumbles, uncontrollable restlessness and successions of strikes fill the air."[15]

Class hostility raged between Conservative and Labour representatives on the local governing bodies. Paddington was by tradition a Tory borough. It almost invariably sent Conservatives to Parliament and to the LCC, several of them hospital governors, including Henry Harben, who represented South Paddington from 1898 to 1907, and Sir Harold Kenyon, who represented the same ward from 1931 to 1946. These men belonged to a small circle that dominated local affairs, including the Borough Council. However, if the Conservatives dominated genteel South Paddington, the slums on Harrow Road returned Labour candidates. Meetings of the Borough Council were time and again disrupted by these Labour men and women. In 1921 during a quarrel over maternal benefits the "Labour Councillors rose, marched into the middle of the Council Chamber, and for a quarter-of-an-hour shouted without cessation at the top of their voices 'Divide, divide!' finishing their turbulence with the lusty singing of the 'Red Flag'... The proceedings ended in disorder."[16] Outside the Council Chamber, the temper was worse. In April a tailor was charged with fomenting disaffection when he mounted a soapbox in Hyde Park and urged the crowd to "throw over the rotten Government system."[17]

The Conservative representatives crushed bolshevism wherever they saw it, and they saw it everywhere. The MP for North Paddington, a furniture dealer named W.G. Perring, told his constituents (at what the *Bayswater Chronicle* described as one of the happiest gatherings ever recorded in the social life of the borough): "It was the thriftless who wanted to undermine the wealth of the country ... It was nothing short of suicidal, said Mr. Perring with marked emphasis, to endeavour to destroy the brawny capitalist class, the men who have risen from the ranks and proved themselves the worthy trustees of the destinies of this country." As an alderman, Perring voted against the appointment of an assistant medical officer of health with the remark that "there was a growing tendency in the borough for people to expect everything that they wanted to be done for them. There seemed the want of a sense of responsibility among them. They looked to somebody else to do for them anything that they wanted to be done."[18]

In the face of such flagrant class hostility, a voluntary hospital could hope for little. Donations to St Mary's, which fell at the end of the war to levels not seen since 1862, did not start to rise again until the mid-1920s. It was another decade before they surpassed nineteenth-century amounts. The polarization of politics also checked an incipient movement towards a state medical service briefly advocated by leading physicians.[19] In 1919 a Ministry of Health was created to promote cooperation between the government departments and extra-government organizations concerned with medical care. However, support for more radical proposals quickly dissolved, while the minister of Health was downgraded and removed from the cabinet office.

Though the bourgeoisie complained in such meetings as the Paddington Primrose League of the insolence and self-interestedness of the working classes,[20] the voluntary hospital found self-interest more reliable than benevolence. If the wealthy would no longer pay for the care of the sick poor, then St Mary's could only fulfil its mission by inviting the wealthy in to pay for their own treatment and spending the profits on the poor. After the King's Fund gave its blessing, in 1930 the governors of St Mary's began to raise funds for paying beds. The campaign stuttered along until one of their number, F.C. Lindo, began the first of a series of donations that finally amounted to above £100,000. This permitted the governors to erect an entirely new wing on the site occupied by the medical school which, thanks to its own fund-raising campaign, had moved across the road. By the time the new wing opened in 1937, Lindo had died, and it was named in his honour. Whereas the previous scheme had merely skimmed a bit of money from ordinary patients, the Lindo Wing charged up to fifteen guineas per week (not including professional fees) for private facilities. The paying wing provided a more reliable source of income than charity had ever done.

A second strategy was the sale of medical services to local authorities. In the wake of the Boer War, when a third of all recruits were found to be unfit, public opinion moved in favour of health care for children so that they might grow into healthy and productive adults. School meals were one result, and state-sponsored clinics to treat common childhood ailments were another. After an approach by the LCC in January 1908, and much negotiation (including a flat refusal to permit the LCC representation on the hospital board), in April 1910 St Mary's established eye, skin, and ear-nose-throat clinics for schoolchildren, reimbursed at two shillings for most visits.

A further pressure in favour of state medical services was the reform of unemployment insurance. Unemployment, not health, preoccupied central and local authorities during the 1910s and 1920s, but health entered the political agenda insofar as it related to unemployment. In the first decade of the century the Royal Commission on the Poor Laws discovered that the poor law was the customary resort for many thousands of English citizens made destitute by age or sickness. Though they disagreed on many points, both the majority and the minority reports advocated medical insurance. In 1911 a contributory medical insurance scheme was introduced, and all workers earning less than £160 were obliged to contribute.[21] The concern was primarily with economic productivity, so workers' dependants were not covered. Nor were hospitals: the service was entirely in the hands of GPs who would have themselves to pay for any referral costs out of the rather small sum allotted them for each case. In 1917, only fourteen shillings sixpence came into the St Mary's coffers from the National Health Insurance Act.

Two Case Studies in State-Hospital Collaboration: Tuberculosis and Venereal Disease

Demand for medical reform sprang from new theories of disease and new treatments trumpeted by the press. By the early twentieth century, syphilis and tuberculosis could be reliably diagnosed and, it was thought, treated. Unchecked, these two diseases posed a threat to public health, but the poor could not afford treatment. The two diseases, thus, became the object of state intervention. Tuberculosis and syphilis provide contrasting case studies in the developing partnership between hospitals and state officials.[22]

Tuberculosis was included in the health insurance legislation passed in 1911. The scheme provided for research into tuberculosis (as seen above) and it provided funds for tuberculosis clinics, to be organized by local authorities. Tuberculosis was thought to be neglected by the hospitals – where it was usually excluded from the wards as a chronic disease – and by retrograde GPs. Much of the pressure for action on tuberculosis was generated by the National Association for the Prevention of Tuberculosis, formed in 1898, which had as its founding president Sir William Broadbent.[23] The disease was a leading cause of death in late Victorian Paddington, claiming 250 people a year, with a mortality rate of 1.23 per thousand persons as compared to 1.74 in London generally. The rate was declining, due in part to sanitary reforms undertaken by the medical officers of health.[24] Paddington MOH Reginald Dudfield strongly believed that overcrowding was a cause, and he produced statistics to show that consumptives lived in the most crowded streets in Paddington.[25] He also agitated for the pasteurization of milk.

Paddington housed the first TB clinic in England, founded in 1908 on Talbot Road as an offshoot of the voluntary dispensary founded in Edinburgh in 1887.[26] St Mary's also took in tubercular patients, and the Inoculation Department made a specialty of tuberculin treatment, often taking the patients into their research beds to ensure perfect bed rest.[27] Paddington could even boast of having introduced the artificial pneumothorax therapy to Britain. In 1911 Claude Lillingston, a Mary's graduate, had picked up the technique – which consisted of collapsing the lung so as to let it rest (and prevent auto-inoculation, according to Wright's theory) – while undergoing a cure himself, and he brought it back to the research beds at St Mary's.[28] So Paddington was well served for tuberculosis even before the London County Council began to fund the two clinics.

St Mary's and the LCC never saw eye to eye on tuberculosis treatment. They quarrelled about payment and the admission criteria for in-patients. The LCC wanted a reduced rate and control over admissions. St Mary's conceded the first point but not the second. With LCC money (about £1,100 per annum), the hospital installed an outpatient dispensary in the basement and equipped it with a nurse and a medical officer, J.B. Porteous, a recent graduate of the school with ties to the Inoculation Department. There were further wrangles about location: Talbot Road managed to claim all the poor neighbourhoods of Paddington, leaving St Mary's to offer free treatment to the lords and ladies of Bayswater. The map was redrawn, but never entirely equitably. The St Mary's dispensary was run on a part-time basis, while that at Talbot Road was full time.[29]

By 1926 tuberculosis mortality was down to 124 per annum in a population of 144,261. This was better than comparable parishes: Hammersmith with 130,295 inhabitants had 141 deaths. To the LCC, the course of action was obvious: one of the Paddington dispensaries should be closed. But which one? Both functioned efficiently, outperforming other dispensaries. They traced more contacts, saw more patients, and performed more home visits than other clinics in London. Talbot Road was the sentimental favourite, but it was badly located on the parish outskirts, with access blocked by the railway yard. The dispensary at St Mary's was well integrated into the hospital service. The fact that students were taught to diagnose and treat the disease was another consideration. Porteous had a diploma in Public Health, and he extended the work of the clinic into the community, though he didn't develop a scientific program of study and published almost nothing.

The question of closure was left in abeyance, while deaths continued to decline, falling below ninety annually by the mid-1930s. By this time, having taken charge of the old workhouse infirmaries, the local authorities were reluctant to cede powers to the voluntary hospitals. The MOH for Paddington, G.E. Oates, refused to build up St Mary's.[30] Moreover, while St Mary's rested on its laurels, supporters of the Talbot Road dispensary moved into action. By 1941 they had raised enough money to resite the dispensary in more central, spacious quarters, complete with state-of-the-art facilities for a lab, dispensary, lecture hall, dental surgery, artificial pneumothorax, x-rays, and UV light. The LCC ended the grant to St Mary's and moved the work to the newly named Paddington Chest Clinic. St Mary's had been caught napping and paid a penalty for assuming that state funding could be relied upon to continue. This was a salutary lesson.

In venereology, the hospital made no such mistakes. In the early years venereal cases were treated in the out-patient department and occasionally in the wards in advanced forms such as aneurysm[31] or haemoptysis.[32] Numerous Mary's men worked at the Lock Hospital on Harrow Road, including three generations of Lanes: Samuel, James R., and James E.[33] George Gascoyen also served as a surgeon, while Sieveking and Chambers were consulting physicians. Gascoyen and James R. Lane practised therapeutic syphilitic inoculation, strangely anticipating that of Almroth Wright. (Gascoyen explained that, because the disease ran a definite course and did not relapse back to earlier symptoms, if the patient's own pus was extracted and inoculated into various parts round the body, the disease would expend itself in space rather than over time, and the healing process would be sped up.) After James R. Lane's career was cut short by syphilis, his son, James E. Lane, took up where he left off. James E. entered St Mary's from Oxford in 1875, qualified in 1880, and was soon on the staff of the Lock and of St Mary's. Thanks to Wright's friendship with Ehrlich, who discovered in salvarsan a powerful new treatment for syphilis, St Mary's pioneered the drug's use in England, and Lane reported 120 cases treated by 1911. Alexander Fleming performed the injections and pathology work at St Mary's, and at the Lock from 1913.

St Mary's also made a substantial contribution to British venereology through the Royal Commission on Venereal Disease which met from 1910 to 1913. James E. Lane served as secretary to the commission, and Sir Malcolm Morris is credited with having instigated it. It was this commission that recommended the establishment of state-sponsored clinics. As with TB, the general hospitals were seen to be neglecting the disease, while salvarsan was deemed too dangerous to be prescribed by GPs indiscriminately. The Wassermann test provided a reliable means of diagnosis, and random investigation of patients revealed that the disease was widely prevalent.[34] One study quoted by the commissioners showed that of seventy-five patients tested in Paddington Infirmary, 18.6 per cent were positive for syphilis. The outbreak of war raised the stakes: venereal disease caused so much incapacity among the troops that it seemed to threaten the country's defence. By 1917 state-sponsored clinics were in operation.

The Lock hospital entered the LCC scheme as one of the leading venerology centres, receiving £7,000 per year by the early 1920s. By the end of that decade, however, the LCC had cancelled the grant after a scandal involving harsh treatment of inmates. The Lock limped along relying on voluntary subscription and finally closed in 1948. The clinic at St Mary's was far smaller at first, averaging six hundred to seven hundred cases per year in the early 1920s. The clinic was marginal to the developing community of venereologists and was staffed by young men like Arthur Porritt who were waiting for general hospital positions. They did not, for example, publish in the British Journal of Venereal Disease founded in 1925.

In 1932 the LCC tried to close the clinic at St Mary's as part of a move towards daytime clinics run by specialists.[35] Some conservative consultants urged closure,[36] but because medical students had to attend venereal clinics, the hospital governors fought them. In February 1933 they resolved to appoint a director "well versed in venereal practice" to attend twenty hours per week for £400 per annum salary and the right to undertake private practice.[37] It was instead the Middlesex Hospital that was deleted from the LCC scheme, while the funding for St Mary's rose to £3,000 per annum. Thus in 1933 St Mary's acquired the services of G.L.M. McElligott, who was then running the municipal VD services in Stoke-on-Trent. This was one of the most successful appointments that Mary's ever made. McElligott studied under Colonel L.W. Harrison, who had organized a model service at St Thomas's and advised the government on venereal disease. Well connected and himself a careful and astute clinical observer, McElligott made the St Mary's clinic a major centre for the practice and the science of venereology.

Venereology changed dramatically during the 1930s with the development of sulpha drugs. Before that, gonorrhoea patients came in daily for irrigation, attended about one hundred days, and often experienced serious complications. Afterwards, a few tablets could cure them in a matter of weeks. Though McElligott started with sulphanilamide rather late in the day, in 1937 he and his assistant, A.J. Cokkinis, provided the first long-term statistics on the therapeutical efficacy of the sulphonamides. Within two and a half months they had three hundred patients under treatment. The following year they reported in the *Lancet* on 633 consecutive cases treated with sulphanilamide, whom they compared to 250 cases seen the previous year without sulpha drugs: after one month, 70 per cent of the treated cases and only 10 per cent of the controls had been cured.[38] McElligott supplemented the treatment with vaccines from the Inoculation Department.

While the number of consumptives declined in Britain during the twentieth century, the number of venereal patients increased. Between 1933 and 1937, patient numbers rose threefold and attendances sevenfold to more than 90,000 per year. This was far more than had attended the old Mary's and Middlesex clinics combined.[39] By the mid-1930s the clinic brought in above £6,000, accounting for more than half of all government payments to the hospital. St Mary's could offer paid employment to a steady stream of young men, including future venereologists R.R. Willcox and F.J.G. Jefferiss.

On his return from RAF service in 1945, McElligott made the department a whole-time one. The "Special Clinic" at St Mary's became the largest in the country, by 1970 treating 10 per cent of all cases of syphilis. But the number of patients attending the clinic began to climb even before the sulpha drugs appeared. Attendances doubled between September 1932 and September 1933. The attraction was in large part McElligott himself. Some venereologists believed that their first duty was to the public. Samuel Lane, for example, had used harsh caustics on prostitutes and supported the Contagious Diseases Act. Like Colonel Harrison, McElligott put the patient first and eschewed punitive or interrogative methods: "In the first place it cannot be too strongly urged that the patient be treated as a patient and not as a penitent or a prisoner, and the first remark of the doctor should be an invitation to sit down. Any unnecessary standing suggests the dock or the orderly room, whereas what is to be aimed at during this first interview, even in the busiest of clinics, is to create the atmosphere of a private consulting room."[40]

In a venereal clinic, courtesy is of more than incidental importance. Patients included ashamed wives and husbands, recalcitrant prostitutes, and homosexual men who faced prosecution if reported to authorities – all of whom would be wary of hostile or discourteous clinicians. McElligott, who himself concentrated largely on the female patients, told the British Society for Venereal Disease. "In his own district, Paddington, which might be called the prostitutes' Paradise, prostitutes attending his clinic were among the best of the patients, and they were most grateful for what was done for them. They put up with more than the average shop-girl, they expected to be hurt, and when this did not happen they were agreeably surprised and very grateful."[41] By contrast, obstetrician W.J. Gow had disliked women altogether. "In the out-patient clinic he was abrupt, impatient with their often ignorant, muddled and nervous accounts of their complaints, and he seemed entirely unsympathetic with them in their troubles. His reputation was well known among the women of Paddington, in fact so few attended his clinic that he was usually finished in half an hour or even less."[42] His successor was also sometimes impatient and once slapped a prostitute when she balked at being examined by a crowd of students. The medical student who witnessed this encounter worked in the venereal clinic and remarked that "we were the only clinic where we were kind to all our patients, so it was said, and things get around."[43]

A courteous reception encouraged patients to report their contacts or urge them to attend. This became of great importance as gay men began to attend the clinic in increasing numbers from the 1940s. Sodomy was illegal, so one could hardly send lady almoners out to do the contact tracing as occurred in the heterosexual cases. Homosexual attendance relied very much on goodwill among patients and word of mouth. As the student said, "things got around." In fact, while McElligott welcomed prostitutes, he was strait-laced in other respects, and a male patient who admitted to homosexual encounters would be chased out of his office with the threat of eternal damnation. But at the door, someone would whisper to him that he should come back in the evening or on Saturday when Jefferiss was running the clinic.

Gradually, without McElligott learning of it, Jefferiss built up an enormous clientele of gay men, both at St Mary's and in his private practice. Being in the West End helped, as did the proximity of Hyde Park. A survey from the mid-1950s showed that none of the extensive patient pool at the Whitechapel clinic admitted to being gay, whereas eighty-four of one thousand male patients at St Mary's admitted to recent sexual contact with another man (there may have been significant under-reporting in both cases). Jefferiss added that he had seen 224 homosexual men over the previous two and a half years, with 477 attacks of disease among them. There was also clinical evidence of an east-west divide. C.S. Nicol, a Mary's graduate who worked at the Whitechapel VD clinic and brought McElligott's system of contact-tracing across with him, remarked in a paper on anal gonorrhoea that the condition was rare among men. A West-End practitioner replied that he saw it often.[44]

Thanks to a liberal grant from the LCC, McElligott developed a large clinic, a fruitful program of research, and stature for himself. He directed the RAF's venereology services during the Second World War and replaced his old teacher, Colonel Harrison, as official advisor to the government on venereology, until his own retirement in 1959. McElligott brought all his old ideas with him to shape national venereal policy, including special attention paid to contact-tracing and a resistance to compulsory methods. Thus, while national policy shaped local services at St Mary's, those same services shaped national policy. St Mary's was both mover and moved.

The Problems of Medicine

The chorus of praise for medicine was one argument for nationalization. A counter-discourse criticizing hospital and medical services was another. Two of the most critical and influential accounts of the medical profession during the first half of the twentieth century were fictional: G.B. Shaw's *The Doctor's Dilemma* and A.J. Cronin's *The Citadel*. Shaw was a socialist and Cronin a physician, yet their complaints were similar. Socialist physicians added their own criticisms, blaming inadequate hospital care and incompetent GP service for rampant ill-health among the British public. St Mary's was in the thick of the controversy. Cronin practised in Paddington, and he set part of his novel there, while the "Doctor" of Shaw's play is modelled upon Almroth Wright. St Mary's also trained two prominent members of the Socialist Medical Association, Esther Rickards and Aleck Bourne.

G.B. Shaw was in his day the leading critic of the medical establishment. He was unconvinced by germ theory and entirely convinced that the political costs of enthroning medicine as a public good were too high. In 1906 *The Doctor's Dilemma* stated his criticisms forcefully. The medical characters include the sensible GP who doesn't fall prey to medical fashion and Harley Street consultants who do. At the start of the play, the "Doctor," Colenso Ridgeon, has just been knighted for developing vaccine therapy. But because Ridgeon has only a handful of beds at his disposal, few patients can be admitted for full vaccine therapy. The play asks whether a physician who has such power can be trusted to use it wisely. Shaw got the idea for the play, like many of his criticisms of doctors, from conversations with Almroth Wright. Shaw was frequently seen at Inoculation Department tea parties, and sometimes at the medical society, where he and Wright twice engaged in debate over female suffrage. Wright admitted to Shaw that he sometimes had to choose between patients for admission to his few beds. However wisely Wright used his power, Ridgeon uses his to personal advantage, refusing to admit a man dying of tuberculosis because he covets the man's wife. To Shaw, who was a Fabian socialist, medicine was either inefficacious and fraudulent or efficacious and dangerous, its dangerousness lying in its unequal distribution.

Shaw's play is complicated and morally ambiguous. More readable and, indeed, read was A.J. Cronin's *The Citadel*, published in 1937 and made into a film two years later. The novel tells the story of an idealistic young doctor whose idealism is ground down by the poverty of his patients and the greed of his colleagues. Practising in a Welsh mining valley, the hero finds he can do little for his desperately poor patients. He manages to obtain higher qualifications and moves to London – to Paddington, in fact – to practise. Slowly he works his way up the ladder, first treating only the local poor, then gradually acquiring wealthier patients and fraternizing with consultants. But he learns that his fellow consultants are incompetent frauds who would rather watch patients die than admit an error. Moreover, he cannot manage to get his poor patients, however ill, admitted into the voluntary hospitals (and St Mary's would have been the obvious first choice). He complains to his wife, "They're not full up. They've plenty of beds at St John's for their own men. If they don't know you they freeze you stiff. I'd like to wring that last young pup's neck! Isn't it *hell* – Christ! Here I am with this strangulated hernia and I can't get a bed. Oh! I suppose some of them are full up! And this is London! This is the heart of the bloody British Empire! This is our voluntary hospital system. And some banqueting bastard of a philanthropist got up the other day and said it was the most marvellous in the world. It means the workhouse again for the poor devil. Filling in forms – what do you earn? What's your religion? and was your mother born in wedlock? – and him with peritonitis!"[45] The novel's finale consists in a confrontation between the idealistic young doctor and the old guard who want his licence revoked for performing the unorthodox therapy of artificial pneumothorax (a routine operation at St Mary's but not at Talbot Road, where the aging medical officer disapproved of it). The young doctor, hauled up before the General Medical Council, vehemently denounces the ignorance and commercialism of the medical profession as a whole. Cronin, unlike Shaw, was a doctor himself, and this very public airing of grievance scandalized the profession.[46]

Another literary critic of modern medicine was Arthur Conan Doyle. Conan Doyle was friendly with the senior staff at St Mary's, who persuaded him to give occasional speeches or papers there, and his son Kingsley attended the school. Conan Doyle turned increasingly to spiritualism, especially after Kingsley died during the flu epidemic of 1918. He was sceptical of "science," which he defined as "the consensus of opinion of scientific men, and history had shewn it was slow to accept a truth." The phrase was quoted at the St Mary's medical society in 1914.[47]

Conan Doyle, Cronin, and Shaw were among the thoughtful literary critics of medicine. Among the others was John Rhode who produced above a hundred murder mysteries, several of them set in Paddington against the backdrop of "St Martha's Hospital," which boasted "Sir Alured Faversham, the world renowned pathologist." Like Bernard Spilsbury, Faversham is a famous forensic pathologist; like Almroth Wright, he invents new therapies. Medical men and their sinister science tend to be the villains of Rhode's novels. In one tale published in 1928, a physician convicted of euthanasia returns to disguise himself as a Praed Street herbalist and kills off half the neighbourhood. In another of 1925, the murderer turns out to be Faversham's chief assistant (Fleming? Freeman?) who murders his uncle by experimentally injecting him with an allergy remedy developed in the hospital laboratory.[48]

Rhode's books hardly constituted a serious criticism of medicine, but they did reflect a wider public uneasiness. Antivivisectionists fanned popular fears of sinister experimentation. Feelings ran high in Paddington, as in 1930 when speakers at a meeting in Bayswater blamed the rise in cancer and infection on inoculation which poisoned the bloodstream and weakened the body's resistance.[49] These were Almroth Wright's arguments turned upside down. During a by-election in South Paddington that year, antivivisectionists mobbed candidates' meetings, heckling them and demanding an end to medical experimentation. At one such meeting held in Paddington Baths, candidate Admiral A.E. Taylor and his fellow Empire Free Trader, the press baron Lord Beaverbrook, stood their ground and refused to support antivivisection. The St Mary's students, recognizing the two men as champions of medicine (and Beaverbrook as the school's benefactor), staged a spectacular demonstration in a fifty-foot mock-up battleship onto which, singing "Glory Hallelujah," they carried the two men.[50] Taylor won the election.[51]

While some bewailed the sinister encroachments of medicine into daily life, others complained that it did not encroach enough, because the benefits of modern medicine did not reach enough people. The British public was at the mercy of GPs who were repeatedly exposed as incompetent. In 1935 a survey by the BMA revealed that over half the fractures treated each year were mistreated, often causing permanent disability. In 1936 another study showed that one out of ten cases of TB was only diagnosed after death because GPs were not carrying out sputum tests.[52] Other studies revealed that ill-health was widespread throughout the country. One study of the 1930s showed that half of the population could not afford a healthy diet with all the necessary vitamins. Another tallied the public cost of ill-health in the hundreds of millions of pounds and criticized the limited response provided by the voluntary hospitals.[53] Previous debates, leading to TB and VD clinics, had centred on protection of the healthy; now people began to wonder why tubercular and venereal patients should receive free treatment while arthritis or rheumatic sufferers did not.[54] Left-wing thinkers, spurred on by the introduction of universal male suffrage in 1918, began to argue that the public had a right to health.[55]

Democratization meant that MPs, county councillors, and guardians had to listen to the demands of the poor as well as the rich. Guardians became more open-handed, defying governmental prescriptions for stinginess and refusing to pay into centralized funds. Paddington councillors registered their protest when the rates doubled between 1918 and 1921, rising from 7s. 6d. to 14s. 8d. on the pound. Most of the money, about ten shillings, went directly to the central administration. Meanwhile, increased relief payments for the unemployed, voted by the councillors in 1921, were vetoed by the minister of Health as infringing on the "fundamental principle" that poor relief must be lower than private earnings.[56] The confrontation between government and boards of guardians culminated in the abolition of the latter in 1929, at the same time as the government stiffened the means test and cut relief payments.[57] Poor-Law hospitals were transferred to the county councils.[58] The Paddington Infirmary, or the Paddington Hospital, as it was renamed in 1921, passed into the hands of the LCC. The separation of health care from poor relief, begun in 1874, was finally achieved and the stigma banished.

Health came to occupy the mainstream of politics. This was in part a consequence of the defeat of the left. Until the late 1920s the political conflict between the right and the left concerned wages and responsibility for unemployment. In the General Strike of 1926 the trade unions were defeated by the Baldwin government. Left-wing politicians then shifted the terms of their critique of capitalism and began to highlight the terrible illness that unbridled capitalism caused among the general population. This is illustrated by the provision of care for expectant mothers. When suffrage was granted to all adult men in 1918, it was also extended to women above the age of thirty. This put women's issues more squarely on the political agenda.[59]

Middle-class women had long since taken up the cause of maternal and infant mortality: as far back as 1863 the Bayswater Bible Society was holding weekly meetings for mothers. In 1895 private benefactors paid the salary of a full-time nurse for the St Mary's maternity service. In the early twentieth century a series of voluntary maternity welfare clinics were founded. The first in England was set up in 1910 by the Women's Labour League in North Kensington, a borough with very high infant mortality rates.[60] The Paddington School for Mothers, formed in 1911, was run by voluntary subscription until 1914, when it began to receive funds from the Board of Education, the Ministry of Health, and the Borough Council. By

1921 the Paddington school employed seven part-time medical officers as well as health visitors, and it provided cheap or free milk and food to expectant or nursing mothers and children. Members of the St Mary's Ladies' Association participated in these enterprises, and in 1916 two women governors moved that the hospital should cooperate more closely with the Paddington School for Mothers.[61]

The women sponsoring the clinics demanded that politicians also concern themselves with lowering maternal and infant mortality. In 1918 an act was passed to provide for antenatal and child welfare clinics, and from 1921 clinics were held at St Mary's and the Paddington School for Mothers. The Borough also began to pay for obstetrical service at St Mary's, sponsoring fourteen beds. And yet maternal mortality rates continued to increase[62] – in Paddington from 2.67 per cent before the First World War to 4.71 per cent at the end of it. After Labour was voted out in 1931 and the new government adopted a policy of retrenchment, a state-run maternity scheme was "clearly out of the question," according to historian Pamela Graves. So from 1932 the Labour women "began to emphasise malnutrition due to unemployment and low wages as a primary cause of maternal deaths and illness." What had been seen as a technical problem – the delivery of medical services to mothers – became an indictment of the inequities caused by capitalism.[63] However, as Lara Marks has shown, maternal mortality rates remained higher in wealthy districts, for clinical rather than socio-economic reasons.[64]

While maternal mortality in Paddington was on par with the national average, infant mortality was extraordinarily high. During the 1920s the rate in Paddington was above seventy-seven deaths per thousand births, as compared to a metropolitan average of seventy-two per thousand. Into the 1930s Paddington had the highest rate in London.[65] Death rates were high in the wealthier wards because most unwed mothers were domestic servants, and illegitimate children died faster than those born in wedlock. The infant mortality rate among legitimate infants in 1901 was 124 per thousand; among the illegitimate, it was 413 per thousand; twenty years later, the rate was 92 and 160 respectively. At one borough council meeting after another, Labour and (conservative) Municipal Reform councillors practically came to blows over the question of who was to blame and how a remedy should be effected. Where conservative councillors blamed "many contributory causes" for the deaths, Labour councillors "contended that poverty was the chief cause" and they objected to "an effort to whitewash the whole problem and to throw the onus on to the mother herself." However, Labour was, as ever, outnumbered on the borough council. Speaking for the majority, Conservative councillor Sir William Perry, MP, blamed "widespread knowledge available these days" (i.e., abortion), and he entirely vindicated both the council and its medical officer of health.

As a parish combining rich and poor residents, Paddington reproduced within itself a larger debate about the causes of poverty and illness. Paddingtonians argued whether, as one letter to the editor asserted, "The slum mind produces the slum, and not vice versa," or whether, as a Labour councillor retorted, it *was* vice versa.[66] They also disagreed about how radical the remedies should be, ranging from stricter surveillance of unwed mothers to municipalizing maternity services. The medical profession was also divided. Located near Harley Street and accommodating one of the great voluntary hospitals, Paddington was a stronghold of voluntarism. Sir Ernest Graham Little, the hospital's dermatologist, waged unremitting war against all forms of state medicine from VD clinics to nationalization of the hospitals. He saw the voluntary hospital as a noble institution: "The voluntary hospital is built upon humanity, and the human interest is what keeps it the fresh and lovely thing it is. All of its component elements give of their best, freely and without reward."[67] To sacrifice noble aspirations in favour of bureaucratic methods would threaten the bonds of sociability throughout society in general. Surgeon Arthur Dickson Wright also denounced nationalization. This was the voice of privilege speaking.

And yet the poor of Paddington were not to be overlooked. They exerted a powerful influence on the middle-class doctors who worked among them, an influence that was all the stronger for being juxtaposed with extreme wealth. In 1930 the bishop of Kensington remarked at a meeting on housing schemes in Paddington, "What we want to do is to make it impossible for people to live happily in Gloucester Terrace or vicinity, while the infantile death rate in Harrow Road is so high."[68] It is doubtless more than a coincidence that the two men who led the campaigns for state action against TB and VD, Sir William Broadbent and Sir Malcolm Morris, were both consultants at St Mary's. Likewise, two of the most prominent figures in the radical left's campaign for a state system of medicine, Esther Rickards and Aleck Bourne, were graduates of St Mary's whose exposure to the Paddington slums served as an education for socialism.

Esther Rickards was born in London in 1893, the daughter of a veterinary surgeon.[69] She was educated at Birkbeck College, then the London School of Medicine for Women, and entered St Mary's in 1917 for her clinical years. She served as a clinical assistant, first in the ophthalmic clinic and then in the VD clinic. After qualifying, she became assistant medical officer of health for Paddington, and in 1925 she became the first female surgeon at the Lock. That year she also obtained her FRCS and moved to Harley Street. In 1925 she obtained a temporary post as assistant surgeon at the new Sussex Hospital for women and children in Brighton. Rickards wanted to be a hospital surgeon but her radical politics[70] – and probably her sex – debarred her. She was a Labour party activist, serving as alderman and county councillor for Greenwich from 1928 to 1946, and in 1930 she joined the newly formed Socialist Medical Association, where she advocated the nationalization of the hospitals.[71] Once the NHS was introduced, she served on the North-West London Regional Health Authority, which encompassed St Mary's Hospital. She was a governor of St Mary's from 1947 to 1971 and chair of the Samaritan Hospital for Women. A loyal friend to St Mary's, on her retirement she was named honorary consulting surgeon.

Whereas Rickards worked behind the scenes, Aleck Bourne went public with his socialism. The son of a Wesleyan minister who earned only £3 a week, he entered Cambridge and St Mary's on scholarships. His autobiography recalled a month spent "on the district" attending obstetrical cases in Paddington, often in "a one-room slum dwelling" where an entire family resided.[72] In his first case, "I found a dirty little room with one double bed covered with newspaper (which is actually a good bed covering if blankets are short). There was a wooden box as a cot for the last baby, probably a year old, and a corner of the room for the elder child, a coal stove and some rickety chairs." The midwife, a "fat old gamp of the old school with no training in cleanliness and certainly without the most elementary knowledge of antiseptics," had to remind Bourne to deliver the afterbirth. Bourne wanted to become a surgeon but the competition was too severe. Gow advised him to try obstetrics instead. He became an obstetric registrar and thenceforth made his journeys to St Mary's and presumably to the slums in a morning coat and top hat. He duly acquired a staff position at St Mary's and another at Queen Charlotte's Lying-In Hospital. By dint of a series of successful textbooks, he became one of the most celebrated obstetricians of his generation. In 1937 a Mary's student prefaced his review of the seventh edition of Bourne's *Synopsis of Obstetrics and Gynaecology* with the remark: "Sixty-five umbrellas, eight bowler hats, a brace of pheasants, and 'Bourne's Synopsis.' This might well represent a day's takings by the Lost Property men of the London Passenger Transport Board. The book is endemic in the buses and tubes, and reaches epidemic proportions about four times a year."[73]

As a lecturer in obstetrics and diseases of women at St Mary's, Bourne taught that patients had to be understood as individuals, in the context of their home life and their social and economic circumstances. Even after he graduated to the senior staff, he insisted on working and teaching in the OPD where he could more amply teach social medicine. In the *Hospital*

Gazette during the early 1940s he complained that "the student is qualified without ever having seriously considered the social conditions which produce so much disease and therefore the way to prevent it. The medical student is, in my experience, the least socially conscious of any group of students, and this is surprising considering that he is brought into such intimate contact with the products of bad social conditions. It is due to no lack of sympathy or kindliness."[74] During the early 1940s Bourne delivered a series of lectures at St Mary's that were published in 1942 as *The Health of the Future*. The book was overshadowed by the publication of Beveridge's report a few months later in December 1942; but it was a significant document, helping to bring opinion around in favour of Beveridge's sweeping demands for social reform, and it reveals how politicized some sectors of the medical profession had become. Bourne made a coherent and cogent statement of principle, articulating a social philosophy that would have been unthinkable a century earlier and, while still radical in 1940, became almost a commonplace of postwar politics.

Above all, Bourne argued that people had a right to health. Ill-health prevented humankind from achieving perfection because mind and body were firmly interlocked. Health was a crucial foundation for any understanding of the common good; morals and philosophy were only secondary objectives. Ill-health was "a fundamental evil." It was also, Bourne argued, an extremely prevalent one because many unhealthy people received no treatment at all. Across London in Poplar, he showed, children were malnourished and lived in appallingly crowded conditions and as a result were anaemic. In Paddington, poverty was not so great and the children were not anaemic; they were, however, pale and sickly because many lived in "ill-lit, ill-ventilated, overcrowded rooms, sometimes in a basement." Clinics for mothers and syphilis and tuberculosis were all very well, but they couldn't attack the underlying social problems.

The first half of Bourne's book identified the problem, the second half provided the solution. Medical education had to be revamped to address social concerns and preventive medicine. Bourne suggested that students attend the MOH on his rounds. "If the teacher could show to his students that the real interest of a disease lies not so much in the rarity or complexity of its pathology, but in its capacity to cause disability and distress, the student would regard these conditions as having a social as well as a scientific interest." Bourne then surveyed existing public health legislation and medical services. Only one-third of children were vaccinated against smallpox and only 5 per cent against diphtheria, so that thousands died needlessly. "The knowledge at our disposal is sufficient, if implemented, to form the basis of a policy and service which would produce results far beyond our present capacity." If the state only recognized the citizen's right to health, then it must undertake far-reaching social reforms. State action was required because many causes of ill health were beyond the individual's control. Moreover, "health spells efficiency, energy, happiness, all of which contribute to better citizenhood and therefore to the benefit of the community." The outbreak of war made the matter all the more important: unhealthy men made bad soldiers.

Key to the national health service that Bourne sought was a nationalized hospital system. Charity was failing, and most hospitals had to rely on expensive loans and overdrafts. (That of St Mary's stood at £70,000.) Poverty kept them from providing up-to-date services – and Bourne's long, fruitless efforts to establish an academic unit of obstetrics at St Mary's, stymied for lack of beds, doubtless lent personal vehemence to this argument. "If Health is a matter of such primary importance to the people that it must be the responsibility of all, as expressed through the Government, has not the role of a diminishing and uncertain charity become incapable of sustaining so great a burden? So long as a large part of one of the greatest of all medical activities – the hospital system – is in the care of charity and uncoordinated voluntary service, there is possible a repudiation by the Government of responsibility for the health service as a complete whole, and a sanction for further unorganised development." At the same time, qua consultant, Bourne insisted the nationalized hospitals should maintain their administrative autonomy and liberty of thought.[75] All in all, he presented a thoroughgoing indictment of the existing service. *The Health of the Future* took its place among other contemporaneous works, such as *The Future of Medicine* by David Stark Murray, another socialist, and the Beveridge report, with its sweeping attack on inequity and morbidity.

The Second World War also radicalized opinion, as people began to expect that postwar reconstruction would aim at a better standard of living for the masses.[76] The Blitz forced many people into the hospitals and created a greater public attachment to these institutions. As in 1914, the war effort provoked considerable state intervention into the economy and into medical services. The EMS (Emergency Medical Service) was crucial: the Ministry of Health divided London into sectors, each organized around a teaching hospital, whereby emergency medical care was provided in central hospitals and less serious cases were evacuated outside London. As well, a system of regional blood transfusion services, a national public health laboratory service, and regional specialist facilities in rehabilitation, fractures, plastic surgery, neurology, and psychiatry were set up. The EMS ended the traditional, proud isolation of the teaching hospitals. The system worked so well that many came to believe that a similar system of integration and coordination among hospitals should be maintained in peacetime.[77]

The National Health Service

The government was not deaf to the demands for change. Early in the war Winston Churchill formed a union government with some key Labour figures occupying important offices. Many within this government approved of the principle of nationalization of medicine. At first the government only thought to make permanent the benefits of the EMS by placing hospitals under local authorities, but as pressure mounted from the left, officials proposed a salaried GP service as well. Opposition from hospital governors, consultants, and GPs forced retreat. According to a new scheme framed in 1945, hospitals would be jointly run by traditional hospital managers and local authorities, while GPs would remain independent contractors rather than salaried agents.

Also in 1945, however, a Labour government was elected after it promised a comprehensive health service. The new health minister was Aneurin Bevan, a man well familiar with the inequities of medical provision. Raised in the poor mining districts of South Wales, one of eight surviving children out of thirteen, he had laboured in the mines himself until his eyesight was damaged by "miner's nystagmus," and in 1929, aged thirty-two, he had been elected an MP. Bevan was firmly in the left wing of the Labour party;[78] the fate of the hospitals seemed to be sealed. But many doctors objected violently to the plans proposed. Some, like Graham Little, opposed any encroachment on professional privilege and voluntarism; others protested against municipal control of the hospitals; still others rejected the idea of a salaried profession. The government was prepared to take on the insurance companies, but it needed the good will and cooperation of the medical profession. That good will was marshalled and delivered to them by Charles Wilson, later Lord Moran.

Wilson had distinguished himself as dean at St Mary's, but not as a medical practitioner. While his medical skills and personal qualities were never in question, he had no great enthusiasm for private practice. His finances were often near depletion, and patients sometimes scolded him for failing to bill them. However, Wilson did attract a few important patients. First among them was Max Aitkin, Lord Beaverbrook, a Canadian financier who moved to England and became involved in English politics and, subsequently, journalism. Beaverbrook's son was seized with abdominal pains, and the father was advised to arrange for an appendectomy. Beaverbrook was unconvinced, so he called in a physician, hoping to hear that the operation was not necessary. Wilson advised immediate surgery. Beaverbrook was still not won over and called in a surgeon who agreed that the operation could be postponed. The child worsened and had to undergo an emergency operation that night. Beaverbrook decided that in Wilson he had a medical advisor who was prepared to defy him when need be, a medical man he could rely upon. The two men became friends.

Wilson interested Beaverbrook in his plans to rebuild the medical school and secured liberal donations to that cause. Indeed, Beaverbrook began to think of St Mary's as his own hospital, and in 1932, when he wanted to impress a newly elected Labour MP, offered him the services of St Mary's, writing, "If you have not yet thrown off your trouble, will you let me arrange for the St Mary's Hospital staff to look into it? I have a long connection with that hospital."[79] The object of his benevolence was, in retrospect, an unfortunate one: doubtless the young Aneurin Bevan, who declined the "kind offer," became the more confirmed in his hatred of voluntary hospitals as symbols of "the continued patronage and power of the propertied classes."[80] Beaverbrook was a close friend of Sir Winston Churchill, and at Beaverbrook's suggestion, Churchill made Wilson his personal physician soon after becoming prime minister. For most of the Second World War Wilson led a hectic life as he followed his august patient around the world, battling pneumonia and coronary thrombosis. He was elevated to the peerage for his pains.

Wilson, Lord Moran, had a far-reaching influence on medical politics of the day as president of the Royal College of Physicians from 1940 to 1950. He believed that the members had turned the college into "a club not a college"[81] and had relinquished leadership in medical politics to the British Medical Association. He worked to wrest power away from the BMA during the negotiations with the minister of Health leading up to the NHS.[82] Bevan capitalized on this split between the general practitioners represented by the BMA and consultants represented by the royal colleges and pitted one faction against the other. He did so by introducing the principle of national rather than local control of the voluntary hospitals. There is some suggestion that he did so on Moran's prodding. As Moran later recalled, Bevan asked him how hospitals could be made more uniformly efficient, to which he replied: "'You will only get one standard of excellence when every hospital has a first-rate consultant staff.' Bevan asked how consultants could be persuaded to leave teaching hospitals and 'go into the periphery?' (He grinned) 'You wouldn't like it if I began to direct labour.' Moran: 'Oh, they'll go if they get an interesting job and if their financial future is secured by a proper salary.' Bevan (after a long pause): 'Only the state could pay those salaries. This would mean the nationalization of hospitals.'"[83]

At the college and the House of Lords, Moran spoke strongly in favour of a national service that would place hospitals under regional health boards rather than municipal councils, and teaching hospitals directly under the minister himself. Other plums offered to the consultants were the right to private practice, the right to admit private patients into NHS hospitals, and distinction awards. Agreement between the royal colleges and the government left the BMA out in the cold, so that Bevan was able to take a stronger line on general practice, prohibiting the sale of practices and introducing a basic salary. By the end of 1946 the bill to establish the NHS had been passed, and it only remained to work out the details. The two royal colleges and the BMA were represented in a negotiating committee that included Moran, who successfully mediated between the BMA and the minister of Health. As a compromise, GPs would be paid by capitation rather than salary. Again, in the Lords, Moran spoke warmly in favour of the amendment. Those who admired his interventions and the NHS itself called him "the peacemaker," while in BMA circles he became "Corkscrew Charlie." Anigoni's portrait of Moran in his presidential robes conveys beautifully the impression of a master strategist, a Richelieu for the profession, his sideways look reflecting his circuitous thinking.

Much has been made of the division between consultants and general practitioners that Moran and Bevan exploited.[84] Critics of the NHS have traditionally attacked it as being organized around hospitals and curative services rather than general practitioners and prevention, and much of the reform of the NHS in subsequent decades was intended to redress this imbalance. As the spokesman for the consultants, Moran has been blamed for the NHS's problems, especially after a famous remark he made in 1958 describing general practitioners as would-be consultants who had "fallen off the lower rung of the ladder." And yet this view should be tempered. Moran introduced courses in general practice to St Mary's at the instigation of an energetic GP alumnus, Geoffrey Barber. Moran argued as well that GPs should have access to hospital beds: "I know it will be said that the standard of those hospitals will go down, but I do not think that that should happen if we see that the general practitioners are properly integrated with the consultants already on the staff of the hospitals. It is the bond between these two that will decide the success of this experiment."[85] Arthur Dickson Wright also argued for GP access to hospital beds and closer relations between the branches of the profession.[86] The emphasis on personal relations was characteristic of the atmosphere Moran instilled in St Mary's Hospital Medical School, and it helps to account for the school's renaissance under his direction.

The NHS at Home

St Mary's Hospital changed dramatically during the first half of the twentieth century because the context within which it functioned also changed dramatically. Improvements in diagnostic and therapeutic techniques, here exemplified by venereology, further increased the middle-class demand for a reform of health services, so as to make those services more equitably distributed and less reliant upon uncertain philanthropy. War, depression, and democratization of the public sphere radicalized British opinion. The medical profession took a vital part in public debates over medical services. The staff at St Mary's, informed by their experiences in Paddington, helped to shape the outcome of these debates.

The board of managers of St Mary's played little part in the move towards the NHS. During the 1920s and 1930s it refused to consider nationalization, but by the 1940s it seems to have recognized that the hospital must come under state control. Indeed, Moran, himself a member of the board, had been predicting nationalization for thirty years.[87] St Mary's was perhaps in a uniquely favourable position. Since 1920 Moran had refashioned the hospital – affiliating it with the old infirmary – so as to prepare for the coming of nationalization. During the 1940s he tailored the NHS to accommodate St Mary's so that its status as a teaching hospital guaranteed it and the other teaching hospitals special benefits.

There remained one serious problem. If teaching activities were to be so important, there had to be some guarantee of efficiency. In 1942 the departments of Health and Education set up a committee to investigate existing medical education. This, the Goodenough Committee, reported in 1944 that a comprehensive education could only be provided in hospitals of seven hundred or more beds. St Mary's had only half that number: in medicine, only 47 of the 175 recommended, in surgery only 90 of 175, in obstetrics only 29 of 70, and so forth through all the departments. As the lecturers ruefully remarked, the figures revealed "an extremely serious condition."[88] A "Reconstruction Committee" began to plan for survival. Fortunately, just as St Mary's needed to find more beds, other hospitals in the district had good reason to offer them. Because the teaching hospitals would be self-governing under the NHS, smaller specialist hospitals welcomed proposals for affiliation that would secure them the same benefits. Two children's hospitals – Paddington Green and Princess Louise in Kensington – both agreed to join the scheme, as did the Western Ophthalmic Hospital, the Samaritan Hospital for Women (both on Marylebone Road), and St Luke's Hospital for the Dying in Bayswater. By the appointed day in June 1948 when the NHS took effect, the agreements were in place.

The affiliation scheme was not a panacea. St Mary's could now claim to command more than seven hundred beds, but this was a minimum standard. The ideal set by the government was nearer one thousand. Moreover, though the newest of the teaching hospitals, St Mary's had some of the oldest, most dilapidated, and generally inadequate buildings in London. Long before nationalization loomed, the governors recognized that the hospital

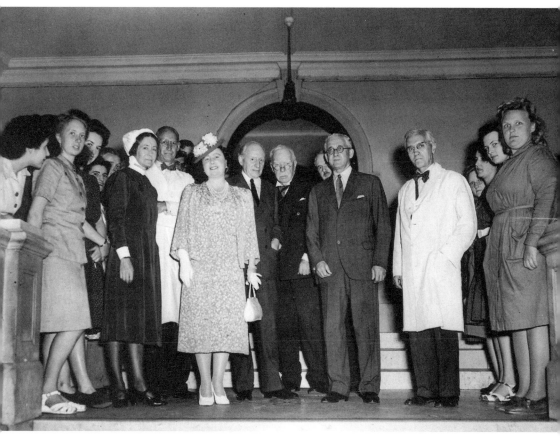

A royal visit to St Mary's. St Mary's Hospital NHS Trust Archives and the Royal
College of Surgeons of England

had to be rebuilt, and they had accordingly planned a public appeal. Early
in 1941 they planned to base the appeal on Moran's special relationship
with Winston Churchill by producing a medal with Churchill's rotund face.
This, they reckoned, would be sure to attract support and large donations
in the United States (not yet in the war). The director of a company producing safety razors had agreed to pay for the costs of the appeal. Churchill
was agreeable, the queen's approval was obtained, but the Foreign Office
vetoed the proposal. Soon, however, another promising basis for an international appeal presented itself: penicillin.

∞ 8

Pathology between the Wars
Wright and Fleming

Wright and Moran: Of Philosophy and Football

DURING THE 1920S and 1930s at St Mary's, Sir Almroth Wright and Charles Wilson, Lord Moran, dominated the scene. They were two very different characters, forced into a shotgun wedding. During the 1920s and 1930s, as the two pushed the school and the Inoculation Department closer together institutionally, they veered away from medicine proper in their outlooks, one towards physiology and philosophy and the other towards politics and sports. Both men were institution-builders: during the late 1920s and early 1930s, they managed to get hold of considerable sums of money and rebuilt their respective institutions in a large shared building facing the hospital. Both were concerned with the impact that institutional structures had upon human thought and behaviour and tried to create institutions that would, by shaping behaviour, perform a kind of social engineering. However, their goals were quite different.

Almroth Wright continued to build up his research institute. He believed that certain social, economic, and intellectual structures needed to be in place for thinkers to reach their full potential and make their discoveries. But the institutional structures were not enough. He had shown how research and therapeutics could be combined and how medicine should be reformed. But people were imprisoned by their irrationality. No matter how well Wright argued, no matter how beautifully his experiments proved his theories, he remained prey to the confederacy of dunces conspiring against him. And so he spent the final decades of his long life writing and rewriting a treatise on logic. His goal was to identify, analyse, and explain the ineffable process of thought and subject it to scientific discipline. He tried to explain to men (he hadn't much hope for women) what they thought and why, so that they might behave more rationally.

Moran, by contrast, was no rationalist. He also studied the human mind, but his concern was with character rather than with thought. He wanted to know what constituted character, whether it was innate or could be built up, and what conditions brought it out. He perceived that the ineffable must be kept ineffable, that character deconstructed is character destroyed: there must always be mystique. One form of mystification was rugby. Moran spent much of his life playing, coaching, watching, and cogitating on rugby. It was a metaphor for life and for professional practice, and it brought out personal qualities of character and collegiality that both demanded. Wright wanted to teach people to think properly; Moran thought that if you could teach them to play properly, the rest would follow, whether they thought it through or not. Wright was an enlightener, a Voltaire, Moran an anti-enlightener, a Rousseau. Like Rousseau, he complained that the existing educational establishment stifled the natural play of mind, and the title of his jeremiad, "The Student in Irons," recalls the Genevan's ringing cry that "Man is born free but is everywhere in chains."[1]

By the 1920s Wright's star was waning. He relaxed his grip on the Inoculation Department and withdrew into philosophy. The clinical elite remained hostile to his work, especially after the dispute over war wounds.[2] He recounted that a visiting consultant told him, "No one in the Profession pays the least attention to these little games that you folks play in laboratories."[3] Wright also lost credit with the pathologists who rejected his opsonic indices. New work forced even him to admit that much of the early work on opsonins had been flawed. By contrast, Moran's star remained high in the heavens. The two men illustrate two different approaches to reforming the medical profession, one rooted in knowledge and the other in social power.

Almroth Wright

After the war the Inoculation Department was less lively than it had been, but it remained a place of serious research, in stark contrast to the medical school. A student of 1919, Ronald Hare, described the two. Hare's father was a country practitioner who treated patients with differently coloured but practically interchangeable bottles of salts. Traditional medicine, as Hare understood it, was virtually powerless against the major diseases. At St Mary's he began to understand why this was so, for, he found, the

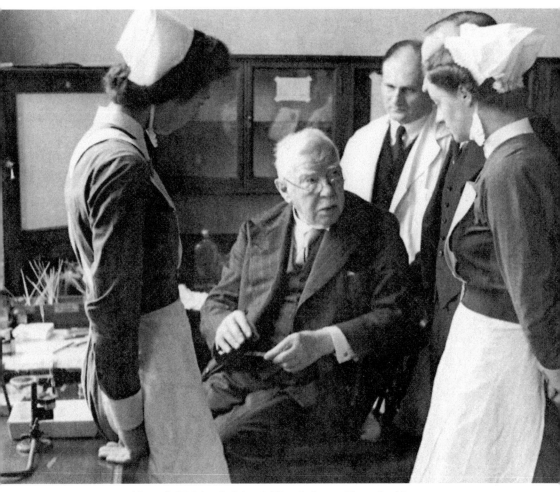
Almroth Wright. St Mary's Hospital NHS Trust Archives

clinicians were too busy with private practice to perform research, and anyway, there was nowhere to do it. "The only laboratory at St Mary's to which they had access was a tiny room in the basement where the medical clerks tested urine. Prof. Langmead had one which was larger because he was professor of medicine, but this was a very recent innovation, and in any event, its one technician and all its resources were occupied in the manufacture of insulin, not yet commercially available. The laboratory occupied by Dr Roche Lynch was also out of bounds. Although it carried out some of the more elaborate biochemical tests needed by the patients, its main activity was the detection of poisons in the bodies of victims of murder."[4] In the school labs, "there was generally only one technician to look after a whole department, the laboratories were stone cold most of the winter, they were thick with dust and there was very little apparatus, a great deal of it broken or out of action."

By contrast, Hare recalled, "I do not think I will ever forget my sight of the upstairs laboratory, into which we could see through large glass doors on the way to the lecture room. There were white-tiled benches at which sat four men entirely concentrated on what they were doing. The room itself was in semi-darkness but their benches were brightly illuminated by shaded lamps. There was a bright fire burning at one end, there seemed to be an abundance of apparatus about, much of it of brass, and all highly polished. The place had an air of real purpose about it." The practical teaching, likewise, was "conducted with an efficiency unknown in the medical school. There were not only several technicians to fetch and carry but some of the men I had just seen in the laboratory emerged to act as demonstrators. What is more, each student's place was properly prepared for him with rows of stains all ready, blotting paper, slides and cultures ... This was the first time I had seen a properly run laboratory in which a real attempt was being made to do research. And, moreover, by men who, when viewed from the back in dim light, seemed utterly devoted to their work." Young Hare determined to join them. After completing his medical qualification, he transferred across to Wright's domain, remaining there until 1929.

Wright continued to study immunity. He attempted "immuno-transfusion," a combination of vaccine therapy and blood transfusion. The sulpha drugs introduced during the 1920s presented themselves as rivals to his vaccines, and he turned his attention to chemotherapy, but he didn't really believe it could substitute for therapies that bolstered the immune system. He developed a new theory of in-vitro immunity after discovering a new bactericidal activity in blood serum, but, Hare remarks, his concepts and techniques were inadequate for the work, and bacteriologists ignored his conclusions.

In the Inoculation Department itself, Wright was and remained the "Grand Old Man." There were still daily teatime gatherings in the departmental library. Surrounded by acolytes, Wright pronounced monologues on philosophy, science, or perhaps his most hated bugbear, feminism. Around such a man, even in his advanced old age, one young medical student recalled, "the waves and currents of hates and fears and hopes eddied ceaselessly."[5] As he saw his work eclipsed, Wright grew ever more determined to prove himself correct. He devoted his final years to writing a theory of knowledge that would give him the last word in all his many disputes. He called it *Alethetropic Logic,* or "the logic which searches for truth," as distinct from the arid logic of mathematicians or, heaven help them, statisticians. He never finished the treatise, and it was left to his grandson, Giles Romanes, to publish it posthumously, with a preface explaining its genesis: "Sir Almroth was constantly applying the knowledge obtained in his large experience of publishing his own experimental results, teaching students and post-graduates, and of persuading those in authority to adopt methods arising out of his work. It was soon impressed upon him that the presentation of the facts is a relatively easy task, but that the recipient of the facts is not necessarily in a frame of mind to believe the truth of the statements. He realised that without recognition and reception of the truth no progress was possible and further that the less palatable the facts were the less likely they were to be believed. He was convinced therefore that men must be provided with the criteria of truth."

The treatise can be roughly divided into two sections, one concerned with the bodily basis of belief and the other with the statistical method. Wright believed that people had a physiological need for belief: exposure to concepts or images created a reflex response in the body and was translated into mental images. In the process of translation, neuronal tension occurred, and it was aggravated if appropriate mental images did not immediately suggest themselves. Weak people, such as women, gave in to this neuronal tension and formed mental images before they had enough evidence for them. The act of belief, by relieving tension, conferred pleasure, and woman in particular "is everywhere a *gourmande* of the pleasures of Belief."[6] Thought required high levels of neuronal tension which the true thinker could channel, without leaping prematurely towards intellectual closure. Wright – an ascetic himself – said he could only write well if his pulse rose to 100. Errors were of two sorts: simple errors, or paralogisms, and fallacies that reflected a particular bias or mental shortcoming. A man could be corrected of his errors but not of his fallacies. The only hope was education: if men were taught logic properly in school, they might be made more reasonable.

Wright's physiological theory had first been aired in *Brain* in 1895 and predated his long years of intellectual frustration. However, the final section of the book addressed this frustration, consisting largely of an attack on statistics. The requirements of statistical method were, he thought, unattainable on ethical, administrative, and cognitive grounds. One problem of statistics was that there could be no genuine comparison between subjects and controls. If a vaccine were being studied, subjects and controls must be exposed to normal and identical levels of infection. But if they were lumped together (to share the same conditions), the controls benefited from the declining incidence of disease in the vaccinated group.

Worse, statisticians prohibited use of retrospective statistics. Major Greenwood, a statistician and ally of Karl Pearson, asserted that Jenner's smallpox vaccine had never been statistically proved to work. Wright was incensed: anyone who had seen a smallpox epidemic knew that vaccination worked. This proved for him the intellectual bankruptcy of the statistical method and the superiority of clinical judgment. When assessing the efficacy of a therapy, you didn't need a control if a patient's condition was desperate, because improvement would be proof enough.[7] Wright, who had revolutionized pathology at the turn of the century by quantifying it, now argued that subjective "certainty" was more scientific than measurement. His slogan, that the physician of the future must be an *immunisator*, seemed to change in emphasis: the immunisator of the future must be a *physician*. Science could improve medicine, but it could not replace it.

By the time Wright's book was published in 1953, the statisticians had carried the day. In Britain the first modern, randomized clinical trial was of streptomycin in 1946. The movement towards more rigorous standards of evidence had been growing since the beginning of the century.[8] To show that Wright and his school (as well as St Mary's Hospital Medical School generally) became remote from intellectual developments in clinical medicine, we take a short detour to follow the fortunes of two of Wright's rivals for the position at Mary's in 1902 – F.J. Poynton and Sir John Broadbent – as they engaged in a dispute about old and new forms of clinical knowledge in respect to cardiology.

Objectivity in Medicine

In 1917 G.A. Sutherland, a physician at Paddington Green Children's Hospital, gave the Lumleian lectures to the Royal College of Physicians on "modern aspects of heart disease." He advocated a "new" cardiology that used instrumental and graphic methods such as the electrocardiograph (ECG), and disparaged the subjective knowledge of previous cardiologists.

(The ECG was developed by William Einthoven, based on the principles of electrocardiography worked out by Augustus Waller.⁹) Sutherland's lecture sparked a long debate in the *Lancet* about the old versus the new school. Four Mary's men intervened, two on behalf of the old school and two, so they thought, on behalf of the new. Poynton (supported by a recent Mary's graduate, H.G.P. Castellain, a medical inspector) reaffirmed the hypothesis of rheumatic infection. He was taken aback when Sir James Mackenzie, the leading cardiologist of the day, joined what had been a minor exchange and denounced Poynton's work as backwards looking and sterile.

Others leaped to the defence of the old school. E.H. Colbeck, a Mary's graduate who practised in London, argued that Sir William Broadbent had been as knowledgeable about the significance of heart murmurs as anyone since. Sir John Broadbent, who had collaborated with his father, joined in to denounce the ECG as giving a misguided importance to the "doctrine of auricular fibrillation." Two points were at issue. The first was whether fibrillation – which had been observed in animals but was not the sort of thing one could observe experimentally in humans – was an important cause of heart stoppage. The second was whether digitalis was a specific remedy for fibrillation (acting by slowing the cardiac muscle as, again, had been observed in animals) or whether it added "tone" to exhausted heart muscle, as Sir John Broadbent argued: "Any clinician knows the extraordinarily satisfactory results obtained from digitalis in cases of heart failure and dropsy associated with mitral incompetence, even when the pulse is quite regular and there is no question of 'auricular fibrillation.'"

This remark was too much for Thomas Lewis, who had trained under Mackenzie and discovered fibrillation in 1909 using the cardiograph. Lewis replied, "It is clear that if *one* clinician has such knowledge, digitalis has the action here credited to it. But the clinician must show the source of his knowledge; he must bring forward the evidence for his faith." Plenty of careful observations "conducted on scientific lines" showed that digitalis acted beneficially in auricular fibrillation; "Casual bedside observations are not to be weighed in the same scale." Lewis demanded hard evidence of the "extraordinarily satisfactory results" that Broadbent invoked.

Broadbent's feeble reply brought stinging retorts from both Lewis and Mackenzie, who implied that, while Broadbent cloaked himself in the outdated knowledge of his father, Sir William himself, were he alive, would have been for the "new" school. Sir John Broadbent lacked the stature to speak for the old school, but Clifford Allbutt, regius professor of medicine at Cambridge, was eminently able to do so. He wrote to the *Lancet* defending the "mass of clinical material" gathered by the great cardiologists of yore, which the new school ignored.[10] For Allbutt the medical profession was like an elderly GP who might know little of pathological processes but had vast clinical experience. The experience of one was the experience of all.[11]

By contrast, the new school showed a Cartesian scepticism for anything it couldn't judge for itself on the basis of evidence placed before it. It demanded to see the raw material of judgment, as well as the judgment itself. Clayton Lane, a Mary's student who joined the India Medical Service, exclaimed during an entirely different debate in 1901, "If a published case is to be any use it must be fully reported so that all who read may form their own conclusions. In no other way can the vexed question of the mode of death under chloroform be finally settled, for no man can be expected to accept unhesitatingly another man's dictum on a questionable point."[12] Likewise, Thomas Lewis demanded evidence for Broadbent's "faith" in one remedy over another. Traditionally, the faith of a prominent clinician had been itself evidence. Prestige and knowledge were intimately connected in a relation of mutual reinforcement, so that to attack the one was to attack the other. By the early 1920s a new set of battle lines had been drawn in the contestation over medical knowledge. The confrontation was between those who sought objective and quantifiable measures of physiological activity and therapeutic outcome, and those who defended subjective impressions formed by great men at the bedside. St Mary's Hospital Medical School was firmly in the second camp. So was Sir Almroth Wright, driven there by his hatred for the statisticians.

Wright's admiration for clinical judgment was not unmitigated and was certainly not at the expense of laboratory forms of knowledge. More certain than clinical judgment, he argued, was the "crucial experiment" obtained by means of "claustration" in the laboratory. The laboratory provided *ceteribus paribus* conditions: it permitted the scientist to screen out complicating factors, especially when using in-vitro procedures. "Many physiological experiments cannot be carried out *in vivo*. And such of these experiments as admit of being carried out both *in vivo* and *in vivo* give always more regular results *in vitro*. And naturally so. For when we operate *in vitro*, we exclude always a number of 'perturbants,' and are therefore always operating in a more fallacy-free environment."[13] However, crucial experiments only suggested, they didn't dictate treatments. Because the lessons were indirect, ordinary practitioners failed to see their relevance and had "absolutely no intellectual regard for, or appreciation of, what is usually called Crucial Experimentation."[14] Even though Wright had obtained in-vitro proof that typhoid vaccine worked, no one had listened.

Wright's Influence

During the interwar period, researchers at the Inoculation Department, as they sat around the slumped figure in the high-backed chair, listened to a continual denunciation of statistical methods. They were told to prefer experiments done in vitro to those done in vivo. If in-vivo experiments were to be performed, the retrospective statistical method – which tabulated probable cures – was preferable to the formal clinical trial.

An example of this orientation can be seen in the work on immuno-transfusion. Wright published a paper on the subject in 1919, and his students pushed the investigation further. They believed that immuno-transfusion worked where vaccine therapy couldn't stimulate depleted leucocytes. Only an infusion of normal leucocytes could save the patient. In a paper published in 1923, Leonard Colebrook and E.J. Storer puzzled over how to prove this. They refused to compile statistics, because, they argued, these cases were too few and it was unethical to withhold treatment. Instead, they invoked clinical standards of evidence. Immuno-transfusion worked when it cured intractable cases. The two men reduced the problem of proof to standards of eloquence and personal reliability: "The difficulty of furnishing convincing testimony of dramatic improvements and cures produced in hopeless cases will consist in the difficulty in finding words (for photographic records will only rarely be available) – words graphic enough to depict to the reader the desperate condition of the patient when treatment was initiated and the resurrectional change that followed. Where verbal description is inadequate and photographic records are not available, the reader will have to be largely guided by his estimate of the trustworthiness and sobriety of judgement of the reporter."[15] Colebrook and Storer classified their cases as "plainly desperate" or "serious but not desperate" and so forth. Their paper sounds like an act of ventriloquism on the part of Wright.

That said, there is also considerable evidence against Wright's domination of the Inoculation Department. Hare says that by the time he joined, one could dare to disagree with Wright's published work, even in print. The Inoculation Department was a warren of laboratories and researchers, some of whom were left to their own devices. During the mid-1920s, these researchers filled journals, especially the *British Journal of Experimental Pathology*, with findings on such topics as "the bacterial factor in the aetiology of dental caries," the structure of salivary gland tumours, and the bactericidal action of merchurochrome, sancorysin, and streptococcal toxin.[16] The loose structure of Wright's empire was recalled by Keith

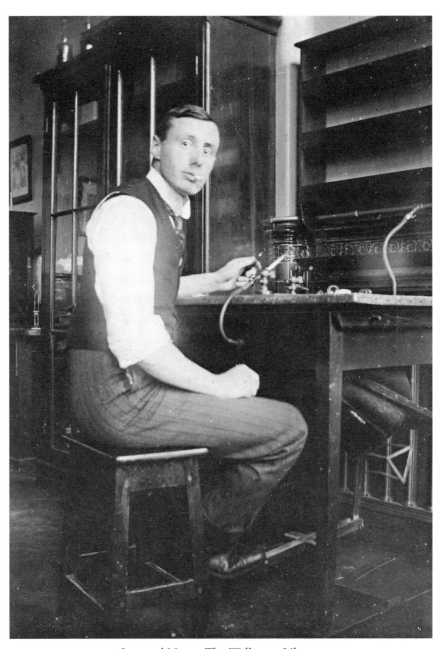

Leonard Noon. The Wellcome Library

Rogers, who entered St Mary's as a medical student in 1929 and moved to the Inoculation Department:

You see, the old man could employ whoever he liked ... There were some extraordinary characters. Have you heard about the Dutchman? God knows where the Dutchman came from, but he had a little room on the first floor, a very small room, it was crammed full of bits and bobs, which he knew what they were for, but no one else did. And he was a pet of the old man's. But I never knew what his job was! And you've come across Lewis Holt? Lewis Holt was engaged by the old man to prove the old man's theory of the cause of scurvy. The old man had a theory that scurvy was caused by acidosis, and Louis Holt had a batch of guinea pigs on the old man's diet ... And he'd just got the guinea pigs to the stage of developing scurvy, and Györgyi wrote up vitamin C, and the whole thing was blown apart![17]

After that, Holt, though he got an MSc for the work, was left to twiddle his thumbs until Fleming put him onto some antitoxin work. As for Keith Rogers, after an eventful few years in the Inoculation Department (where he was treated by Fleming with penicillin to cure an eye infection that threatened to impair his performance at a shooting match) he took up a pathology position in Birmingham.

In 1938 Wright decided that the Inoculation Department lacked a virologist, and he told John Freeman (always his intermediary in school matters) to sort it out. Writing to Lord Moran, Freeman was pithy as always: "Dear Wilson, Wright asked me to tell you he would like Dr F. Himmelweit's name to be put down if possible as Lecturer in Filter passing Viruses & Virus Diseases. I think this subject may develop into as big a thing as bacteriology, & it would be well to be in early on it. Yours J.F." When Moran failed to act, Wright himself wrote five weeks later asserting that "all the men in the National Institute" thought highly of Himmelweit, and that the interests of the school and "my personal feelings are engaged in the matter."[18] Himmelweit was appointed. A year later Freeman tried to convince Moran that Himmelweit should teach (smallpox) vaccination, commenting, "I won't burden you here with the technical reasons for this choice of man – they are ready on demand." These letters beautifully characterize the informality of arrangements at St Mary's. Even more characteristically, Moran scribbled rugby scores on the back of them.[19]

The mainstay of the Inoculation Department remained the manufacture and administration of therapeutic vaccines. Wright placed this work in the hands of Freeman and Fleming, his two right-hand men. Freeman ran the allergy clinic and investigated allergic reactions. Fleming was production manager for the therapeutic vaccines; his own research interests, where they diverged from questions raised by his chief, concerned bactericides which he discovered: first lysozyme and then penicillin.

The question of Fleming's independence and his standards of knowledge are controversial because they relate to the discovery of penicillin. André Maurois argued that Fleming failed to turn his chance discovery into a practical therapy because Sir Almroth Wright disapproved of chemotherapy, and his domineering control of the Inoculation Department prevented Fleming from studying penicillin independently.[20] Others reply that Wright was neither so hostile and nor so domineering.[21] Some have suggested that the obstacles were merely technical: Fleming himself blamed the fact that chemists couldn't purify the mould sufficiently to inject it into the bloodstream of animals or humans. Some blame Fleming's preoccupation with the test-tube, which blinded him to the possibility of therapeutic trials. Although Fleming's innermost thoughts remain inscrutable, connections between his practices can be traced. What he could or couldn't do was determined by the resources available to him at St Mary's. Medical theories count as resources just as surely as do chemists, for a particular conception of the role of the clinic or the laboratory will determine the equipping of it. Before looking at the discovery of penicillin, therefore, let us step back and survey the resources at St Mary's.

During the early 1920s Wright undertook at least two projects aimed at improving and integrating clinical and laboratory research at St Mary's. Both were inconsequential, but they do reveal his conception of the Inoculation Department and its relationship with the school. These projects also reveal his attempts to place research on a sound financial footing. Until 1920 Wright channelled funds towards the school by providing cheap pathology teaching. From 1920 he began to sponsor the school more directly. The heads of departments in both institutions formed themselves into a research entity called the Pathological Institute. The effect was to highlight the research activity of both institutions, giving it formal recognition and an institutional basis. The Pathological Institute consisted of separate departments of Anatomy (J.E. Frazer), Experimental Pathology (Collingwood, the physiology professor), Special and General Pathology (Kettle), Chemical Pathology (Willcox), Systematic Bacteriology (Fleming), Clinical Bacteriology (Freeman), and Immunology and Vaccines (Wright), with Wright as the director of the institute.

The Pathological Institute was largely funded by the Inoculation Department, which provided £1,000 per annum for research, £400 of which went towards research scholarships. Wright had received a scholarship from the Grocers Company in 1887 which, he attested in 1903, enabled him "to devote my whole time to study and research ... Without it I should hardly have been able to survive at science."[22] His scheme enabled him to recruit new researchers to the Inoculation Department at a time when visitors were dropping off. It was well justified by the calibre of students who took up the fellowship and then went on to careers in research. Ida Mann, later a fellow at Oxford and a prominent ophthalmologist, recalled, "My first paid award was a studentship in the Institute of Pathology and Research at St Mary's. This was officially under Sir Almroth Wright, but was awarded me on condition that Professor Frazer kept me incommunicado in the Anatomy Department and never let me set foot in the hollowed masculine territories of the Institute itself."[23] Ronald Hare was another early beneficiary: "And so, without benefit of even an internship and still less a postgraduate qualification, but far, far more important, when only 25 years old and still possessing the youthful enthusiasm the modern system of training so effectively dissipates before a man starts his life's work, I entered the laboratory that was to be my scientific home for the next 6 years."[24] Hare went on to work with Leonard Colebrook on protonsil (the first of the sulphonamide drugs) at Queen Charlotte's Hospital, then to produce penicillin during the war; he was appointed the first bacteriology professor at St Thomas's in 1946.

The Pathological Institute also supported lectures on applied research. This was (and remains) a very distinguished lecture series, because Wright had very distinguished friends. The first line-up of speakers was Wright himself, Archibald Garrod (regius professor at Oxford), G. Elliot Smith (professor of anatomy at UCL), Sir W.B. Leishman (director of pathology in the Army Medical Services), E.H. Starling (physiology professor at UCL), Sir A. Cruickshank (chief analyst to the Metropolitan Water Board), William Bulloch (professor of bacteriology at the London), and Sir Berkeley Moynihan (professor of surgery at Leeds).

The remaining funds of the Pathological Institute paid for departmental research projects. Regular payments were made right up until the outbreak of World War II. An example of how this functioned is provided by some correspondence on chemical pathology. In February 1921 Willcox complained that, due to the pressure of routine work, "it was impossible for the Staff to undertake any research work."[25] The Pathological Institute resolved that if the hospital would create a new appointment in that department (at £170 p.a.), the institute would contribute £100 for research, conditional upon annual reports showing that valuable research was being performed. The hospital governors were agreeable, but demanded that the top-up be guaranteed rather than conditional. They remarked that "Sir

William Willcox has given his personal assurance to the Board that valuable research work under these conditions would be carried out by the department of Chemical Pathology." This was good enough for the institute, which replied "that this Committee, having Sir William Willcox's assurance, were *quite satisfied* that the proposed grant would be spent on *Chemical Research*"; they were prepared to guarantee the payments so long as they had funds. A gentleman's agreement was formed, and each year the grant was indeed renewed.

The Pathological Institute has been derided as a paper entity that didn't have any real existence.[26] To some extent, lack of resources was to blame. The pittance that the Inoculation Department could devote to research in the medical school was not enough to implant a research culture. The Inoculation Department had never generated enough money to fulfil all Wright's ambitions for the reform of medicine. The sums became more obviously inadequate during in the 1920s and '30s, as other, better-funded institutions were established, including the MRC research establishment at Mill Hill and such American institutes as the Rockefeller Institute and CalTech.[27]

Wright was keenly aware that his Pathological Institute was falling behind. In October 1925 he drew up an application to the Rockefeller Foundation for a grant. The Rockefeller had already invested many thousands of pounds in other schools, above all the London School of Hygiene and Tropical Medicine and University College, London. Wright decided it was his turn. The application consisted of a short statement, claiming that "for 25 years or from the very outset of the modern movement in medicine the Governing Board and Staff of St. Mary's Hospital have fostered Medical Research and the more scientific methods of treatment that have sprung from it." While the bacteriological departments were "self-supporting and a little more than self-supporting," other work was "totally unprovided for ... There is here need of laboratory accommodation, of equipment, and of assistants and subordinate staff to take some of the burden of the routine work and make the prosecution of research work possible." If funded, the other departments would "be able to draw up level with the productive bacteriological departments. And we would add that if the laboratories of all the various departments could be assembled under one roof – and there is a site available which would permit of this being done – a powerful impetus would be given to the development of scientific medicine and higher medical education."[28] The document, which fitted onto one page, was signed by the entire roster of St Mary's officials: the dean, the chair of the medical committee, the chairmen of St Mary's Hospital (Arthur Prideaux) and the Inoculation Department (Lord Iveagh), and Wright himself.

Wright did not get his funding. The Rockefeller archivist can find no sign of the application, so it is possible that he never submitted it. It is also possible that the Rockefeller refused to grant the money. Moran later remarked to Carmalt Jones, "Almroth Wright, in my time when I was Dean was nothing else than a handicap to the School. He was uncooperative, very unpopular with the grant giving bodies, in spite of his ability."[29] Certainly the document would have been easy to refuse. It seemed to say "give us the money and trust us to use it well." That might work for an interdepartmental arrangement but would hardly impress the Rockefeller Foundation.

Wright became a scientist before there existed much in the way of philanthropic or state funds for research. The Brown Institution and the Grocer's scholarship were mere pointers in the path. He successfully built up a thriving research institute by assuming a certain intellectual arrogance, a lordly air, among the lords and businessmen from whom he solicited funds. He was a scientist speaking to laymen and, in the first decade of the twentieth century, it was not fitting for medical reasoning to hold itself accountable to lay opinion. As government and philanthropic foundations to sponsor research were slowly established, mechanisms of peer review were introduced to overcome this problem, and scientists were required to defend their work before fellow scientists, in a formal rather than informal manner. Wright never adapted to these new forms of accountability.

It is instructive to contrast the application made by Howard Florey at Oxford to that same Rockefeller Foundation in the late 1930s for funding for investigations into bacteriology and pathological chemistry.[30] Both applications could be said to involve penicillin. Wright applied for money to prop up the other departments, and an obvious desideratum was a skilled chemist. As Hare observed, the pathological chemistry department was wholly given to forensic toxicology, so Fleming had to enlist medical students to try to purify the mould. A top-rank chemist might have been able to purify penicillin in 1928, though the techniques and instruments were probably still too crude.[31] The task was quite beyond a student. By contrast, as Howard Florey told the Rockefeller Foundation, he had a first-rate chemist in Ernst Chain to work on purifying bactericidal substances. Florey wrote fifteen pages detailing past and future work to prove that the project was feasible and that Oxford was well equipped to do the work. Fourteen years lay between the two applications, years in which applying for research grants had probably become an established genre.

Fleming was left to muddle through. To his mind, that was not entirely a bad thing. He remarked that, had he been a member of a large research team, he would not have been able to drop everything to pursue penicillin. Thus, while lack of funding may have prevented the early purification of penicillin, that same lack permitted its initial development.

The Discovery of Penicillin

The life of Alexander Fleming exemplifies the opportunities and obstacles that a place like St Mary's could put before an intelligent, observant, and nimble-fingered young man at the turn of the century. The combination of a deeply traditional teaching hospital and an innovative research lab enabled Fleming to undergo a gradual transformation from an ambitious shipping clerk to a Nobel laureate. Raised on a farm in the Scottish highlands, in 1895, aged fourteen, Alexander joined his elder brothers already living in London. He left school at fifteen and became a clerk in a shipping office. He didn't enjoy the work, and when his father died in 1901, he used his legacy to apply to medical school. First he studied the necessary preliminary courses at the London College of Preceptors. His previous schoolwork had been desultory, but now he made an effort and distinguished himself. He applied to St Mary's in part because it was nearby, and in part because, as a member of the London Scottish Regiment, he had played water polo against the school team. He was the prize student of his year, with Charles Pannett following him in second place. Both worked towards higher surgical qualifications, but, after Fleming qualified in 1906, he was invited to join the Inoculation Department. The invitation was arranged by John Freeman, another student of 1901, who wanted to keep him at St Mary's for the sake of the Rifle Club, to which both belonged. Once in the Inoculation Department, Fleming never left it, becoming Wright's right-hand man. His main task was to oversee the production of vaccines. He also helped Wright in his researches and developed his own lines of investigation, including, as seen, war wounds.

Fleming spent much of the 1920s studying lysozyme, a mildly bactericidal enzyme found in such bodily fluids as nasal mucus. It had not been noticed previously because it lyses only some bacteria, and it was something of a fluke that a vulnerable bacteria and the bactericide happened to meet on one of Fleming's culture plates. Fleming thought that it might be an important biological defence, but the fact that, as other researchers found, it was not present in all animals and all fluids, militated against this argument. He studied the substance for most of the 1920s, creating a mini-research paradigm for students such as Frederick Ridley who, in 1928, published a study of the action of lysozyme in eye infections.[32] By the end of the decade Fleming had turned his and his students' attention to penicillin, for which lysozyme proved a practice run.

The exact process by which Fleming discovered penicillin has been disputed. He could not have discovered it in the manner he described.[33] It was thought that a spore of penicillin had drifted onto some plates cultured with staphylococcus which he had left lying about for cleaning. In fact,

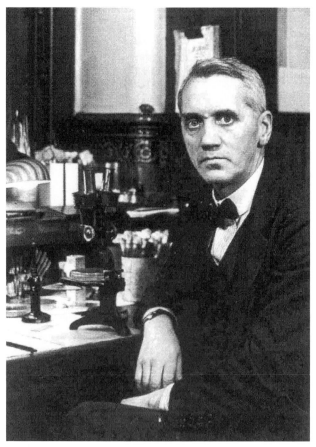

Alexander Fleming. St Mary's Hospital NHS Trust Archives

penicillin has no effect upon mature bacteria but instead causes a fatal mutation in growing bacteria, so that the penicillin had to grow on the culture plate before the bacteria were implanted. Moreover, the two cultures grow at different temperatures, penicillin preferring a cooler temperature. So the plate had already been contaminated when Fleming seeded staphylococcus on it. Returning from holiday, he glanced at it and stacked it with a mass of other plates in a tray of chemical bactericide for cleaning. It was sitting there, not quite submerged, when Fleming haphazardly pulled it off the top of the pile to show to a passing researcher. Glancing at it a second time, he said, "That's funny," and began to investigate what he had seen, namely, a staphylococcal culture which had been lysed in the vicinity of a fungal growth. So struck by it was he that he fixed the culture plate permanently, and it still exists in the British Library. He showed it to everybody else in the lab that day, but none saw anything remotely interesting in it. Only Fleming, who had seen such lysis before with lysozyme, realized there might be something in it.

In the next few months Fleming established that the mould could destroy cultures in vitro. He also discovered that when it was injected into the

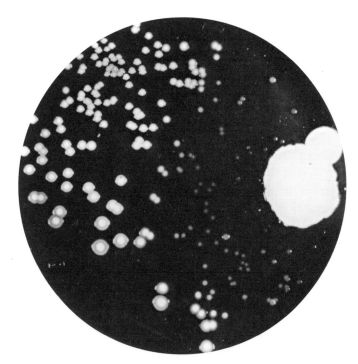

Fleming's culture of penicillin.
St Mary's Hospital NHS Trust Archives

bloodstream of animals, it disappeared within minutes, quickly becoming unmeasurable. Because of this, he apparently concluded that this new bactericide would be clinically useless in its current form, though he did speculate that it might have clinical and bactericidal uses in the future. Moreover, he was unable to get a pure culture of the fungus that could be safely injected, free of pyrogens or impurities that might cause serious illness.

Even the medical students, to whom Fleming taught bacteriology, heard this account. Felix Eastcott, who entered in 1936, recalled, "He would talk about different sorts of cultures, separating bacteria on a culture plate, and he would mention penicillin. And every group of students always asked the same question: 'So, this sounds as though it might be good for treating patients.' And he would say, 'Yes, it could be. But the chemists can't get it in sufficiently pure amounts to do it.'"[34] But, Hare and Macfarlane show, Fleming made only desultory attempts to purify it. He did try it out clinically, daubing it at surface infections. But the mould culture couldn't cure long-standing boils, and Hare has suggested that Fleming may have lacked access to deep-seated wound infections where penicillin might have proved more effective.[35] He did cure the eye infection of Keith Rogers, a worker in the department, but he didn't test it on other eyes.

Wai Chen, following Macfarlane, has argued that, raised in an environment geared towards the production of vaccines, which he oversaw as a kind of production manager, Fleming concentrated his efforts on applying penicillin to the vaccine work.[36] One serious problem with developing cultures for growing vaccines was opportunistic infections like streptococcus, which would contaminate, say, a whooping cough culture and make diagnosis and the development of an autogenous vaccine difficult. Penicillin neatly inhibited the secondary cocci, leaving only the *H. pertussis* – against which it was ineffective – free to grow. In 1937, I.H. Maclean published an article arguing that the use of penicillin in whooping cough cultures permitted a heavier implant of the whooping-cough culture, facilitated the process of swabbing, and improved a positive-culture rate of about 14 per cent to nearer 80 per cent.

Wright's lab was overwhelmingly devoted to in-vitro research, and it did establish the in-vitro properties of the mould. The question remains whether, given the superb laboratory and clinical facilities of the Inoculation Department and its history of practical therapeutics, more could have been expected. Also at issue is the assessment of Fleming's character as a scientist: was he rigorous or negligent? Ronald Hare (speaking frankly for television) called him a "damned good technician" but a "third-rate" research scientist.[38] Certainly Fleming was among the most manually deft workers Mary's has ever known. He counted opsonic indices with a facility that other bacteriologists couldn't imitate. Fleming was a master of lab techniques and ward techniques alike – he could inject a vein that no one else could find.

Fleming remained, in some respects, a surgeon manqué. He followed his chief's example of in-vitro quantification to the nth degree, as well as disregard for in-vivo statistics. In a textbook survey of vaccine therapy published in 1934, he fell entirely back on clinical authority of the most traditional sort in his advocacy of various vaccines. Thus, for example, in comparing stock and autogenous vaccines, he remarked, "Except for an interval during the war, the author has been in charge of such a [vaccine] clinic for some 20 years, and has arrived at certain conclusions." Qualitative assessments then followed, characterized by nothing more quantitatively rigorous than references to "many" or "some" patients. Or, "In the Out-Patient Department at St. Mary's Hospital the writer has on many occasions treated patients in the first instance with stock vaccines and, when the improvement was not marked, has used autogenous vaccines with the result that a very definite improvement in the condition was manifest. Of course, this did not happen in every case, but it was sufficiently frequent to be significant."[39] Fleming did give some clinical statistics, but all were drawn from the literature, none compiled at St Mary's. A pamphlet published in 1931 to raise funds for the hospital listed the numbers saved by typhoid vaccine but then, moving on to vaccine therapy, had to fall back on the apologetic remark: "It can only be described in scientific terms [inaccessible to the laymen to whom the pamphlet addressed itself] and no mass statistics are available to prove its value; but most people know that advantage is being taken of it either by themselves or their friends."[40]

Like Almroth Wright, Fleming had had his own run-ins with statisticians. In 1909 he had introduced to England a modification of the Wassermann Reaction – a diagnostic test for syphilis – which, by using very small quantities of generic serum, placed the test within the reach of even those hospitals without a licence to perform vivisection. However, a group of pathologists at the London who tested the modification found that it gave wrong results one-quarter of the time, and they blamed the fact that the quantity of serum was too small and undetermined, in contrast to the "known quality" and "well-adjusted and uniform quantities" of the Wassermann. They called on Fleming to prove that his technique worked "by publishing a suitable series of cases and investigating more thoroughly those in which his test appears to be wrong." When Fleming did no such thing, they set the problem to a research student, R. Donald, who concluded against the modification.[41]

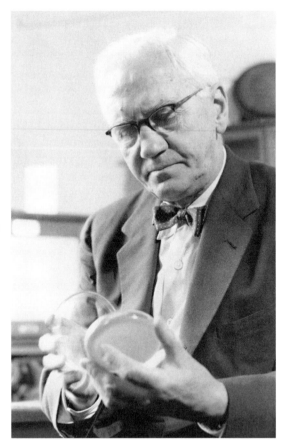

Fleming looking at his
culture plate. St Mary's
Hospital NHS Trust Archives

Fleming's laboratory reconstructed. St Mary's Hospital NHS Trust Archives

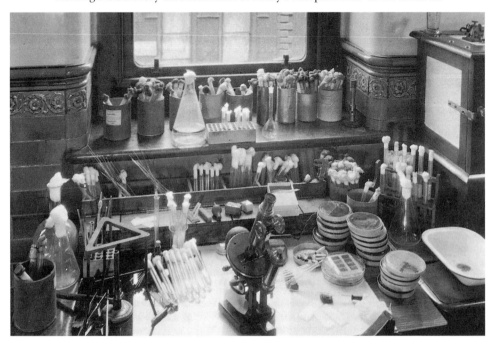

Throughout 1912 the controversy raged in the pages of the *Lancet*. Fleming and a handful of defenders argued that Donald's techniques rather than the modification itself was to blame: he hadn't performed a saline wash of the serum, for example. The London crowd insisted that Donald had followed Fleming's published instructions "precisely." They complained, "Anyone who may desire to gauge the value of these tests honestly is in a difficult position. He follows the directions of the author exactly and then learns that his results are considered to be valueless because he has not adopted some trivial procedure which is considered to be essential by someone else, but which has never been published in the detailed manner which is indispensable for scientific purposes." Two experienced bacteriologists jumped to Fleming's defence. D'Este Emery remarked, "Two observers may honestly believe they are carrying out a complicated technique like the Wassermann exactly similarly, but unless the process has been described in the utmost detail, small but important differences may creep in. One may centrifugalise his corpuscles to constant volume, another may not; one may accept any antigen which gives a negative result with a normal serum and a positive one with a syphilitic serum, another may test it still further, and so on. My explanation is a possible one. Can anyone suggest an alternative?" P.W. Bassett-Smith insisted that the technique required experience and therefore the first hundred or so cases were statistically unreliable. Bassett-Smith had once himself criticized the modification, but now having performed more than nine hundred tests, he concluded it was almost always correct.

The dispute probably taught Fleming that number-crunching required identical circumstances of replicability, but that genuine identity was a chimera. Tellingly, his ultimate defence of his test was clinical judgment. If, he argued, his modification were anything like as unreliable as the Londoners suggested, his twelve thousand diagnostic tests performed at St Mary's between 1909 and 1912 would have produced nine hundred false positives and "the method would have been absolutely discredited by the clinicians of St. Mary's Hospital, from whom I have had almost all my material." Thus, while laboratory precision and statistics provided a more rigorous standard of certitude than a nebulous and unquantifying clinical judgment, their very rigour made them unobtainable in 1912 as in 1902 and even 1934. By comparison, clinical judgment looked sound.

Absolute precision in vitro and vague gestures to in-vivo performance also characterized the work of Wright's second chief assistant, John Freeman, who ran the allergy clinic. Much of the early work was done with Leonard Noon who was, according to Freeman, one of the best brains ever to grace the Inoculation Department. It had been established that when pollen was scratched into the skin of a hay-fever sufferer, a large weal resulted, and that no such weal was to be seen if there were no allergy. Pollen sensitivity was the model, but the principle applied to all manner of allergies from animals to foodstuffs. Noon realized that prophylactic vaccines could be applied to allergies; that, by a process of gradual desensitization obtained by exposure to very small and gradually increasing doses, the allergic reaction could be stifled.

Noon died in 1912 of tuberculosis, leaving Freeman to run the clinic. Before he took over the Allergy Department, Freeman had been mostly distinguished by his rugby playing. If Fleming brought a surgeon's sensibilities into the Inoculation Department, Freeman brought those of a GP. He was, one junior reminisced, incapable of research. This seems surprising, given the value Wright placed on his services, for example, in 1917 asking the army authorities to send over this "old and trusted pupil" who had "a talent for research and laboratory work."[42] However, it should be recalled that one of Wright's persistent concerns was that experiments and practical work should be done exactly according to his own specifications, with machine-like precision. Freeman could be entrusted to carry out his instructions to the letter, without trying to vary them according to his own lights; indeed, for half a century he followed the procedures that Noon had worked out in a few short years.

Freeman wrote a few early articles on desensitization procedures, but his magnum opus ("B.B.," or the "bloody book," as he called it) did not appear until 1950.[43] Like Fleming, Freeman made little attempt to quantify his clinical experience, beyond providing a summary list of one hundred cases in which the allergic reaction had been triggered by emotional shock or tension. The tone is that of the avuncular GP who gets to know his patients in their idiosyncrasies, often visiting their homes, and then finds himself primarily treating these idiosyncrasies and reasserting a moral order in the pathological household.[44] Freeman blamed bad mothering for most unhappiness, and his case histories were also moral homilies: "Mother insists on visiting boy's bedroom against his wishes," or "Boy of fifteen sleeps with mother." As family size shrank, he argued, mothers cosseted lone children excessively, causing allergies. Freeman's insistence that mind and body acted together and must be treated together was a hard-won, valuable clinical insight, but it was not the sort of hard bacteriological data one might expect of a disciple of Almroth Wright.

In short, Wright surrounded himself with men who did not perform serious clinical research but instead relied upon traditional forms of retrospective clinical judgment. Despite his pronounced intentions of reforming medicine, he nurtured within his institute a fifth column of clinical traditionalism. There was a logic to this progression, one that reflected the crossed fortunes of Wright's bacteriology and bacteriology generally. At the turn of the century, he had been at the cutting edge of the science. His methods were foundational, and his students filled positions around the world. But within a few years, bacteriology had emancipated itself from his influence. Researchers using his methods arrived at conclusions very different from his own, and they developed their own techniques that further undermined his findings. Ronald Hare and Parry Morgan left the Inoculation Department because they could no longer subscribe to Wright's opsonic theory.[45] Pathologists also rejected the research program that he spelled out in such detail to the MRC in 1914. There were too many other interesting questions to study. Wright was no longer a powerful resource on which bacteriologists could draw, and likewise, he could no longer draw upon his fellow bacteriologists as supporters for his programs.

By the time he lost the pathologists' support, Wright had attracted many clinicians to his camp. As shown, many of the younger clinicians at St Mary's took up his work. Wright's methods were always designed to serve clinicians as much as bacteriologists because he thought clinicians should do their own vaccinating. For example, H. Warren Crowe, a student who entered St Mary's in 1902 and subsequently became a practitioner in Devon, produced at least thirty-one articles and books, most of them arguing in favour of vaccine therapy. (He was still treating rheumatism with vaccines into the 1940s.) These included an article in the *Lancet* in 1912 entitled "How to Fit up a Laboratory for £10," using a soup ladle to sterilize syringes and a thermos to grow the cultures for vaccines.[46] This kind of make-do laboratory bricolage had been taught at the Inoculation Department from the beginning. Likewise, while top bacteriologists denounced Fleming's simplification of the Wassermann as bastardization, others defended it as practically useful to smaller clinics.[47] By the interwar period, clinicians were becoming more dependable allies for Almroth Wright than the bacteriologists, and he repaid the compliment by throwing his weight behind clinical judgment.

The proximity of the St Mary's medical school probably influenced the development of Wright's thinking. It was not merely that both Freeman and Fleming were graduates of the school with its long established "practical" orientation. Wright developed a genuine respect for clinical judgment as on the whole far more functional than the standards of scientific judgment that were formally challenging it. His theory of creative logic revolved around two models of thought: the crucial experiment and the clinical diagnosis.

He argued that the act of diagnosis which doctors regularly performed was a better example of creative ratiocination – of alethetropic logic – than the sterile mechanical forms of formal or statistical logic. As for the rough body of knowledge, the rule-of-thumb maxims that doctors had collectively accumulated over time, Wright argued that it was methodologically inefficient compared to the crucial experiment, and could provide only rule-of-thumb guidelines. Nonetheless, he believed that the content of this reservoir of knowledge was fairly sound.[48] Thus, the exchange of values between laboratory and school ran in both directions. Just as the new laboratory pathology shaped the culture of the hospital and the medical school, so too these institutions shaped the culture of the pathological laboratory.

9

Moran's Mary's

IN FORMAL STRUCTURE and in philosophical outlook, the medical school and the Inoculation Department moved closer together during the interwar period. They did so physically as well. During the 1920s, Charles Wilson, the future Lord Moran, took a leaf from Almroth Wright's book and began to market the medical school to prominent businessmen and public figures as an *avant garde* philanthropic cause. He raised enough to build a new school on a separate site alongside the hospital. When it became evident that Moran's grandiose plans had actually borne fruit, Wright casually passed the hat around his sponsors and built the Pathological Institute as one wing of the new school building, though still keeping it separate administratively and financially. By the early 1930s St Mary's had a state-of-the-art medical school and medical science complex. Wright could draw upon his old supporters (Iveagh alone gave £40,000 of the £100,000 needed to rehouse the institute). But Moran was doing something new. Selling medical science was not new, but selling St Mary's as its exemplar did require imagination and ingenuity.

That the school needed rebuilding was undeniable. W.W. Sargant, who came as a student in 1928, said "St Mary's was in a terrible way when I arrived ... The Medical School was simply a house near the Paddington Canal, and the students' dirty recreation rooms were in the hospital cellars and disgracefully furnished."[1] A modern school needed more and bigger teaching laboratories, seminar rooms, student facilities, and a library. But there were obstacles. Most medical philanthropists donated to the hospital.

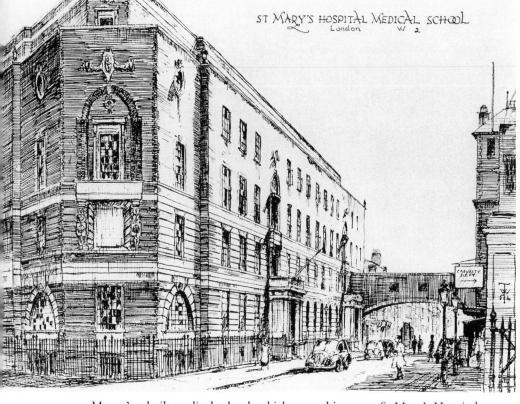

ST MARY'S HOSPITAL MEDICAL SCHOOL
London   W 2

Moran's rebuilt medical school, which opened in 1933. St Mary's Hospital NHS Trust Archives

In the early 1930s Moran tried to obtain a separate charter, but the governors squashed that particular "home rule" movement dead at a board meeting which Moran couldn't attend because he was called to a patient. Hospital, school, and institute all needed rebuilding funds, and each feared the other might queer the pitch. Some of the consultants also resisted Moran's plans, notably Broadbent, Warren Low, Willcox, and Wright. Others were sceptical or simply bored by them. J. Ernest Frazer, the anatomist, complained, "That Wilson has the drive of the devil. He won't let us alone to do our work. It's all committees and appeals and plans, plans, plans."[2] The physics lecturer, W.H. White, declared himself to be "inured to Mary's bleat of poverty a good few years now," having done more than his share by accepting its paltry remuneration over the years.[3] White was a sardonic and popular lecturer who finally left St Mary's for a position at the University of Saskatchewan.

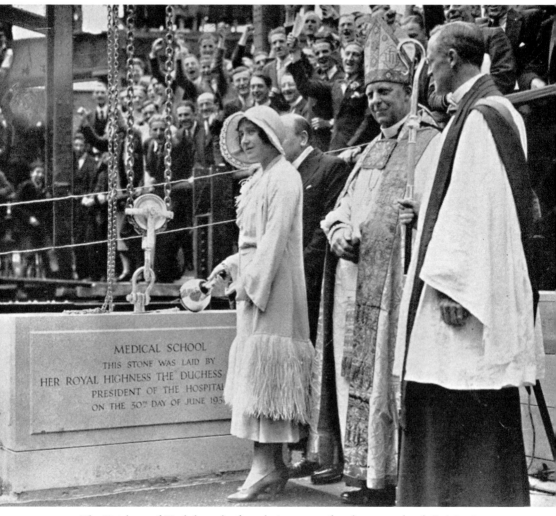

The Duchess of York lays the foundation stone for the new school. St Mary's
Hospital NHS Trust Archives and the Royal College of Surgeons of England

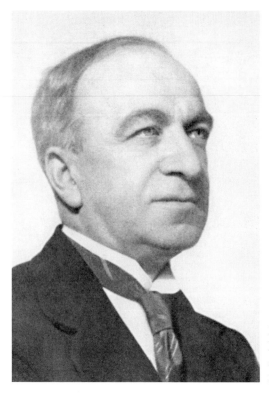

Zachary Cope. St Mary's
Hospital NHS Trust Archives
and the Royal College of
Surgeons of England

The greatest handicap to the appeal was that it couldn't point to any out-standing *medical* research going on at St Mary's. Moran could invoke Wright, but that coinage had become tarnished; moreover, Wright didn't want to be invoked. In the spring of 1929, just as Moran's fund-raising reached high gear, Wright launched an attack on Moran in the hospital boardroom, insisting on the separation of their two projects. Wright frankly told Moran, "I would like to warn you off from making any use of my work" for "propaganda" purposes because "I have no confidence in your discretion. Further I understand perfectly that you do not hold my work in any esteem, that being so you ought not even to visit to make sure of it, you ought to leave that to those who do."[4] Despite this incident, Wright did feature prominently in Moran's many printed appeals.

The clinicians were generally less promising as "propaganda." Gordon Mitchell Heggs, who entered St Mary's as a student in 1923, recalled: "Research was then undertaken by a few dedicated men and women who were rather isolated from the others. The Honoraries wrote descriptive articles, published comprehensive books and provided clear and practical teaching ... They taught and practised the up-to-date medicine of the day laced with the milk of human kindness."[5] Heggs instanced Zachary Cope, who joined the staff in 1911, as an outstanding example of this traditional orientation. Several St Mary's consultants, and especially surgeons, produced standard textbooks that went through many editions, including Bourne's manual of obstetrics and *The Essentials of Surgery* by Handfield-Jones and Porritt. Others built up a reputation for a particular technique performed with consummate skill. Wilfred Harris treated trigeminal neuralgia with an injection of alcohol straight through the face into the sensory ganglion of the trigeminal nerve at the base of the skull, an intervention that required such cool daring and steady hands that few other neurologists attempted it. Duncan Fitzwilliams wrote a definitive book on the breast, largely a plea for radical mastectomy. Cope had begun his classic works of differential diagnosis and in particular on *The Acute Abdomen* and actinomycosis.

Charles Pannett had established a reputation for gastric surgery and published continuously, including three dozen papers during the interwar period alone. The new assistant pathologist, W.D. Newcomb, later recalled, "We had an awful lot of stomachs from Pannett coming down." It was primarily Pannett's meticulous surgical skills, rather than any flair for research, that won him the respect of his surgical colleagues. Arthur Dickson Wright remarked approvingly that Pannett "was a splendid professor not being side-tracked by obsession with research and foreign travel, so often

Charles Pannett operating. St Mary's Hospital NHS Trust Archives and the Royal College of Surgeons of England

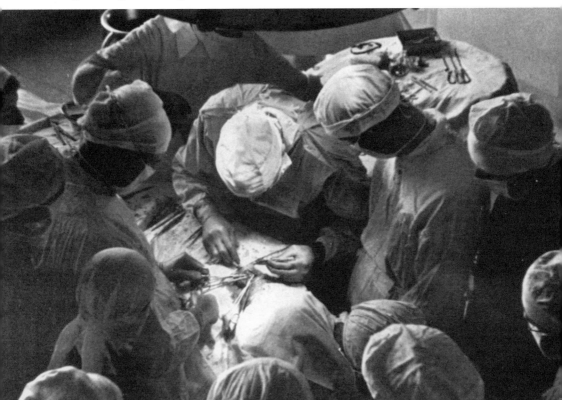

futile where the education of the student is concerned. He did a great deal of teaching and had a very good collection of classified lantern slides." Retirement gave Pannett the opportunity to take up experimental research performed in the Pathological Institute. In 1964 the eighty-year-old surgeon published a paper in *Nature* suggesting that irradiated bacterial culture inhibited the growth of implanted mouse carcinoma.

St Mary's physicians contrasted poorly with the surgeons and with emerging academic medicine elsewhere in London and provincial universities.[6] Langmead produced less than a dozen articles on such homely topics as habitual constipation, chronic dyspepsia, and injuries from toy pistols. Moran had abandoned his research into gastric function, undertaken primarily to obtain his RCP membership, to write almost exclusively on political matters during the 1920s and 1930s. Aleck Bourne undertook a variety of investigations, often collaborative, into puerperal fever and sex hormones, but he too is best remembered for his political activism, both as a socialist and for challenging the abortion law with Rex v. Bourne. The law prohibited abortion in any but life-threatening cases, and Bourne flouted it openly in 1935 when he performed the operation on a fourteen-year-old girl raped by guardsmen. He was prosecuted but not convicted.[7] His was not a name to bandy about among capitalists who might be convinced to sponsor medical education, thereby, as Moran wrote to Beaverbrook, "building up a position in the affections of the people."[8]

During the mid-1920s, thus, the reform and rebuilding of the school could not be done on the basis of its academic staff. Indeed, once the clinical units had been installed and teaching affiliations had been formed with the Paddington Infirmary, Queen Charlotte's Hospital, and the Lock, all accomplished soon after the First World War, the teaching structure largely stultified. Specialization might not have existed for all the influence it had upon St Mary's between the wars. Obstetrics provides a case in point. Bourne didn't obtain beds until 1934 when he became the senior obstetrician, whereupon he shared out his few with his juniors. He tried to establish an academic unit, but St Mary's didn't have enough beds to spare for the specialty. Practical midwifery was taught at Queen Charlotte's Hospital, where Bourne did have beds. Moreover, his colleagues were vehemently opposed to the idea of academic obstetrics. He noted that no research emanated from the obstetrics department between the wars.[9] Yet obstetrics was the best of the special subjects; the others had even fewer resources.

Moran's brave new medical school thus could not be sold to benefactors on the basis of its teaching or research. It had to be a different kind of school, organized around a different kind of driving force. For Moran, this was the students. His greatest insight, the one that informed everything else, was that the quality of medicine rested on the quality of the medical practitioner. He disagreed with Wright's theory that the reform of medicine would be through the laboratory, as he told Lord Beaverbrook: "I might even convince people that it is no good offering prizes for such things as cancer research but that the only method is to get better brains into medicine and the rest will follow."[10] But Moran distrusted braininess. He was indifferent to specialist training for the same reason that he dismissed – in sweeping terms reminiscent of Norton's half a century earlier – state schooling: they encouraged a narrow intelligence at the expense of character. Moran pinned his faith on the public schools, insisting that the only way of getting the "best of a bad lot socially is through the public schools."

Moran's plan to reform St Mary's emphasized teaching, with research being an almost incidental by-product. This was evident when in 1935 he asked for advice from A.V. Hill at UCH on hiring a physiologist: "I don't want a dreary pedagogue pouring out at the prescribed hour his piece. If we can get the right man I don't think he will grumble that we are not prepared to give him what he wants. I want a producing department with someone at the head who will ask himself if he can do anything to make his subject the language in which a substantial minority of the students think." He had to be "someone with ideas, who will plunge into the game of experimenting how best men can be induced to use their wits. I don't suppose he will discover any new educational methods because we have nothing that the Greeks had not but in trying he may throw off some sparks. And if he is intelligent enough to do this he may want to find out things for himself." Moran brought in an outstanding teacher and researcher, Arthur St George Huggett, despite misgivings (not unfounded, as it turned out) that he might be difficult. Again, in 1939, he brought in the most academic man he could find to fill the chair of medicine: George Pickering.

Moran expected to reform British medicine through the reform of St Mary's, by making the School "an English Johns Hopkins." Johns Hopkins was founded in Baltimore in the 1890s as the first graduate school of medicine, requiring that all students hold an undergraduate degree. Hopkins set a new standard that other ambitious schools had to meet. Moran decided to introduce the same policy for St Mary's, or as near to it as he could accomplish, which emphatically did not mean ruling out boys coming straight from the public schools. Instead he tried to require that they matriculate for a university degree rather than just a conjoint diploma. He told Beaverbrook, "the idea of an Honours School grows in my mind." Beaverbrook donated £63,000 towards the new building.

The banker John Barings, Lord Revelstoke was the other great benefactor of the school. On his death in 1929, Revelstoke left £25,000 (about 1

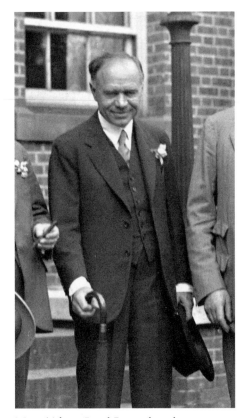

Max Aitken, Lord Beaverbrook.
University of New Brunswick Libraries,
Archives and Special Collections. UA PC
25 no. 1 (2). This photograph has been
altered from the original.

per cent of his estate) for rebuilding. Moran sold the project to him as serving both public health and science. "I had said to him that there was a
growing feeling among thoughtful people that the only really hopeful
method of working for a healthier race was to increase the facilities for
medical education and research at the medical schools." He pointed out to
Revelstoke, who was surprised to hear it, that the vast sums subscribed for
medical care could not be diverted to medical education and research. Revelstoke was so struck by this disparity of funding that he suggested Moran
draw up a scheme like the King's Fund, but for schools rather than hospitals. Moran had no intention of sharing the kitty. He convinced Revelstoke
that such a fund would be a failure until public opinion had been educated
to support it, and this would occur only if a model were placed before them.
He craftily invoked the Haldane Commission report's remarks to this effect.

Again and again Moran insisted that reform rested on the support of "the few thoughtful people" rather than "modern publicity methods," appealing to an elitist streak in his benefactors. Another interested party was told, "We have found so far that these plans interest people in direct proportion to their ability and we feel that it is from the leaders of industry and finance that we must look for our support rather than from the general public."[11] Nor did he scruple to play upon nationalist prejudices. The Rockefeller had already set up an example of just such a school at University College, but Moran argued that "we require the scheme to be planned on English lines and supported by English people."[12]

It was just barely plausible in 1929 to take Johns Hopkins for a model for St Mary's. To Englishmen, Hopkins was associated with illustrious name of Sir William Osler who had come to personify the ideal of the "great physician," one who knew his science but was more remarkable for his personal qualities and bedside manner. Witnesses trying to convince the Haldane Commission that physicians didn't really practise science instanced Osler who, though one of the greatest physicians of the day, had no reputation in chemical pathology or bacteriology: "No one would pay the slightest attention to his opinion on that, if he expressed it."[13] Thus, the clinical teaching at St Mary's – everywhere conceded to be excellent – could be seen to support the idea of a Hopkins honours school although, in fact, Johns Hopkins had always attracted leading scientific researchers. By the time Osler had left Baltimore in 1904, he was under attack by these scientific types who considered his day to be over. However, in England, the ideal of practical clinical teaching still reigned sufficiently supreme that Moran's scheme sounded viable.

But, however hard Moran tried, he couldn't sell the idea of scholarships to benefactors. With his usual acumen, Lord Beaverbrook identified the problem. Initially, in 1929, he approved of the project: "Now that the building is assured, I hope the Board will make every effort to populate it with brilliant students, with plenty of scholarships for those entitled to them." A few years later, however, when Moran applied to him for money, his old benefactor, himself a law-school dropout, turned him down. Writing to Moran's wife, Dorothy, he said that he could not "see any use in subsidising any of them [the students] with scholarships. If I can find some other way of helping the School I mean to do so. But his brats brought in from the Provinces, with no particular ability and no great prospect of doing any useful work, will not be benefited by making their lives easier during their schooldays." "Brats" was a strong choice of words (and "brats from the Provinces" especially so, coming from a Canadian), but it was hard to deny that medical students of the 1920s and 1930s didn't look like scientific research students, and Moran's choice of medical students perhaps least of all.

Moran's scholarships attracted notoriety when they were sneeringly labelled "rugby scholarships." The game enjoyed a new popularity in the 1920s, when 231 new clubs were founded. Ross McKibbin has argued that the "rush to rugby" was "an overt statement of deliberate class-differentiation."[14] Whereas soccer was a mass, popular sport, rugby smacked of the public school. Richard Holt has observed that it "seems to have promoted a strong male group conformity and a certain social conservatism wherever it was played."[15] Moran, seeking to build up a public school spirit, believed that if St Mary's could win the hospital rugby cup, the school's popularity at Oxbridge would be assured. It was said that he was so rugby-mad that he turned the school into a rugby-team-producing machine – that he brought in professionals wherever he could; that he would prolong the academic life of hopeless students so as to keep them on the team; that he stood on railway platforms to waylay well-known rugby players and convince them to change tracks to St Mary's; and that he broke the amateur code by offering players scholarships. Most damning, he was said to have arranged to have women students prohibited from the school so as to get a better standard of rugby. Moran denied the charges and blamed them on jealousy. Thanks to his policies, he claimed, "Sixty boys each the outstanding men at Oxford and Cambridge were so monopolised by St. Mary's that the older schools got alarmed and sought to discredit the scholarships by caricaturing them as a search for footballers."[16]

Matters came to a head in 1932. The *Daily Mail* in September 1932 aired the story that one hospital in particular had been attracting rugger players "by means foreign to the spirit of true amateurism." Later that year, Sir Farquhar Buzzard, the regius professor at Oxford, criticized not only the rugby scholarships but the whole system of pushing St Mary's. This included motor buses sent to Oxford and Cambridge to entertain students in London and "inspired" articles in the university papers, tactics that would be "most harmful and most undignified" if other schools were to use them. "I don't think the Middle Temple would adopt similar methods for attracting law students," Buzzard concluded chillingly.

John Freeman, Moran's ally in fund-raising, penned a spirited reply, arguing that most of what happened in medicine went under the heading of advertising: the "chief value of any scholastic or professional success is – advertisement, if you insist on it; the motive behind most of the papers in the *Lancet* or BMJ is – just advertisement; and often attendance at and speaking at medical meetings has no better motive. Who then shall 'scape whipping?"[17] This hard-headed interpretation of professional activities, usually described with such adjectives as "noble" and "devoted" and "self-sacrificing," could hardly have endeared the Mary's school to the spokesman for untarnished Cambridge ideals.

Moran's views were formed before the war, though his wartime experience gave them new direction and force. When Moran entered St Mary's as a student in 1901, the school had been newly and briefly a power in the world of hospital sports. In 1900 St Mary's had won the rugby cup for the first time, and had enjoyed success in football, cricket, swimming, and athletics. But already the *Hospital Gazette* was worrying that unless the school obtained a decent playing pitch, it would lose the Oxbridge students. Not until the mid-1930s was the problem resolved, when Moran convinced Beaverbrook to purchase a field at Teddington. Hospital sports advertised the school and the fine qualities of its graduates. The first volume of the *Hospital Gazette* argued that sports trained the student to become a "good doctor and a gentleman" by teaching chivalry and the pursuit of excellence.[18] Moran flourished in this atmosphere. He came from a soccer school, but at St Mary's he switched his allegiance to rugby and, despite his light weight, even found a place on a county team. For him, rugby was the queen of sports, and sports were one of the great and serious things in life – perhaps as great and serious as medicine itself. He began to write for the *Hospital Gazette*, first short, descriptive pieces about matches, but then he became the journal's editor and began to advance a coherent philosophy of education, medicine, and sports.

Moran's was a manichean view of the world as ruled by opposing forces that were exemplified by democracy and rugby. In 1910 he wrote an editorial – which got him into trouble with the school authorities – predicting the nationalization of the voluntary hospitals and the medical schools, as an inevitable consequence of increasing democratization. State-managed schools would lack a school spirit and become mere qualifying shops, dominated by exams and compulsory attendance. Medicine would become a mere trade. By contrast, at Rugby School, Thomas Arnold encouraged responsibility rather than docility in the face of compulsory rules. Responsibility, argued the young Moran, made men (by which he meant that it made them "manly," a word often on his lips).[19] Two decades later he repeated the gist of the argument: "We are dealing with an adult Englishman and to get the best out of him we must appeal to the best that is in him. He will not be policed; he must always rebel against the whole system of small insurances that we take out against the natural waywardness of youth."[20]

In the democratic world of the future, where merit and mediocrity would do battle, Moran believed that the medical profession would have a special place. The old elites would succumb, and doctors would assume greater importance as exemplars of such moral attributes as chivalry, valour, and self-sacrifice. Medical students might learn these moral attributes on the wards, but a surer route was to let them teach themselves in the rough and tumble of the rugby match. After World War I, sport was to Moran related in some important way to war: it brought out in young men the qualities they would need to survive as soldiers and as men in the trenches. Before the war, however, he was scornful of the toy soldiering of the army reserves. "The fascination of Rugger is its reality. The absence of this makes amateur soldiering unpopular."[21] Already in 1908 he had argued that the medical school's shortage of students should be met by rugby, "the great recruiting sergeant ... for rugger alone makes any appeal beyond the players and is generally the standard by which the hospital is recognised as a force." The school where men made the "sacrifices" that rugby required "has a finer spirit and a pleasanter atmosphere than one in which the individual reigns and keeps his eyes glued to his own future." It was in this article that Moran made his first public suggestion for sports scholarships, a suggestion which the editor, Zachary Cope, firmly squashed as being unlikely to attract "men of the greatest intellectual promise."[22] Another correspondent in the *Gazette* wrote an insightful sketch of Moran's character, criticizing his "crude cynicism" but praising his "settled aim and ideal" of "backing and fostering the public school spirit ... You aim at a school which shall be first. You know it is not a dream but a possibility. It is to your credit that you see clearly the means to that end." The commentator concluded, "Your work is only incidentally concerned with games. You have persuaded many that character is the great recruiting sergeant for a school, that quantity follows quality."[23]

Moran spent World War I as a regimental doctor in the trenches, keeping the regiment at fighting pitch. This required him to judge whether men were fit to go to battle or whether they might break down. He had to develop a calculus of mental strength. The problem fascinated him both during the war and for many years afterwards. Courage he defined as "the expression on the battlefield of character." Character and courage were largely innate qualities and couldn't be created from bad stock, but where the germ existed, proper encouragement could bring them out. In the trenches, all the old competitiveness and individualism was banished: "Nobody there bothered about getting on in life; they were content if they were not pushed prematurely out of it. Money no longer meant anything except to pay for a meal in an estaminet. In that life men only demanded two qualities – that a man should control his fear and that he should be unselfish. We came to exalt courage because it stood between us and the utter ruin of our cause. We came to demand that a man should play for his side and not for himself."²⁴ Moran was in no way militaristic: war was for him primarily a suitable culture for growing interesting specimens of humanity.

Into the interwar period, Moran maintained that moral virtue could be reinvigorated because it sprang from the depths of human nature. He did not publish his *Anatomy of Courage* until 1945, when another war had made the questions it posed current once again. Nonetheless, his views never changed. As dean, he was less interested in producing modern scientists than in producing manly young men. They were not far removed from the gentlemanly ideal of the mid-nineteenth century, save that they were more willing to get their hands dirty, on the rugby pitch, in the trenches, or at the bedside. Death, violence, pain – their own or that of others – were never far away. They confronted these demons with a laugh and a joke and got on with the job.

If a preoccupation with one's own health was sapping and softening society, these virile young men, even as they purveyed health, provided the counterweight. They were like the guardians of the Plato's Republic, being both courageous and philosophic, kind to citizens and fierce to strangers. The metaphor may be somewhat strained, but it becomes strengthened, perhaps, when Moran's public work is taken into account, namely, his contribution to the NHS. With the introduction of the NHS, health moved to the very centre of British political life, where it has remained, with doctors being the guardians of this system of values. Doctors have had their political and financial setbacks, but this too is entirely Platonic, for Plato warned that the guardians must be kept in a constant state of deprivation as the price of power.

Moran thought that a greater dispersion of public school values would elevate the medical profession. Others feared that his cut-price gentlemen would debase the profession. The genuine aristocrats of medicine, the standard-bearers of Oxbridge like Buzzard, complained of the methods that Moran used, which smacked too much of the assembly line. By offering scholarships, he was enlarging and diluting the category of gentleman, effectively debasing the coinage.²⁵ Though he never obtained anything like the £150,000 endowment to which he aspired, he was able to offer scholarships to a few picked students each year. The scheme proved extraordinarily successful. By the mid-1930s, applications for the public school scholarships ranged between forty and sixty, and the two university scholarships drew about ten applications. Meanwhile the St Mary's rugby football team had become the mightiest in London. Before Moran became dean, St Mary's had won the United Hospitals Cup only once in almost half a century. Half a century later, St Mary's had won the cup more often than any other team and attracted some of the outstanding sportsmen of the day

– not only rugby players but also Olympic athletes such as Jack Lovelock, who won a gold medal in Berlin in 1936.

The first two university scholars were D.N. Rocyn-Jones and Tommy Hunt, both rugger men. Rocyn-Jones became an orthopaedic surgeon and sheriff of Monmouthshire. Hunt's father was a clergyman who couldn't afford to send him to medical school so the boy relied on scholarships and teaching posts to study at Oxford and St Mary's. Hunt was among the first clinicians to treat Addison's disease with suprarenal cortical extracts, which he extracted from pork suprarenals purchased from the butchers in Edgware Road. He joined the staff in 1930, and as senior physician after the Second World War, he was an invaluable intermediary between the NHS consultants and academics.

Many others couldn't have entered medicine without the scholarships. Stanley Peart, the son of a professional footballer from Newcastle, was one. The fleet-footed younger Peart played a wing position. Moran invited him to an interview and, ignoring his grades, asked, "How fast do you run the hundred yards?" Peart brazenly took nearly a quarter second off his fastest time and "lo and behold" he was offered a scholarship. "And that meant that it was possible to go, and so I went." His academic accomplishments considerably exceeded those of the rugby field: he became Sir Stanley Peart, FRS and professor of medicine at St Mary's.

Those public school men who did come to Mary's on scholarships were atypical. George Bonney, the son of a GP, went to Eton on a scholarship. His father's sudden death seemed to rule out a medical education, but his uncle, the gynaecological surgeon Victor Bonney, arranged an interview at St Mary's. Rugby wasn't much played at Eton, but Moran asked George searching questions about his position in the Eton crew ("If I'd said 'Bow,' maybe I wouldn't have got in!"). Bonney became a consultant in orthopaedics at St Mary's. Denis Brinton, another of Moran's picked scholars, went to Eton because his father taught there. Brinton would later replace Wilfred Harris as the hospital neurologist and Moran as dean of St Mary's. B.E.C. Stanley, the son of a Wesleyan minister, was another rugby player who could not, his obituarist remarked, have entered medicine without the scholarship that St Mary's awarded. Jack Suchet, born of a family of Russian immigrants, also came to Mary's on a rugby scholarship. William Sargant, whose father faced bankruptcy in the slump of the late 1920s, has said, "Financially, I just scraped through my medical student days because of my games scholarship."[26]

Felix Eastcott, yet another future consultant, also squeaked in on a rugby scholarship of sorts. He recalls his interview with "Sir Charles Wilson, as he was then": "'Ah, Eastcott,' he said, 'I've got your Headmaster's Report. Oh, you've done a bit better lately. And what position do you play?' I thought 'Well, Sir, it's inside right.' 'Oh, soccer, I suppose.' 'Well, I'm afraid, yes sir, it was a soccer school.' 'Mmm,' he said, 'But' I said, 'I'm organising a rugby team, just informally.' 'Ah good,' he said, 'Matthews, give him a 15 per cent reduction.' So I got in! That was just about the length of the interview!"

Not all of Moran's picked men were rugby players or even sportsmen. Tom Kemp (a scholar and rugby international) remarked of Jack Litchfield, the son of a schoolmaster, "If athletic prowess got him in he has concealed it brilliantly ever since." Litchfield himself insisted he was given a scholar-ship "Because I was bright."[27] Litchfield, who became a consultant at St Mary's, chose that school because Moran didn't examine candidates; he in-vited them to lunch.

On the outbreak of World War II, the young men of St Mary's, as of the other schools, marched off to join the war effort. Some performed extraor-dinary acts of heroism and self-sacrifice. Two in particular have entered the annals of the school's history, Ivan Jacklin and Peter McRae. Both were scholarship boys and great sportsmen, rugby players and all-rounders. Both served in the Royal Naval Volunteer Reserves and both were lost at sea, Jacklin in 1943 and McRae in 1944. Jacklin was a South African, educat-ed in Cranleigh, where the headmaster described the seventeen-year-old as

The seven asides rugby football team in March 1941: Carl Young, Ivan Jacklin, Cocky Cockburn, Peter McRae, Tom Kemp, Moran, and hidden behind him, John Graham Jones and A.W. Young. Collection of Tom Kemp

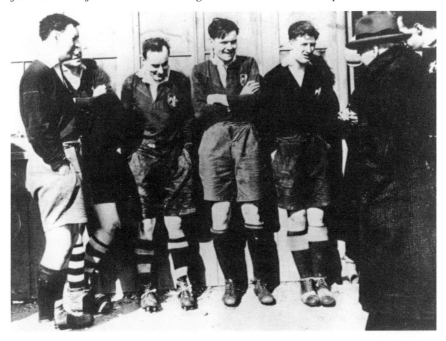

"a gentleman by birth, breeding and instinct." As his obituary observed, a man of such character, finding himself on a torpedoed liner short on lifeboats, had little likelihood of survival. While the ship went down, he swam to and fro, helping service women to the rafts, before the waters finally closed over his head.

Peter McRae, who captained St Mary's in rugby, cricket, squash, and tennis, was a "happy, charming fellow," who lived with an aunt in Taunton but had, in the Jacklins, a London home. In 1944, when his destroyer was hit by a torpedo while engaged in a Russian convoy operation, the men lined up on the side to leave it, whereupon another torpedo threw them all into the sea. McRae and seventeen sailors made their way onto a tiny float that threatened to capsize. McRae was heard to say "I seem to be in the way here" and disappeared over the side. The others were rescued.

Altogether 640 students of St Mary's served in World War II. Twenty-one died in action (less than half the toll of World War I), twenty-six were taken prisoner of war, and fifty-one were mentioned in dispatches. Eleven received the Military Cross, four the DSO, and four the George medal.[28] Several of the prisoners of war were incarcerated at Changi and at other Japanese camps. John Diver wouldn't leave his patients and died of beriberi. Others survived, including A.W. Frankland, later a consultant allergist. In Changi, Frankland was startled to see another player on the pitch wearing the St Mary's fleur de lys. Another survivor was Courtney Lendon, who produced an MD thesis on "Disease among Prisoners of War," in which he recorded in dry, objective tones the enormous suffering of the prisoners, particularly from dysentery, cholera, and deficiency diseases.[29] E.E. Dunlop wrote a preface for the thesis that praised his scientific detachment, dignity, and restraint amidst the "appalling desolation of rain, mud, and jungle" and for taking even this opportunity to reflect, observe, and research. Dunlop was a famous Australian rugby international and an honorary Mary's man who had worked at the hospital in 1939 and played rugby at St Mary's and in Changi.

On the western front at Arnhem, John Graham Jones, a member of the legendary rugby team of the late 1930s, was one of the parachutists who descended to find a German panzer division waiting below. He was sent to a large hospital that received prisoners of war from across Germany and soon found himself so busy and so interested in the work that "I didn't even realise I was a prisoner." Conditions were not so very different from a demanding house job. Having been taught to grow penicillin cultures by Fleming, he arranged an informal clinical trial of that drug which was supplied by the Red Cross. During an epidemic of pneumonia, there was only enough to treat one side of the ward; Graham Jones observed that the other

side, treated with sulpha drugs, was visibly worse off. Another rugby player, a South African called Lipmann Kessell who came to St Mary's in 1935,
was also at Arnhem. He escaped and spent three months hidden by locals
before finally getting away. He was somewhat familiar with the territory,
having been on a rugby tour to Amsterdam in 1936.[30]

World War II vindicated Moran. Afterwards, he continued to argue for
character and courage as the best bulwark against the newest enemy – the
Cold War. He spoke widely on behalf of such institutions as Outward
Bound, insisting that sports and other tests of endurance supplied a lack
among civilized nations that had been the birthright of primitive peoples.
Once again his ideas became anachronistic. In 1969 he took part in a BBC
discussion of courage. A few heroic men and women were interviewed, and
the elderly Moran and W.W. Sargant, among others, traded arguments. Sargant was one of Moran's rugger scholars – he used to joke that he found a
five-pound note in his boots after each game. He aspired to a medical consultancy but, after espousing a brand of hormone therapy that became discredited, turned to psychology and became a consultant at St Thomas's.[31]
Sargant attributed his physical approach to psychology – heavy on electro-
convulsive therapy and lobotomy – in part to the "practical" approach to
medicine he learned at St Mary's.[32] Where Moran identified character
with courage, Sargant firmly dissociated them. Weak, cowardly, even insane people could display courage, he argued. For Sargant, courage was
fear expressed physiologically, a protective inhibition or clamping down of
response to stimuli.[33]

Moran's scheme for St Mary's was a shotgun wedding of meritocracy and
elitism. But his project of social homogenization was only possible if certain unassimilable groups were shut out altogether, namely blacks and
women. Moran believed that the school he entered at the turn of the century was one of the best in the country. Its students won sporting trophies
and academic awards. But over the next decade the number of students fell
off and so, he argued, did the quality: "If you go just before the first war
you find that our entry was about 19 of whom eight or nine were black.
Moreover the attitude of the senior staff was one of 'I just don't care.' It
would last their time."[34] It is impossible to know what Moran meant by
"black" and impossible to verify the statement. Nonetheless, the student
register does indicate a strong international contingent: of the fifty-five students who entered between January 1912 and August 1914, twenty-three
were not born in the U.K.: most came from India, Sri Lanka, and Egypt, but
Russia, Lagos, the West Indies, New Zealand, France, America, Argentina,
and Eastern Europe were also represented. One student who applied in the

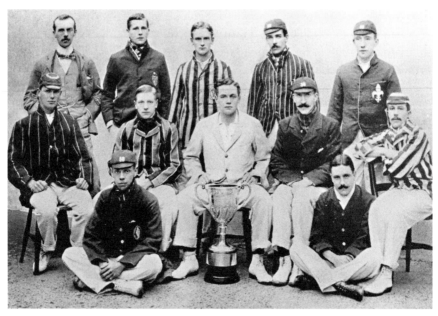

Cricket team. St Mary's Hospital NHS Trust Archives

summer of 1914 was Arthur Dickson Wright, the son of a London panel doctor (and distant relation of Sir Almroth) who later recalled, "St. Mary's was desperate for medical students at the time and I was welcomed like a millionaire in a night club."[35] A comparison with Moran's cohort, taking from January 1900 to August 1902, shows ninety-seven entries with only fifteen born abroad: five in India, four in the U.S., three in Canada, one in the Cape Colony, and two part-course students from the continent. The students from India in 1900–02 tended to have Anglo-Saxon names, such as "Nicholson," and "King," while those of 1912–14 bore such names as "Biswas" and "Padmanji."

It should be emphasized that some of these early non-Caucasian students at St Mary's were extremely able and had very distinguished careers. In 1899 The Lien Wu entered as the first student from the Straits Settlement. He was at Cambridge before coming to St Mary's, entering both institutions on scholarships, and then joined a pathological institute in Singapore. Within a decade he was serving as director of the Imperial Army Medical College and was chief MO to the Manchurian Plague Service, as well as physician to a series of political leaders. Wu became a distinguished historian of Chinese medicine.[36]

But non-white students were probably more tolerated than accepted. Songs like "The Happy Little Nigger" continued to figure in the annual minstrel show, as much a necessary part of the entertainment as cross-dressing. Admission of non-white students caused administrators some anxiety. On 15 October 1912 the minutes of the Medical School Committee record: "The question of the admission of Oriental students was considered, in view of the fact that several Indian & Egyptian students had applied for admission during the present year. Statistics showed that during the past year the number of oriental students working in the school was 5% of the total. After consideration of the question, it was decided that no restriction upon the entry of Oriental students be made at present." The following year Broadbent again raised the question of "Oriental" students "in view of their increased numbers."[37] With the outbreak of war, the number of foreign students remained high until April 1916, whereupon they disappeared almost completely. The war doubtless impeded travel. But a more compelling reason for the eclipse of foreign students is revealed by the appearance of twelve women's names in the register for April 1916.

The Admission of Women

The decline in student intake, long a problem, became acute in World War I. James Garner, who has written an account of the "Great Experiment," notes that by late 1915 the school's current account was overdrawn by more than £1,000, and bankruptcy loomed.[38] Meanwhile the London School of Medicine for Women had far more applicants than it could accommodate at the affiliated Royal Free Hospital. In December 1915 St Mary's staff voted against admitting women, and instead each paid over £20 from his own pocket. The following month, however, Broadbent joined negotiations with the London School of Medicine for Women. Four months later, women began to walk the wards at St Mary's.

This wasn't the first time that women had approached St Mary's. In 1873 a group of women applied to St Mary's, as to all the other schools, and were uniformly rejected. However, sympathetic staff including Norton, Owen, and Cheadle helped to found the London School of Medicine for Women. Their strait-laced colleagues censured their action: in 1874 a majority of fourteen, with eight against, declared that "it is not expedient that teachers in St. Mary's school should connect themselves as teachers with the London School of Medicine for Women, such connection being deemed to be highly injurious to the interests of St. Mary's school."[39] Decades later the first to introduce female doctors into St Mary's was, ironically, the school's most notorious misogynist, Sir Almroth Wright, who publicly denounced female suffrage and debated the matter against G.B. Shaw before the medical society. However, in June 1906 the medical school committee resolved that "ladies be admitted to Dr. Wright's special course of lectures on opsonins to be given in the Library during June and

July." The *Hospital Gazette* was amused when one qualified female practitioner doing research in the Inoculation Department brought in her husband to supply the necessary blood samples.[41] In February 1914 the
hospital board resolved to accept qualified women along with men in a
venereology course, though the fact was not advertised.[42] Once war broke
out, the widow of the physiology lecturer was paid to prepare classes,
though not permitted to teach. Women were, thus, gradually insinuating
themselves into St Mary's. They had been eligible to serve on the board
since 1910 and had actually begun to serve from January 1913 (prompt-
ing Almroth Wright and Luff to resign from their seats). But female board
members were prohibited from deliberating on issues regarding the school
or the duties of the consultants.

It was still a leap to admit women as equals with the male students. This
was, moreover, an extraordinary batch of women. Ida Mann, who came to
St Mary's in 1917, remarked that the first women "were chosen for their intelligence, ambition, and academic record. They were supposed to create a
good impression among the men students. Of course these were horrified.
All the keen young men had escaped to the war, with only the lame ducks,
the persistent failures at exams, and the elderly men students left. The girls
were so clever, worked so hard, were no good at Rugger, didn't want to indulge in sport, even of the bedroom variety, and were a dead loss all round.
Indeed they rather showed up everyone's inefficiency."[43] Yet to everyone's
surprise, the arrangement seemed to succeed. After eight months the dean,
Sir John Broadbent, reported to the University of London that "there had
been no objection on the part of the men students, and they had had absolutely no friction of any kind."[44] Financially, the school was saved. Kettle
had to repeat his pathology classes because the rooms couldn't accommodate all the students. Other schools followed St Mary's example, and by the
end of the war seven accepted women. In 1920 St Mary's scrapped its relationship with the London School of Medicine for Women so that it could
train women for the full five-year course and charge the full fee.

But the atmosphere had already begun to sour. At the end of the war male
students and qualified men returned to demand their proper place be restored to them. In the hard times of the 1920s they resented female competition. There was also an element of cultural shock between these hardened
veterans and the women. The war had been conducive to misogyny in general, with much resentment felt towards the civilians, so many of them
women, on whose behalf soldiers had ostensibly fought. In 1919 anti-female
complaints began to be voiced in the *Hospital Gazette*. Women crowded to
the front during clinical demonstrations. Their presence curtailed the old
trial by humiliation, an important mechanism of student bonding.

It was in this atmosphere that Moran became dean. Was this self-styled apologist for the masculine culture of the trenches himself a misogynist? He had no personal antipathy towards brainy young women, for he married one: Dorothy Dufton was a Cambridge scholar working on metabolism when they met, and while she gave up her laboratory research, she canvassed for the school all her life. On the other hand, repelled by a plain-featured and "voluble" female pathologist who asked him "how Basal Metabolism was done," he "discouraged her."[45] But personalities aside, Moran entertained a more politic view towards female physicians as a whole. In an undated letter to Dorothy, he dismissed complaints against the women students: "I regard all this as the growing pains of co-education. The male students are very much against the female & it will all affect entry of former for a bit. Some of the arguments against were more amusing than weighty. The surgeon complained bitterly that female house surgeons got 'cold feet' during night & called him out of bed & Harley Street, a trivial provocation. The whole feeling was that they were a necessary nuisance because of the money! So their chivalry wears at the touch of a working day. Doesn't it underline wisdom of keeping them in cotton wool & glass cases in the administration of all?"

Nonetheless, Moran's views changed while he was dean. He aspired to be, to use Stalin's term for the poet, an engineer of human souls. However, his philosophy was rooted in a belief that men must be taken as they are. He might be able to manage student opinion at St Mary's, but he could hardly affect that at Oxford or Cambridge, where an atmosphere of misogyny prevailed during the 1920s. These students preferred medical schools like St Bartholomew's that did not accept women. Indeed, the University of London had predicted in 1917, "If women were admitted to only a few Schools, there is reason to believe that those Schools would lose men students and would become mainly Schools for women."[46] If Moran wished to attract students from Oxford and Cambridge, he had to conform.

The provocation for the exclusion of women was a petition that a number of male medical students signed, asking that women no longer be accepted. As James Garner notes, the petition began: "The recent, but apparently habitual defeat of St Mary's in the Rugger Cup-tie, calls for serious consideration," and it concluded: "The men do not want the women, they have no wish to be friends, or to co-operate with them in any way." Garner describes the document as "a clever piece of targeted psychology, designed with Charles McMoran Wilson in mind."[47] This probably does Moran less than justice. A man who could bring the BMA to heel was unlikely to be stampeded by a few medical students. A counter-petition signed by thirteen male students argued that "the anti-feminine feeling among the men students is largely worked up by a few enthusiasts, and is not the result of mature consideration by the majority. Accordingly this feeling could be reduced by less undesirable measures than that proposed." Moran could have neutralized the hostility but chose not to. More likely, he orchestrated student opinion with some judicious asides. A month previously he had asked the hospital governor, Colonel Parkes, to investigate whether the school could afford to eliminate the women students. He was told, yes, barely, though the reserves might diminish.

The petition demanding the exclusion of women was drawn up in March 1924, and exclusion was formally adopted in May. First, the petition was presented to a specially convened meeting of the hospital staff, which interviewed two male medical students and then voted to exclude women. The Medical School Committee met and failed to come to any conclusion. Sir Almroth demanded exclusion, but others defended the women or the fees they brought. The matter was returned to the hospital staff; this may have been done to circumvent the pre-medical teachers who tended to support the women. The consultants reaffirmed their earlier stand against women by twelve to six, and the school formally adopted that policy. On April 8 the matter was sent before the hospital board, which had the final say. The board apparently rebuffed the resolution, perhaps thinking of its female subscribers, so the resolution was returned to a joint meeting of the medical staff and lecturers. On a motion by Moran, the meeting voted to exclude women from clinical studies and to review their admission for the five-year term that autumn. The resolution was returned to the board on 12 May. Objections by governors Lady Harris and Mrs Harben were silenced by the old regulation preventing women governors from voting on school matters, and the board confirmed the resolution of the staff.[48]

The women protested the underhanded way that the thing had been pushed through and passed the hat around the Medical Women's Federation, which came up with £810 as an initial contribution towards establishing entrance scholarships, "modestly" modelled on the Rhodes scholarships, to attract public school girls. They offered Moran control of the fund. Moran wrote a cold little reply, saying that, because the board had made no final decision, the MSC could not entertain the "generous offer." This was blatant obstructionism, given that the point was to influence the board's final decision.[49] The female medical students wrote to the hospital board complaining that the dean's rejection of the scholarships was "puzzling." Equally so was his complaint that, in attending only for clinical studies, women repelled students from Oxford and Cambridge who themselves came only for clinical studies. The letter concluded, "We are reluctantly forced to the conclusion that the new policy is due not, as we were asked to

believe, to financial but to some other reasons." That these reasons consisted first and last of rugby they knew only too well.

Though they might meet the financial objection, the women were unable
to overcome the rugby objection. Not that they didn't try: they pointed out
that King's College admitted women and still won trophies. Their male supporters appealed to the spirit of "true sport, which does not consist in
wanting other people to come and win your games for you." (These men
tended to be scholarly: W.C. Faull and G. Douglas Robertson were FRCS in
1923; R.B. Bourdillon was a Oxford chemist of some standing when he
came to St Mary's for medical studies; and R.M. Fry, who ignored Fleming's warning that the petition would attract the wroth of Wright, became
director of the research labs at Queen Charlotte's Hospital.[50]) James Garner confirms the women's claim. From 1910 to 1914 St Mary's won 35 per
cent of their matches, and from 1919 to 1923 they won 60 per cent, including, in 1923, the united hospitals cup itself, for the second time in the
school's history. It was probably this win that suggested to Moran he could
aim higher than a mixed school.

A note of incredulity permeates the women's protests. These were bright
and hard-working individuals, committed to improving public health.[51]
They were doing a public good, yet they were to be chased out of the school
for what must have seemed a very trivial reason. Were there not any authorities responsible for medical education who might also consider this a
frivolous reason? That fall they wrote to the Board of Education, pointing
out that Moran had demanded funding for his academic units on the
grounds that Mary's admitted women. Women in the Labour Party, meanwhile, approached both the board and the Ministry of Health independently. The Board of Education replied that it was a matter for the chancellor
of the Exchequer, who could only ask the University Grants Committee to
take the matter into consideration.[52] Time had now run out for the women
at St Mary's. On 16 October, after hearing petitions from fifteen women's
organizations, ranging from unions to the Empire Guild of Women, and
after rejecting countervailing motions by Lady Harris and Mrs Harben, the
St Mary's board voted to exclude women.[53]

Moran worked to contain any unpleasant fallout. He told potential
women donors that the objection to women was purely financial and that a
hefty endowment would overcome it.[54] He also silenced angry female doctors. In May he had called a meeting of the female students in the library
and addressed them frankly. He told them, "I have not the slightest sympathy with the extremists on either side," and reiterated his personal approval
of the principle of co-education. Then he got down to brass tacks. The
women were worried that if the school repudiated them, they would lose out

on house jobs. Moran responded with a thinly veiled threat: "He did not see why they should be in any way prejudiced if the question was allowed to remain a business proposition, and if they did not allow themselves to be associated in any way with an attack by the Press on the School ... There would be no difference as to posts unless they attacked the School."[55]

House jobs were only the tip of the iceberg. In their correspondence with the Board of Education, the women spelled out the effects of repudiation. The female students must be "seriously damaged. They can no longer claim to be graduates of any school, for they have been disowned – they will have none of the support which a powerful school always extends to its graduates, and this is an actual deprivation quite apart from the psychological effect of such a calamity upon the individual." The women had, further, the right to think that this support "would be always available to them," for that was the unspoken contract between student and school. Female GPs were equally at risk: "The friendly welcome which old St. Mary's men in practice have in the past given to women settling in their districts would be replaced by a most awkward situation. Women would feel like outlaws if their School has cast them adrift." Thus, if those women who had acquired professional standing – such as Marguerite Kettle (née Pam) who wrote for the *Lancet* – made a fuss, the young female students with their career still to make would suffer for it. Co-education at St Mary's passed quietly into history.

The petitions framed by the "outlawed" women of St Mary's pointed to an important fact. The activities that went on beneath its roof were only a small part of the life of the school. A school owed its position as much to the promises it extended to former students as to the amenities it could offer the incoming batch. The bigger the school, the more influence it could exercise. St Mary's, like the Athens of antiquity, existed not only in stone walls but also in the minds and hearts of men and women who planted themselves around the world.

Mary's in the World

The career trajectories of the 255 women who passed through St Mary's were assessed in 1936 by Marguerite Kettle.[56] She was addressing critics who argued that it was hardly worth educating women to medicine because most of them left the profession to have children. Many did leave – often because employers like the LCC refused to hire married women. But Kettle's statistics, and others published by women's organizations, showed that the wastage wasn't much greater than among men. Twenty-five of the women did not complete the course (four had died). Sixty per cent qualified with a conjoint diploma, 40 per cent with an MB BS, and a third completed higher qualifications. Three-quarters were still in employment at the time of the survey, and half of those were in general practice, usually in the provinces. Thirty-two had hospital appointments.

Some women achieved real prominence. Kettle made a name for herself as a journalist and an activist, rising to be vice-president of the Medical Women's Federation. She killed herself in 1939 after her husband died. Another who died prematurely, aged forty-seven in 1944, was Jean Orr-Ewing. A bacteriologist of note, she was a fellow of Lady Margaret Hall in Oxford in 1929 and joined Florey's team working on the use of penicillin to treat war wounds. Ida Mann was another early fellow at Oxford, though she had to conceal her marriage to hold the position. Mann became a leading ophthalmologist and is credited with saving Moorfields Hospital after it was damaged during the war; she emigrated to Australia in protest against the coming of the NHS. Esther Rickards, by contrast, battled for the NHS through the Socialist Medical Association. But often the accomplishments of these women disappeared from the historical record. Rickards's death passed almost unnoticed in the medical press, despite her having acquired a Fellowship of the Royal College of Surgeons and an OBE. Even the Royal College of Surgeons' obituary emphasized her needlework. Similarly, in 1951 when Gertrude Eleanor Harre retired as assistant curator at St Mary's, her "gracious personality" and domestic ways were most missed: "It was she who presided at four o'clock tea and managed to provide cake for the guests even in the time of scarcity during the war."[57]

Five of the female graduates of St Mary's had moved abroad by the mid-1930s. This was a path that many male graduates also took. One of the most eminent, Sir Leonard Rogers, also reflected on the school's influence over his career. Born in 1868, he came from a professional family: his father was a naval captain and his great-grandfather had been president of the Royal Society in the 1820s. As a student, Rogers made ends meet by working as a demonstrator. In 1893 he entered the India Medical Service and went to Netley, where he studied bacteriology under Almroth Wright. A career in the IMS was difficult for a Mary's man, he observed, because St Bartholomew's dominated the service. Others complained of army service that "leave is almost unobtainable; pay is very small (commencing with £50 a year less than any Army Veterinary Surgeon gets), and any non-routine allowances extremely difficult to recover; also the work is greatly increasing and nearly all one's service is spent abroad." Conditions were such as to reduce "a body of gentlemen into a mob of discontents."[58]

But Rogers did well in the IMS. In the late 1890s he undertook studies of outbreaks of kala-azar, malaria, and dysentery. At the end of six years he returned to London, obtained an MD and MRCP, and transferred to the civil wing of the service. Working in the pathology lab of the Calcutta medical school, in 1903 he discovered that potassium permangate could cure viper bite, and in 1904 he was the first to see flagellae in the organism causing kala-azar. He published several monographs and a hundred scholarly papers in his lifetime. After consulting with his old physiology teacher, Augustus Waller, he developed a treatment for cholera that remains in use today: hypertonic saline solution. Previously, most cholerics died of dehydration, made worse by the bloodletting that was the treatment of choice for much of the nineteenth century. He also developed a treatment for leprosy and showed that when restricted to nerve lesions, the disease was not infectious. In 1911 he became professor at Calcutta and in in 1916 he was named FRS. Returning to London in 1920, he taught tropical medicine at the London School of Hygiene and at St Mary's, served on the medical board of the India Office and raised interest in research into tropical medicine.

Rogers was at the beginning of a tide of Mary's graduates who became prominent through colonial service. He advanced some of them personally, including his successor as pathologist in Calcutta and as head of the new School of Tropical Medicine, R. Knowles. Others who qualified during the decade after 1895 included J.B. Addison, who became chief medical officer of Hong Kong and a member of the legislative council. A.F. Cole became editor of the *China Medical Journal*, R.W. Dodgson the director of the Government Research laboratory at Cape Town in 1901, W. Fletcher the director of the Institute for Medical Research in Kuala Lumpur and secretary of the Colonial Medical Research Committee, A.E. Horn principal MO in German East Africa and an advisor to the Colonial Office. J.W. Hunt served on the legislative council of Fiji. S.P. James became a statistical officer in India, then an advisor to the Local Government Board on tropical disease and was elected FRS in 1931. F.C. Madden became professor of surgery, dean of the medical faculty, and acting rector of the state university in Cairo. E.R. Rost helped found Rangoon Medical School.

Many entered the India Medical Service or the Colonial Medical Service from weakness rather than strength. Not having enough money to buy a practice, they fanned out around the globe, spreading the medicine that they learned at St Mary's. Early editions of the *Hospital Gazette* were full of hair-raising tales, like those of Felix Roth, a surgeon on the Benin punitive expedition, who described horrible scenes of massacre and crucifixion in terms that struggled to be reassuring: "All the white men who were massacred behaved well."[59] Rost in Burma told homelier stories of using his bicycle tyre to inflate a rectum and remove a bladder stone suprapubically.[60] At the Chinese hospital that he ran, Cole told the *Gazette* in 1913,

"humbly and at a very great distance we follow in the steps of the Therapeutic Inoculation Department, where the sound of blood dripping ceases
not day or night."[61] The full weight of Almroth Wright's methods was
brought to South Africa in 1911 when he accepted an invitation from the
Witwatersrand Native Labour Association to combat pneumonia among
gold and diamond mine workers. Conditions for these workers were appalling. Wright and his team collected samples of the different species of
pneumonia and produced vaccines that were used in inoculations. Two
years later the legislature prohibited the recruitment of "tropical" natives –
those shipped in from the north – and the vaccines were never really put to
the test. Some of Wright's workers stayed on and founded the South
African Institute for Medical Research.

Mary's men pursued distinguished careers in the Royal Army Medical
Corps (RAMC). St Mary's trained two successive director-generals of the
RAMC. Alfred Keogh did some post-qualification work at St Mary's: with
Haldane and Balfour, he reformed the medical service, bringing in modern
science and specialization, as well as Wright's typhoid vaccine.[62] When
Keogh stepped down in 1918, T.H.J.C. Goodwin, who qualified at St
Mary's in 1892, replaced him. Goodwin came from a family of army doctors; his brother William, who also trained at St Mary's, served as assistant
director in the late 1920s. As befitting a peacetime director-general,
T.H.J.C. Goodwin gave many speeches, at St Mary's and to other schools,
in which he urged listeners to join in sports that imparted manhood to them
and strength to the nation.[63] Late in life as governor-general of Queens-
land, his presence graced many a sports stand.

For every CMS or IMS or RAMC man who rose to prominence in the service, another returned to England a shattered wreck. A.P. Boon lost his savings in a tornado, then died of malaria in 1892. In the early 1920s
thirty-six-year-old C.G. Galpin died of dysentery picked up in the Dard-
anelles, the third rugby captain from St Mary's to die from war service.
C.H. Brodribb joined the IMS in 1903 but was forced out by ill health and
established a sanatorium in Penaenmawr offering treatment "based on the
production of autoinoculation, produced by means of graduated walks of
great beauty controlled by rest and careful clinical observation."[64] He died
in 1927 after "years of ill health bravely borne." Another foreshortened life
was that of R.B. Anderson, who qualified in 1869 and became a GP in Tobago, where he rose to become a JP and member of the legislative council
by 1889. Then he quarrelled with a patient, refusing to attend her, and was
sued for malpractice, a charge the court upheld. Though English courts reversed the decision, Anderson lost everything. According to the *Lancet*, he
"spent the remainder of a most unfortunate life in resenting the position to

which the unjust and drunken colonial judges had reduced him." With his death at age fifty-three in 1900 was closed "a lurid page in the constitutional history of this country."[65] The story was hardly an advertisement for colonial medical service.

Most Mary's men abroad or at home lived more happily. Often they inherited a practice from their father. Sometimes they formed veritable dynasties, as did the Maurice family of Marlborough. James Blake Maurice came to St Mary's to study in 1858. He sent three sons to St Mary's, in 1885, 1888, and 1891. Subsequent generations took their place into the next century, with admissions in 1905, 1934, 1938, and finally, 1965. The family ran a flourishing practice in Marlborough, provided medical services to the public school, and in 1859 helped to found one of the earliest cottage hospitals in the country.[66] Many other GPs were prominent men in their local community – James Blake Maurice became a JP and mayor – but this was a quiet and local prestige. *The Hospital* remarked of his funeral in 1912, one day after that of Joseph Lister: "Here, then, we have presented on succeeding days two great contrasts: the eminent surgeon and scientist on the one hand, and the great general practitioner and surgeon on the other. The memory of the first was commemorated in the most impressive manner in the Abbey of Westminster. The second found his resting-place in a simple country churchyard in the centre of the district where his life work had been accomplished. The work of both men was excellent. The example they set their fellows was great and far-reaching, and the admiration and confidence which each inspired were evidenced in an equally striking and touching manner."

Some Mary's graduates of the first half of the twentieth century did rise to national or professional prominence. Fifty years on Zachary Cope surveyed the career of one hundred consecutive entries to the school at the turn of the century, excluding a very few who didn't stay long enough to sit an exam, or colonials who registered only to take the final exam.[67] Eleven died prematurely; two never practised; nine had poor success; nineteen had moderate success; thirteen had good practices; thirteen did well in teaching, administration, or the services; and fourteen obtained real distinction. These included three pathologists who obtained an FRS, three clinical professors, and The Lien Wu.

This sort of survey tells us much, but not enough. Did a St Mary's education enable its graduates to rise to the top of their profession? To answer this question, it is useful to focus on a few individuals who came very near to the top, to illustrate the identity of a Mary's man and the nature of elite medicine. But a distinction must be drawn between the school as a place of training and the school as a place for a career. Some of the Moran scholars, like Denis Brinton, were appointed to the hospital while Moran was still dean. But most who qualified at the end of Moran's regime had to make careers for themselves in the very different world of postwar Britain. Assessment of their successes and failures must be seen in that context. One measure of the change was the publication in 1955 by a Mary's graduate, Peter Williams, of a book entitled *Careers in Medicine*. Williams invited prominent consultants (including eighteen from St Mary's) to describe the road to success in their field. Such an abstract and objective statement of the conditions for advancement would have been almost unthinkable before the Second World War.

There is some evidence that, between the wars, St Mary's did not attract or hold intellectually ambitious men. They gravitated to the Inoculation Department or left Praed Street altogether. Three examples are provided by Tom Kettle, S.C. Dyke, and Charles Singer. Tom Kettle came to St Mary's while Moran was still a student, soon distinguished himself as a clinical pathologist, and on Spilsbury's departure in 1919, took over that department. He was an outstanding experimental pathologist, particularly interested in the pathogenesis of cancer, silicosis, and tuberculosis. In 1924, three years after Moran became dean, he left St Mary's for a post in Cardiff; in 1927 he took up a university chair at St Bartholomew's, and in 1934 became chief pathologist at the new Royal Post-Graduate Medical School in Hammersmith. The department would become one of the finest research departments in the country, but Kettle was not there to see it; soon after receiving his FRS in 1936, he died of a gastric ulcer.

S.C. Dyke was another prominent clinical pathologist trained by St Mary's, yet so tenuous was his connection to his old school that the *Gazette* did not publish his obituary. Dyke came from Oxford on an open scholarship in 1913, but his interest in clinical pathology only developed after he left St Mary's. He published dozens of articles on questions ranging from blood typing to diabetes to wasp stings. He also wrote political pieces urging the establishment of clinical pathology as a specialist field in its own right, and he was a founder of the Royal College of Clinical Pathology.

Charles Singer, the son of a Hebraist, qualified from St Mary's in 1903 after doing preliminary studies at Oxford. He held the positions which ambitious doctors held: house physician, resident obstetrical officer, and resident anaesthetist. In 1910 he lost the medical registrarship to Moran. That year he married Dorothy Cohen, a historian of science, and began to grow more interested in history than in clinical medicine. After the war he became a lecturer in medical history at University College London; in 1932 he acquired a DLitt from Oxford and became a professor at UCL, doing much to establish medical history as a scholarly discipline.

Kettle, Singer, and Dyke threw off their ties with St Mary's. And, apart from pathology, St Mary's did not produce any outstanding clinical researchers during the early twentieth century. Those who remained and pursued careers there tended to be solid generalists with good social connections rather than intellectuals. During the interwar period, St Mary's Hospital appointed nine general physicians and surgeons; eight were graduates of the school and the ninth, George Pickering, was a university appointment who was automatically given honorary status by the hospital. Three more were appointed physicians to the hospital at the end of the war: Jack Litchfield, Tom Kemp, and Carmichael Young, all good generalists. The latter two were rugby players (as was Lloyd Owen, who was named honorary anaesthetist to St Mary's in 1946).

Prestige and tradition reinforced one another: the favoured students were encouraged to become general physicians and surgeons, and they ensured that an ethos of generalism was perpetuated. In the special departments the record was more mixed: ten were Mary's trained and nine were imported. Anaesthetists came from the London, obstetricians from University College and the Middlesex, the venereologist from St Thomas's, the orthopaedic surgeon from St George's, and even in paediatrics St Mary's was unable to raise a successor to Langmead and so imported Reginald Lightwood, a graduate of the Westminster Hospital Medical School. Those specialists who were trained at St Mary's usually did not distinguish themselves academically or by publication, save for textbooks. Postwar specialist appointments to the school did, however, distinguish themselves by academic publications and advanced research.

Some of Moran's scholarship students achieved academic prominence after 1945. Four were outstanding, becoming professors and FRS. Though all four obtained medical qualifications, three were really physiologists. Two, Henry Barcroft and G.W. Harris, severed their ties with St Mary's after qualifying. Henry Barcroft was the son of the Cambridge physiologist Sir Joseph Barcroft, and after completing his preliminary training at Cambridge, entered St Mary's in 1929. On completion of the course, he moved to University College as a lecturer in physiology, where he studied blood flow, working with some of the leading clinical and physiological researchers of the day, including Sir Thomas Lewis, Pickering, C.R. Harrington, and John McMichael. In 1935, aged thirty, he was named to the physiology chair at Belfast. Thirteen years later, now an FRS, he returned to London with a chair at St Thomas's.[68] G.W. Harris had already begun research into the pituitary gland of the rabbit when he came to St Mary's for clinical studies in 1936. His obituarist remarked, "It must have been quite an experience at the School to receive a student who certainly knew more about the pituitary than any of his teachers."[69] Harris continued to dissect under Huggett and subsequently became a lecturer in physiology at Cambridge and the Maudsley Hospital, then a professor of anatomy at Oxford in 1962, having acquired his FRS in 1953 as a founder of neuroendocrinology.

The other two Moran scholars who achieved academic prominence, A.D.M. Greenfield and Stanley Peart, became professors at St Mary's. Greenfield recalled, "I came from a soccer school and was useless even at that."[70] Trained by Huggett, he succeeded him as professor of physiology during the 1960s. Stanley Peart stands out as the only Moran scholar who returned to St Mary's and pursued a successful scientific career there with feet firmly planted in both laboratory and clinic. However, it should be noted that Peart was not a product of the generalist clinical school that dominated St Mary's during the Moran years. Rather, he was trained by George Pickering who came to St Mary's in 1939. Greenfield and Peart belong properly to the later history of St Mary's, which was transformed during the Second World War to become a place of serious research.

Innovation in surgery requires qualities very different from innovation in medicine. Scientific credentials only began to figure at St Mary's after the Second World War, and these men were imported. Moran's Mary's tended to produce surgeons who achieved lucrative practices and public honours. Arthur Porritt has been described as "an archetypal surgeon of the old school."[71] A Rhodes scholar from New Zealand, by the time he entered St Mary's in 1926 he had already won a bronze medal in the 1924 Olympics in the famous "Chariots of Fire" race. He came to St Mary's for the scholarship,[72] though he had to give up rugby after an ankle injury and so never played for the school. Like Pannett, whom he admired, Porritt became a generalist with an interest in gastric work, to which he added a second specialty, trauma, during World War II. He qualified in 1928, gained his FRCS in 1930, and joined the hospital staff in 1937. He was an enormously popular teacher and, with another Mary's-trained surgeon on staff, R.M. Handfield-Jones, wrote a surgical textbook that went through several editions. But his greatest successes were outside the surgical field, and resulted from the friendships he formed easily. At the end of the war he arranged an exchange program with colleagues at the Peter Brent Brigham Hospital in Boston, a program destined to have far-reaching effects for the later history of surgery at St Mary's. In 1960, the year he was made baron, Porritt presided over the Royal College of Surgeons and the British Medical Association simultaneously. He owed much of his professional success to an early appointment to the royal household, named surgeon to the Duke of York (by Bertrand Dawson and Thomas Horder) when Edward VIII was already on the throne and expected to keep it for many years. But within a year George VI was king. Subsequently, Porritt became governor-general of New Zealand and a life peer.

Quite a different kettle of fish was Arthur Dickson Wright, one of the greatest surgical operators St Mary's has known. After qualifying from St Mary's, he went to Singapore during the 1920s and there, at the age of twenty-six, he became a professor of clinical surgery and gained wide experience operating on a population he described as given to stabbing one another.[73] After four years a vacancy in the surgical unit at St Mary's brought him back, and he started up a special clinic for varicose veins. As he told a houseman, "When I was appointed … they asked me what I wanted to do, and I said I wanted to do neurosurgery. And they said I couldn't, they didn't want a neurosurgeon, because that would have put them all in the shade. So when the question came up again, I said I'd like to specialise in varicose veins, and they said yes, because they didn't think I could make my name, or threaten them in any way, by doing varicose veins. I proved them wrong!"[74] While in Singapore, he had developed a surgical technique for stripping varicose veins to treat rickshaw drivers who couldn't stop to have the veins cut out and then convalesce. His varicose clinic attracted patients from across the country.[75] He filled the Lindo Wing with his private patients, and he also convinced these wealthy patients to donate large sums to St Mary's and to the Imperial Cancer Research Fund. Dickson Wright was an extremely fine operator: when scolded for slapdash aseptic preparations, he replied that he didn't need asepsis; that was for the cruder surgeons who left dead or damaged tissue behind. From the 1940s to the 1960s Dickson Wright performed something like 30,000 operations in the Lindo wing with hardly a case of sepsis.[76] The sister who nursed his beds in Lillian Holland ward recalled with admiration and affection, "His clean surgery, wonderful technique and routine were excellent. It is amazing that I saw more septic wounds in Chepstow Lodge in one week than I saw in Lillian Holland in the twenty-two years I worked for Mr. A. Dickson Wright. His ward rounds were absolutely hilarious at times. We had lots of laughs as well as lots of beatings and bashings."[77]

Though Dickson Wright's skill was never in question, his judgment sometimes was. As his obituarist remarked, "He was a pioneer of many techniques, although not all remain today." Surgical treatment of hypertension was one that has not survived. Ultimately, his presence slowed the development of specialist cardiac and brain surgery at St Mary's. He was the only general surgeon on staff who ventured into the brain, and there would be no specialist neurosurgeon until he retired. One member of staff recalled that "when they had a case that needed neurosurgery, they would slip it out

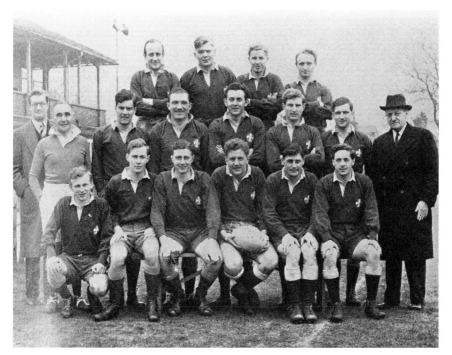

Rugby football team, flanked by Tom Kemp (secretary) and Arthur Dickson Wright (president). St Mary's Hospital NHS Trust Archives and the Royal College of Surgeons of England

to Queen's Square, without telling him." Jack Litchfield, a chest physician, observed that "Dickson Wright was quite prepared to do anything on any part of the human body, and he could do it very well, but not with much judgement ... I wasn't really prepared to unleash Dickson Wright on cardiac surgery!" When asked about his results, Dickson Wright replied, "My patients send me Christmas cards. I get lots of Christmas cards." He abhorred committees and avoided them whenever possible, so his name is almost absent from official hospital and medical school records. But he taught surgery to generations of students, chaired many of their clubs, especially the rugby club, and filled them with stories of St Mary's old and new. He could be vicious to students and nurses he didn't like, and his irascibility and sharp tongue cost him the highest prizes in his profession: a knighthood and presidency of the Royal College of Surgeons. But staff at St Mary's turned to him when they needed an operation.

Pannett, Porritt, Dickson Wright, and their colleagues provided incoming students with an outstanding surgical education, a mix of tradition and iconoclasm. They produced some outstanding, innovative surgeons. J. Crawford

Adams, Felix Eastcott, Kenneth Owen, and Lance Bromley entered St Mary's in the 1930s (Owen and Eastcott on scholarships) and became consultant surgeons at their old school. Adams became an orthopaedic surgeon, Eastcott took up vascular surgery, Owen moved from vascular to genito-urinary surgery, and Bromley became a thoracic surgeon. These men produced classic textbooks and laid the foundation for the international reputation that St Mary's acquired in these fields in the 1950s and '60s.

Moran undoubtedly established St Mary's as one of the leading medical schools in the country. As a boy he came to St Mary's because someone unconnected with the place told him it was the best school in London, outstanding in games and in work.[78] When he became dean two decades later, the school was in a state of decline, reduced by a broader crisis in medical education and by a series of bad appointments. He built it up again, not by making judicious academic appointments (for he couldn't control hospital appointments) but by making it one of the most popular schools for students. Using scholarships and publicity, he gave the school a reputation for being a place where manly virtues like camaraderie, boisterousness, and toughness were cultivated. Right up until the words "St Mary's Hospital Medical School" disappeared from the University of London calendar, his influence continued to be felt. Long after his retirement the school continued to attract world-class athletes, including Roger Bannister, who ran his four-minute mile while a clinical student (and later became the consultant neurologist), and J.P.R. Williams, one of Wales's finest rugby players.

Serious science was not debarred, and a few eccentrics actually pursued it, but the atmosphere of the school was more conducive to producing good general physicians, surgeons, and general practitioners. They were well-rounded and sociable individuals who got on with people. And they had a self-confidence that enabled them to confront difficult clinical problems and the changes that the postwar world would usher in. According to John Graham Jones, "most Mary's people of the vintage that I'm talking about, when they left Mary's, just expected to do a good job and not make a fuss about it. To get on with it." He himself became an industrial physician in Ebbw Vale, Nye Bevan's own constituency, where he saw scientific medicine reach the poorer regions of Wales. Although not a scientist himself, he said that St Mary's taught him how to cope with science. Asked whether the bacteriology he learned there helped him in later life, he replied: "Oh yes. Well, you know, one was quite confident. At the time, you don't think anything of these things, you think, 'What a stupid waste of time.' But they're there in the background, and you fall back on them, and get into a discussion on the pathology of something, and someone tries to blind you with science, about cultures, and this was when you could up them one! ...

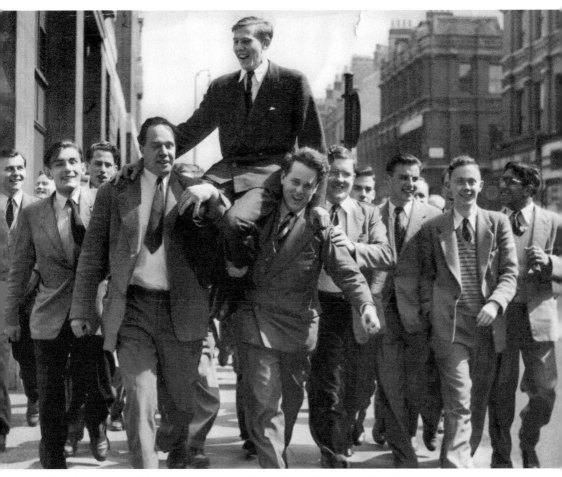

Mary's students with Roger Bannister. Collection of Sir Roger Bannister

We all did it, I'm sure: 'Professor Fleming and I used to …' It's another thing one learnt at Mary's!"[79]

The anecdote raises the question of the relationship between science and social authority. Medical authority can be seen as having two constituent parts: a social aspect and an intellectual aspect. As shown earlier, one can often be converted into the other. Intellectual mastery of a subject can command respect. Alternatively, social status can bolster one's intellectual authority. Medical advisors to the government arranged for Almroth Wright to receive a knighthood because they thought that this would make it easier to introduce routine typhoid vaccination into the army. Moran placed the emphasis on the social side of the doctor's identity, knowing that if doctors had a strong corporate identity and displayed the manners of the upper classes, they would exercise considerable intellectual authority, both over patients and in the political arena, as he had done.

But there is a diminishing return on this mutual reinforcement between intellectual and social authority. The more profound one's knowledge of a subject becomes, the fewer will be the people with enough knowledge of the area to recognize its profundity. Renaissance and Enlightenment scientists wrote for a general public; even Almroth Wright was read by statesmen; but most articles by modern scientists are intelligible only to their peers, who are "in on" the specialized language, concepts, tools, and genres. Specialized knowledge of this sort can be threatening to the traditional generalist who doesn't understand it, and to the public, and on both counts the social prestige of the medical profession as a whole can suffer. Certainly St Mary's harboured many self-styled traditionalists who were scornful of what consultant physician Sidney Phillips called "test-tube doctors."

Although Moran had to work with these traditionalists, he had a healthy respect for science and scientists and helped to inculcate that respect in the next generation of doctors. He and his cohort were probably influenced by Wright who, if he taught them nothing else, taught them to respect science, both as an intellectual pursuit and as an avenue to social and political clout. The glittering parade of celebrities and statesmen who came to the Inoculation Department for treatment and for tea must have convinced even the most traditional physician or surgeon that here was a force to be reckoned with. Thus, while Wright established scientific research at St Mary's, it was Moran who opened the door of the medical school to science and, with the appointment of Pickering and Huggett, ushered it in. He gave the school a strong corporate identity, but one flexible enough to encompass the new categories of doctors and scientists that proliferated after the Second World War. St Mary's was known as the friendliest school in London ("tribal," to its critics), and that circle of friendliness could be stretched to encompass even those eccentric Mary's men who took up science. And while women and ethnic minorities were initially debarred from this circle, they too began to be admitted after the war, and they too found themselves at home, full members of the St Mary's community.

THE RISE OF SCIENCE

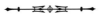

10

The Rise of Clinical Science

MEDICINE CHANGED A great deal in postwar Britain. The NHS was one engine of change, scientific advance was another, and demography yet another. Thanks to the labours of public health doctors and nurses, a rise in the standard of living, and a decline in overcrowding, people began to live longer. The fatal infectious diseases of childhood were all but wiped out, and those remaining were much less severe. Tuberculosis seemed to be beaten by better working and living conditions and by antibiotics. Although new diseases and antibiotic-resistant strains of old diseases appeared, their death tolls remained below those of the old killers. More Britons began to reach old age and to suffer from chronic rather than acute infectuous diseases.

Coinciding with this new morbidity profile, medical research became increasingly physiological. In its early years, laboratory-based physiology was too crude to have much clinical application. One could ligate an artery or inject a chemical and watch as the animal died or recovered. Moreover, British physiology lagged behind continental physiology. In Europe, research was organized on a university basis, whereas British medical training and research remained largely rooted in the proprietary teaching hospitals. British medical researchers and practitioners depended upon public goodwill – in the form of lay governors or private clientele – for their livelihood and they were, therefore, more likely to uphold dominant values, including a widespread repugnance for vivisection.[1]

After an anti-vivisection pamphlet appeared in 1901, many subscribers cancelled their subscription to St Mary's Hospital.[2] Vivisecting staff had to justify themselves to the governors, as in 1904 when they were asked for an account of their practices. The governors were told that no animals were killed for teaching purposes; that the physiologist, Alcock, only rarely (twice in six months) performed experiments; that the animals were fully anaesthetized and immediately killed; and that Almroth Wright had reported "no vivisection experiments, as ordinarily understood, have been carried out during the past few months; only inoculations – in which Bacteria, or their products, are introduced beneath the skin." Laboratory animals were merely injected, just as patients were injected. Wright admitted, however, that some cases involved "the subsequent deaths of the animals inoculated."

In twentieth-century Britain, first physiology, then medicine were put on a more academic footing, and researchers sequestered in universities lost their repugnance for animal experimentation. Through experience, they refined their techniques. By mid-century a rabbit could have a renal artery blocked with a metal clip, the other kidney removed, and still be returned to health (albeit just long enough for a post-mortem to prove health). The new techniques permitted isolation of enzymes and peptides and chemical messengers like vitamins and hormones. The urge was always to narrow the level of reduction and analysis ever further, so as to identify the ultimate causes of physiological events.

The rise of medical science can be illustrated by the development of electrophysiology and cardiovascular science at St Mary's. The work began in the physiology department, at the fringes of medicine, and grew to become a leading activity of both hospital and school. As a case study, the cardiovascular work also provides a good introduction to postwar medicine. Previous chapters have emphasized the social context of Mary's medicine. This chapter provides a more inward-looking case study in intellectual history, so as to illustrate the internal dynamic of medicine – the quest for better understanding and more efficient control – that distinguishes it from the other liberal professions. In this era medicine truly took up the methods and concepts of physical science.

At St Mary's, subjective impressions formed at the bedside remained the standard of medical knowledge until the eve of the Second World War. From the 1940s a paradigm shift occurred, and the new standard of medical knowledge rested on a more objective calculus of certainty. New knowledge-making practices differed in shape and texture from old. This chapter outlines the development of objective analysis of the human body: firstly, as a physical object susceptible to laboratory investigation, and secondly, as a social object, to be compared to other bodies operating under the influence of complex social and environmental factors.

Following the work of Thomas Kuhn, many historians view modern science as guided by scientific research paradigms: patterns of theories and facts that define scientific communities.[4] Members share a language, basic premises, and basic methodologies. The usefulness of the notion is that it forces historians to look at the processes by which knowledge is created, ordered, and transmitted through social groups. More recently, Andrew Warwick has insisted on the need to study schools, textbooks, examinations, and other aspects of pedagogy.[5] Following this line of enquiry, previous chapters have showed that, while early clinicians at St Mary's did study and speculate about their patients, their work was idiosyncratic and did not reflect generalized research paradigms. The first research school was introduced to St Mary's by Almroth Wright, who created a paradigm that other pathologists and bacteriologists joined when they began to test his findings in his and in their laboratories. Ultimately, researchers rejected Wright's opsonic paradigm as unfruitful. His research institute attracted fewer recruits and went into decline. Wright's theories and practices continued to appeal to an aging generation of clinicians who had learned medicine while he was at the height of his influence. However, a new generation of pathologists and clinicians pursued other, newer lines of research.

By this time, clinical medicine had begun to develop a scientific paradigm of its own. A small group of medical reformers possessing all the ideological zeal of the Grand Old Man himself aggressively promoted a new approach to the clinic, rooted in new apparatus of investigation – above all, the electrocardiograph – and they called it clinical science. Like Wright, they combined research and pedagogy to develop theoretically fruitful, clinically effective, and institutionally powerful research programs. Infiltrating St Mary's in 1939, they made it a stronghold of the new clinical science, reconfiguring medical knowledge at the hospital, beginning with clinical medicine and extending the research paradigm into other clinical departments.

Early Cardiology and Clinical Science

While measurement of the heart's action began with William Harvey, the development of refined instruments for the task began in the mid-nineteenth century, with Jules Marey's sphygmograph, which measured arterial blood pressure while leaving the skin intact. Physiologists who brought these tools to Britain included John Burdon Sanderson, who used the sphygmograph to show that patients with Bright's disease had high blood pressure.[6] Pressure was one measure of cardiac performance; another was rhythm. Using the capillary electrometer that Gabriel Lippmann developed during the 1870s, Sanderson measured the electrical activity of mammalian hearts. The capillary electrometer worked by drawing leads using sulphuric acid and mercury which met in a tube. Fluctuations in the point of contact measured electrical activity. Because the electrometer had to be applied directly to the exposed heart, human experimentation was out of the question. Then, in 1887, A.D. Waller found a way to use the capillary electrometer to measure the heart's electrical activity in the unexposed heart. The account was first published in the *Physiological Journal* in 1887 and was the subject of his inaugural lecture at St Mary's in 1888. Usually inaugural lectures were platitudes about the need to study hard and play hard; there cannot be many that appear in surveys of foundational medical texts, but Waller's lecture was such a one.

At the turn of the century William Einthoven constructed a string galvanometer, a more efficient version of the electrocardiograph with three different leads, though at five hundred pounds it was too clumsy for ordinary clinical use. At University College London, Thomas Lewis obtained a galvanometer in 1913 and developed a broad program of research around the kind of investigations that it permitted, including fibrillation and the propagation of the electrical excitation of the heart. It was thanks to Lewis's work that Einthoven was awarded a Nobel prize in 1924. Waller might have shared the prize had he not died in 1922.[7]

St Mary's remained hostile to the new cardiology in the 1910s, though Alfred Hope Gosse introduced a galvanometer the following decade. Another decade, and St Mary's leaped to the cardiological vanguard when, in 1939, it appointed Sir Thomas Lewis's top student, George Pickering, to the chair of medicine. Through the influence of students like Pickering, Lewis refounded clinical research in Britain. He also established journals – *Heart*, the standard-bearer of the new cardiology, renamed *Clinical Science* in 1933 (and subsequently edited by Pickering) – and a Medical Research Society, to bring together serious researchers across London.[8] University College dominated the society, with nine members in 1937, while St Mary's had only two: Pannett and Langmead.[9] Lewis's arguments were controversial, especially when he advocated experimentation on patients, but wherever first-rate medical research was performed in England at mid-century, Lewis's influence can usually be traced. It is worth pausing, therefore, to identify his conception of research.

In 1930 Lewis complained that experimental science was "delegated more and more to the laboratories," while medicine remained mired in its "ancient, traditional method" of observation.[10] The problem was structural: only academics freed from the constraints of practice could perform serious research. Clinicians had to practise on unselected cases, so they couldn't control the questions presenting themselves to their minds. They pursued "clinical omniscience," a superficial familiarity with the known, whereas research faced the unknown. Worse, Lewis added, they were publishing (publication having acquired "a recognised commercial value" in the career structure) and swamping good work in a mass of bad, "pseudo-scientific" rubbish. Even the academic units, supposedly the trojan horse of scientific medicine, were bogged down by clinical routine.[11] Lewis repudiated wholesale the existing medical knowledge:

Clinicians who record facts and views are not chosen, as for the most part are physiologists, for their ability to use precise methods of observation and of thought; in medicine inaccuracies in statement of fact are, owing to the material used, more difficult to detect, penalties for mistakes are less severe; the standard of truthfulness ... is far less rigid, than is the case in physiology. A very grave defect in medical publication, from the standpoint of progress, is the dearth of systematic statements of evidence. In a very large proportion of instances, satisfactory and recorded evidence for current clinical beliefs is either most difficult to discover or is non-existent. Far too much stress is laid upon suggestion; far too little upon proof. In this relation it is sufficient to mention therapeutics, but the defect is not confined to this branch. There is a great work to do in close and critical revision of present beliefs in every branch of clinical medicine.[12]

Of course, one could hardly jettison the old vocabulary or the old concepts to start entirely anew. Knowledge was a compromise. Michel Morange, a biochemist and historian, likens research to building a house "with only rotten planks available, with a non-negligible probability that they will give way." Some buildings collapse, others become more solid as the work progresses.[13] Lewis could no more recreate clinical knowledge *de novo* than Almroth Wright could scientific language. Nonetheless, Lewis did introduce a new orientation into British medicine.

Sir George Pickering

George Pickering trained at St Thomas's before coming to work with Lewis, drawn by the MRC funding that Lewis could dispense. Pickering studied blood pressure and particularly its pathological form: hypertension. Essential hypertension was first identified by F.A. Mahomed, a physician at Guy's, who found high blood pressure in patients with no other signs of disease. He predicted that chronic high arterial pressure must lead to hypertrophy of the heart and thickening of the arteries. Mahomed, who died prematurely of typhoid, worked briefly at St Mary's as pathologist in 1876, invited there by William Broadbent.[14] Broadbent was an authority on

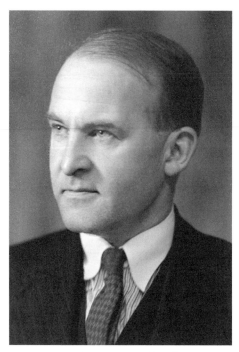

Sir George Pickering. Royal College of
Physicians of London

hypertension at the turn of the century, with an influential book entitled
The Pulse which rested on clinical or observational knowledge, though it
hypothesized an invisible constituent in the blood, "a glandular secretion
or product of metabolism or mineral matter," as the cause of hypertension.
Broadbent prescribed a therapy to eliminate the constituent: fluids, reduced
salt, and hot baths or exercise to induce perspiration.

Early twentieth-century researchers were divided on the causes of the
vasoconstriction causing hypertension. Some suggested a nervous cause,
possibly overactivity of the vasomotor nerves. During the 1930s Pickering
disproved the nervous hypothesis and arrested the practice of treating hypertension surgically by cutting the nerves. Convinced that the cause was
chemical, he performed a variety of experiments with such hormones as
adrenaline and histamine, the results all negative. In May 1938, lecturing
in San Francisco, he reviewed these failures and then, in closing, raised the
possibility of "a protein-like pressor substance" shown to exist in the renal
cortex. In 1898 two Germans had shown that the blood pressure of rabbits
increased when they were injected with kidney extracts, which they named
renin. Renin was extremely difficult to work with, so even careful experiments gave wildly varying results. During the mid-1930s, however, it began
to attract attention once again after a group of researchers showed that
constricting the renal arteries of dogs produced persistent hypertension,

due to the release of a pressor substance, and that injections made from the kidneys of dogs with hypertension produced a greater rise in blood pressure than injections from healthy kidneys. In a paper given to the Physiological Society in 1937, Pickering and Prinzmetal confirmed the 1898 experiments and showed the pressor effect of renin injected into a rabbit's ear. They blamed the delay on the action of anaesthetics, which reduced the effect of renin on animals. The two found other methods of desensitizing the rabbit's ear.[15]

Almost immediately upon the rediscovery of renin, its role in hypertension was found to be complicated by a second substance. In 1939 and 1940, two independent teams, one in the United States and one in Argentina, showed that renin did not itself affect blood pressure, but rather it was an enzyme acting on a constituent of the plasma globulins in such a way as to produce a third substance, which was the effective pressor agent. However, almost nothing else was known of this third substance, for it eluded isolation, though some properties were identified: it was stable to heat, soluble in alcohol, and destroyed by peptic or tryptic digestion. Some called it "hypertensin" and others "angiotonin"; in 1958 all agreed on "angiotensin." The race was now on to find out more about these elusive substances, renin and angiotensin. This was roughly the condition of knowledge when Pickering moved to St Mary's. At that time he was completing experiments involving prolonged infusion of renin into rabbits to produce hypertension and then trying to reverse this effect.

The experiments that he performed on pressor substances appear both complicated and simple. In their formal structure, many of these experiments seem as simple as those of a Sibson or a Maguire: inject something interesting and then watch for the results. But there were considerable differences. Pickering and his students were comfortable performing vivisection and became very skilled at it. The scale of reduction permitted greater generalization from animal to human. In many ways rabbits did not resemble human beings; however, an injection of histamine lowered their blood pressure just as surely as it did that of humans. This was a new licence for vivisection on a large scale. Another great difference with the desultory experimentalism of earlier ages was conceptual agreement. Researchers were engaged in a "very intense rivalry"[16] that increased the standardization of methods and meanings as they pored over one another's writings. Many of these writings had two or more authors. Researchers also visited other laboratories to learn techniques and concepts: Pickering picked up a good deal in the United States in the late 1930s. He and his peers and students were engaged in the sort of puzzle-solving that Thomas Kuhn describes as normal science.[17]

When Pickering moved from UCL to St Mary's in 1939, he moved from a stronghold of laboratory medicine to a deeply traditional teaching hospital. The academic units had failed to implant an ethos of research, and the staff were, one Pickering student recalled, "actually undoubtedly enemies of clinical research."[18] Sir Thomas Lewis, on hearing of Pickering's appointment, added to his congratulations the remark: "I am quite sure that there is an unusual opportunity at Mary's to develop teaching on real University lines; there is no tradition there except one of high standing & one that they do not want you to follow; I am looking toward confidently to your building up a great show."[19]

Pickering had been hired at the insistence of Moran, who was determined to bring the new clinical science into his school. As Pickering recalled the interview, Moran "asked me not a single question but devoted the interview to a homily on how to be a professor of medicine. In essence he said a professor of medicine can do anything he wants provided he carries his constituency with him. His constituency is his students."[20] The two men shared a keen interest in pedagogy. Some of the honorary consultants opposed Pickering's appointment, doubting his clinical abilities, but others warmly welcomed him.

His arrival coincided with the outbreak of war and the evacuation of students and teachers to medical schools and hospitals across the country, the preclinical students going to Manchester and others to hospitals in the sector chosen "more or less at random." Pickering was sent to Harefield Hospital, an old TB sanatorium without any laboratory facilities. He later recalled, "It was evident that with no staff and no laboratories, continued research on renin was out of the question, so I turned my mind to peptic ulcer."[21] Together with George Bonney, a surgical student, he studied the role of intra-gastric acidity in peptic ulcer. Later, with three other students, he resumed his work on nephrectomy and hypertension in rabbits (the animals kept in an old stable). He also threw himself into the life of the school, singing songs at student entertainments, speaking at the medical society, performing on a school brains trust, and presiding over the tennis club.

Pickering's appointment marked a turning point for St Mary's. One medical student, Stanley Peart, declared that "The great turning point in my life was when I met Pickering, for this was my first encounter with a really critical mind." George Bonney told me, "He taught you to think, to think from first principles. And he taught that most of what was written in the text books was absolute balls, which, of course, it was!" According to Peter Sanderson, traditional but vacuous clinical terms such as "shock," and "vascular spasm" provoked outbursts, while "a history torn up in public on a ward round because it had been carelessly written was an experience that few risked repeating." Tommy Hunt recalled that the question "Why do you think that?" was often at Pickering's lips. Felix Eastcott also drew a vivid contrast between the old and the new regimes: the old-style teacher would lecture that "'the causes of a lump here are such and such,' you know, that kind of teaching, which is very good, and you needed it. But Pickering used to say, 'Now, it depends on what you mean by a lump.'"[22] The mass of students wanted old-style dogmatic teaching to get them through examinations. They wanted their lumps. Licensing exams, conducted by senior statesmen of medicine who had written the textbooks, were no place to question first principles. Eastcott, Hunt, Sanderson, Bonney, and Peart became consultants and scholars, but Pickering's methods were probably not appropriate for all students. Most preferred the first-rate practical teaching of the honorary consultants.

The best students, those not wooed away by the glamour of surgery, were brought into the medical unit and co-opted as researchers on the hypertension project. Roger Bannister, who had begun research while in Oxford, had his first house job under Pickering. Tom Kemp credited Pickering with introducing post-graduate work to St Mary's: "Before George Pickering came to St. Mary's in 1939, there was no tradition of post-graduate study, it was self education or nothing."[23] Like Almroth Wright, Pickering also brought in post-graduate workers from further afield. Sanderson, who spent his life in the medical unit, recalled that after Pickering visited Australia, a succession of bright young Aussies passed through, including Richard Lovell, later the first professor of medicine in Australia. After another stint in America, Americans flooded in. Godfrey Bond, speaking at a memorial service, described the group characteristics of "Pickering's young men": they became professors, asked penetrating questions, mocked pomposity, and when they met obtuseness in students, were liable to walk off whistling audibly "O God, our help in ages past."[24]

Sir Stanley Peart

Stanley Peart, who entered St Mary's on a rugby scholarship, began his scientific career with a house job on the medical unit, followed by a stint as "penicillin registrar" under Fleming in 1946.[25] As Peart considered his next move, Pickering suggested he might obtain an MRC studentship to work with Sir John Henry Gaddum in Edinburgh. Gaddum was an FRS, a pharmacologist with one foot in the basic sciences and another in clinical medicine, who laid the groundwork for much of modern bioassay.[26] Peart accepted with alacrity and moved to Edinburgh, where he began to investigate sympathins. Sympathins were released by the liver, upon stimulation of the sympathetic nerves, and they caused smooth muscle to contract. Peart's task was to isolate them.

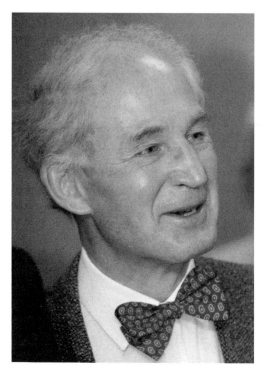

Sir Stanley Peart. The Wellcome Trust

He set to work gamely but soon got bogged down. At first he couldn't keep cats alive during the process of drawing blood from the liver. Shed blood was hard to work with, as it caused violent vasoconstriction. He began to experiment with the blood itself, and, one day, while perfusing a rabbit's ear, he found that ergot blocked the vasoconstriction (subsequently shown to be due to serotonin). Ergot provided a stable background, so that he could then measure and assay the vasoconstrictor substances in the blood. But already one year's funding was up. With Gaddum's approval, he applied for another and turned his attention away from the troublesome liver to the spleen. Splenic blood was much easier to collect without injuring the general circulation. Now the results began to come more easily. He found a substance that inhibited the rat colon, caused vasoconstriction in the rabbit ear, and stimulated the nictitating membrane of the cat; subsequent experiments proved it to be noradrenalin. Peart later described the work as having "nearly killed me experimentally and as a test of my stickability."

In 1950 he was invited by Pickering to join the medical unit as an assistant. The position was a humble one, paying £900, but Peart accepted eagerly, glad to join what had become a lively research team. "Everywhere you looked it was interesting." The assistant director of the unit was Peter Sanderson, who joined the school in 1939 and, upon qualification, moved into the medical unit, rising to assistant director in 1949 (at £1,100 salary).

Sanderson developed an alkaline milk-drip treatment for ulcers, and then began to study the effects of alkalis and calcium in the blood. His forte was the technical side of the research, in the design of the increasingly intricate equipment that the unit needed. He moved the unit into the postwar age of flame photometry when, unable to obtain a colorimeter "for love or money," he built one. He went to Bruges to study one and, with another worker bent on the same task, "We just threw it together." The machine permitted more sophisticated and independent methods of assay. He also made the first machine to measure plasma chloride.[27] As Sanderson's work shows, there was and is no clear-cut division relationship between "science" and "technology." High-tech research is as much a matter of adapting appropriate instrumentation as devising clever theories to test. Bad instruments can be blamed for negative results, and better instruments can confirm a vulnerable theory.[28] Many of the papers produced at the unit at St Mary's appeared in pairs: one paper would set forth a new method of assay, and another would give the results obtained with it.[29]

Just as a scientist like Sanderson could be part technician, so too technicians were scientists. Francis Diggins was born in Wales, but his family came to London when his father found work as a porter on Edgware Road. He began at St Mary's as a page, then cleaned glassware and benches in the physiology department. Later he learned to cut sections in morbid anatomy; still later he learned bacteriology from Fleming. He began to attend evening classes in science, but the war and then tuberculosis prevented him from pursuing higher studies. Diggins spent three years at the Government Lymph Establishment, then the Lister Institute's MRC Unit, and in 1948 he returned to St Mary's to become senior technician to the medical unit. Diggins reflects that "this word 'Technician' has caused an awful lot of trouble for us. I eventually moved over into full time university lecturer [in Surrey], but if you're a technician, you were somebody who came to fix the fridge, whereas I was a good analyst, biochemical analyst."[30] Within the unit, Diggins was one of the team and co-author of some of the papers.

The essential identity of research and mechanical tinkering is also well illustrated in the work of the young Stanley Peart. Just as in Almroth Wright's day even simple laboratory supplies had to be made, nothing could be bought. As he recalled, "We used to make our own exchange resins, you see. I mean, you couldn't buy them off the shelf, you know, you just made them. And the recipes for making them were available in the literature, and you just made them. Starch gels, which were the old-fashioned method of separating proteins, you just made them ... and you took a pride in making a good gel."[31]

First, Peart had to gather his materials: a source of renin – kidneys – and a source of angiotensin – blood. He obtained kidneys from Northumberland where thousands of rabbits were trapped nightly for the London markets. After three days Peart would return with two thousand frozen kidneys. Once home, he would slice them, then dry them in crude alcohol; then they could be ground up into powder, the renin precipitated out as needed with ammonium sulphate. Blood could be obtained in any quantity from slaughterhouses. What he really needed, however, was pure plasma, so he had to pass the blood – hundreds of litres of it – through a centrifuge, a long and tedious procedure. One happy day, driving past a firm that produced milk separators, he pulled in and found for £35 a machine that could produce plasma by the dustbin-load. The next stage was easy: the plasma and the renin were mixed together, and the pressor substance was created, but it remained in the mass of plasma. Charcoal was widely used for clarifying beer and maple syrup and as an absorbing agent, so Peart decided to try it here. The charcoal certainly picked up the pressor substance, but then he couldn't get it off again. The milk separator merely clogged up. Using filters and acetic acid, he was able to remove the pressor substance from the charcoal, but then he had to remove the acetic acid. He found that by adding salt and then mixing it with butanol, he could push the pressor substance into the butanol. At last he had the active principle, but it was still very impure.

He continued to draw a salary from St Mary's, but he undertook the research at the National Institute for Medical Research at Mill Hill. Archie Martin, head of the physical chemistry department, assigned him to Rodney Porter's lab. Porter was a biochemist, trained in Liverpool, who had come to Mill Hill in 1949 and was himself, in 1952, trying to purify gammaglobulin, separating it from the other plasma protein. The two men struggled side by side although, according to Peart, Porter did so with much greater competence. When asked in an interview if the research could have been done at St Mary's, Peart replied with an unusual hesitancy, perhaps born of diplomacy: "Oh yes ... no ... yes ... it was just quicker."

There were many ways to separate molecules. Peart tried partition chromatography. Chromatography consists of placing a solution on a strip of filter paper and then dipping the paper into a solvent, so that the solution flows along the paper. Molecules of different solubility flow at differing speeds and so become separated. Partition chromatography on a larger scale replaced the paper with sheet cellulose which absorbed the stationary phase of the alcohol/water mixture, and the column was eluted with the mobile phase (usually the alcohol). Large-scale partition chromatography permitted the researcher to separate large amounts of applied substances. Fraction collectors collected the substances eluted from the column, which could then be analysed chemically or physically.[32] At Mill Hill, Archie Martin had co-developed the technique of partition chromatography, but by the early 1950s he had become more interested in the promise of electrophoresis – the use of an electrical field to separate biological components – and he urged this upon Peart. Peart couldn't make it work, whereupon Martin grew irritated and "gave me up as a bad job." Rodney Porter, having his own troubles with purification, was more tolerant. Peart returned to partition chromatography and finally achieved success, discovering the correct sequence of ten amino acids that comprised angiotensin. The findings were announced in *Nature* and in the *Biochemical Journal*, edited by Alfred Neuberger, who was also at Mill Hill. With the amino acid sequence established, a Swiss biochemical team quickly synthesized angiotensin the following year, in 1957. The production of substances to reduce blood pressure by blocking the body's production of angiotensin – angiotensin-converting enzymes, or ACE inhibitors – has since become a million-dollar industry.[33]

Peart enjoyed his two years at Mill Hill tremendously, learning from some of the best minds in the business, but he missed working with patients. Pickering offered him a senior lecturer's post at St Mary's but then in 1956 was himself named Nuffield professor of medicine at Oxford, later becoming regius professor. At age thirty-three with an important scientific discovery behind him, Peart was appointed to the vacant chair at St Mary's. Between them Pickering and Peart did much to work out the renin-angiotensin system that underlay hypertension and to establish that field as an important area of basic research in Britain. And finally by introducing modern research to St Mary's, they made the school a leader in clinical science.

Hypertension and the Rise of Epidemiology

Pickering had hardly been idle in the meantime. He wrote the leading textbook *Essential Hypertension* and engaged in a celebrated medical controversy about the causes of hypertension. As J.D. Swales remarks, the controversy owed much of the interest it generated to the stature of the combatants: Sir Robert Platt was elected president of the Royal College of Physicians the year after Pickering became regius professor at Oxford.[34] Pickering was the champion of academic medicine in the tradition of Thomas Lewis, while Platt, professor of medicine at Manchester, remained loyal to standards worked out when he was a general practitioner and criticized academic medicine as narrow. In 1947 Platt published an article entitled "Heredity in Hypertension." Investigating 116 hypertensives, seventy-eight of them cases of essential hypertension, he found that hypertensives were twice as likely to show a family history.

Pickering and his colleagues at St Mary's – M. Hamilton, J.A.F. Roberts, and G.S.C. Sowry – were unconvinced by Platt's arguments for dominant

INTRODUCTORY ADDRESS
ON
THE ELECTROMOTIVE PROPERTIES OF THE HUMAN HEART.

Delivered at St. Mary's Hospital Medical School, at the Opening of the Session, 1888-9.

By AUGUSTUS D. WALLER, M.D.,
Lecturer on Physiology.

THERE is a growing disposition to regard introductory lectures as a survival—a survival unfit for the times. But, like all other customs, this custom, having had its particular reason of being in the past, lives on with altered ends and in changing shape. In its primitive shape, as a general guidance address to those who have just enlisted, it may be no longer necessary nor acceptable, but it certainly cannot be unfitting in any time that each member of a teaching body should in turn be called upon to say, in the presence of his fellow-workers, that which he thinks to be the best worth saying. My particular task on this occasion has been made easy by my colleagues; it was suggested to me that I should speak about physiology, and I am very willing to do so. Let me at once explain why.

The St. Mary's Hospital Medical School is at present rapidly growing, not merely in size, but in complexity; and she has within the last few years developed two entirely new organs, a physiological and a pathological laboratory. It is not unnatural that those who are most responsible for the development should be glad to hear something about the functions of these organs, and should expect from me as the person responsible for the physiological laboratory some report of progress during the last four years. I am on my side very willing that my duty as your introductory lecturer should take this form, which will allow me, not, indeed, to report progress in its full and formal sense, but to report on an item of progress; and I shall, therefore, occupy the greater part of the thirty or forty minutes allowed me, in describing a new bit of knowledge, and how it has been obtained. Our new bit of knowledge is about the human heart, not in a metaphysical or figurative sense, not its motives, not its action, not its power, but its electrical potential. Put into a single sentence, I am going to describe how the heart of man can be shown to act as an electrical organ, and what we learn from such action.

It is a well-known fact that every beat of the heart is accompanied by an electrical disturbance; the nature of this disturbance has, moreover, been studied and understood with the assistance of cold-blooded animals, and in this laboratory in particular an investigation was carried out to learn whether or no warm-blooded animals manifest similar electrical disturbances. These I will not now enter upon, and will only make the passing remark that, while to all appearance the electrical disturbances are similar in the two classes of animals, they are not identically so; these seem to indicate that the contraction, which at each beat of the cold-blooded heart runs down from the base to the apex, runs in the opposite direction in the warm-blooded heart. But this is only by the way, and I make no attempt to explain. It is to the next step that I invite your attention to-day, namely, to the human heart.

Led on from thought to thought it occurred to me that it should be possible to get evidence of electrical action on man by connecting not the heart itself, which is obviously impossible, but parts of the surface of the body near the heart with a suitable instrument; having verified this supposition, the next step was to see whether or no the same evidence can be obtained by connecting the instrument with parts of the body at a distance from the heart, with the hands or feet. The answer was, as you will see, satisfactory. Finally, I tried whether two people holding hands and connected with the instrument, gave evidence of electrical shocks through each other, and I found they did.

The only portion which I wish to explain in any detail is the second step in these experiments, namely, the analysis of the results which are obtained when a single individual, whether man, horse, or dog, is connected with the electrical indicator.

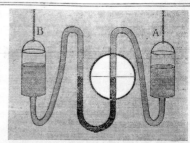

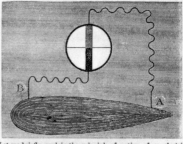

Let me briefly explain the principle of action of an electrical indicator by referring to this diagram, in which the effects of water-pressure are compared with those of what I may call electrical pressure (potential is the correct term, but I take it to be part of my task to-day to avoid technical terms).

A and B are two bottles of water, each connected by flexible pipes with a bent tube half full of mercury. If the two bottles are at the same level, the mercury in the bent tube remains at zero, and it is evident that this is still the case if both bottles be raised together or lowered together. But if the bottles be moved unequally, either up or down, the level of the mercury will alter. It is obvious that if A is lower than B, the mercury in this limb of the tube will move upwards, whereas if B is lower than A it will move downwards. And if we imagine everything hidden from us by a screen with the exception of this portion of the tube which we can view through a circular opening, it is obvious that we shall be able to tell by the movements of the index, whether A is below B or B below A. If the mercury goes up A is below B, if it goes down B is below A.

Now this is precisely what happens when the two ends of an electrical indicator are in connection with any two points A and B of a living body. When A and B are at the same level the index stands at zero, and it does not move if the two points are raised or lowered together to an equal amount. If the index moves up we know that A is lower than B, if down that B is lower than A.

Let us now apply our instrument to the heart. This, which seems rather a bold proposition, is really a very simple and easy matter. We need simply dip the two hands into two basins of water which are in connection with our indicator, when we shall see that the mercury beats up and down with the pulse. These movements of the mercury are due to the electrical changes which occur with every beat of the heart; or we may dip a hand and a foot each into a basin of water with a similar result, only it must be the right hand, the left will not do. This difference, apparently so curious and puzzling at first sight, which seemed unsymmetrical and irrational, is in reality most reasonable, and

Medical science in 1888:

proved to be the master key which threw open the meaning of every subsequent experiment. The difference depends upon the unsymmetrical position of the human heart, which is tilted to the left side somewhat, as shown in this diagram.

Allow me to return for one moment to the physical A B C of the subject. The points A and B are respectively applied to the apex and base of the heart; and if with the contraction of the organ these two portions undergo any electrical change, the change will spread over the whole body in accordance with known laws. I will say no more than that. The form of the change is represented by these oval lines; if the electrical level falls at A it falls over the red area (see note and fifth diagram), which, as you see, includes the left hand and foot and the right foot. If the electrical level falls at B it falls over this blue area, which includes the right arm and the head.

Now it is obvious that the two ends of the indicator must be connected with A and with B before it will indicate any difference between A and B. If both ends are connected with A, or both ends with B, nothing will be seen. This was precisely what we got when the left hand and a foot were connected with the instrument, which begins to pulsate as soon as the right is substituted for the left hand. I might multiply instances, but will only just mention one. If the mouth and right hand are connected with the instrument, its index does not move, but it does so as soon as the left hand is put in the place of the right one. You must connect up a blue and a red point; two blue points or two red points are ineffectual.

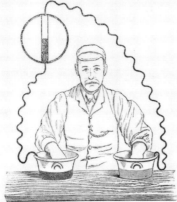

But this evidence does not stand alone. Cases every now and then present themselves with a transposition of the viscera, which are in such people situated just like those of a normal person as they would be viewed in a mirror. The heart, among other organs, is reversed, and, instead of pointing to the left, points to the right. As regards the electrical relations which I was following out, they were precisely as expected. The left arm was in this case the exceptional limb, and formed an effectual couple with any one of the other three limbs, but was ineffective in combination with the mouth. To make a long story short, the results were throughout as indicated in the diagram; any two blue points or any two red points in connection with the indicator were silent, but as soon as connection was made with a red point and a blue point then the index moved with each pulsation of the heart.

Let us hear one more witness. The heart of a quadruped (dog, or cat, or rabbit, or horse) is placed far more symmetrically than in man; it is very nearly in the middle line, so that the changes of electrical level whose foci are at A and B spread straight up and down the body, not obliquely, as in man. The upper half of the body is under the influence emanating from B; the lower half under that emanating from A. Unlike what occurs in man, the

two front paws coupled with an indicator are silent, while either front paw taken with either hind foot gives us the now familiar answer.

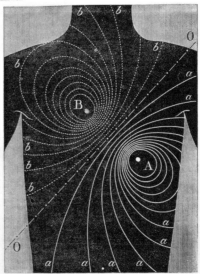

These are the principal facts. What can we learn from them with regard to the normal action of the heart? I must be content with simply stating the answers.

The fact that each beat of the heart gives an electrical change, beginning at one end of the organ and ending at the other, proves that the contraction does not occur throughout the mass of the heart at one and the same instant of time; if the two points A and B rose and fell together, there would be no alteration of the index. The movements of the index show that there is a fall of A at the beginning of the contraction, and a fall of B at the end of

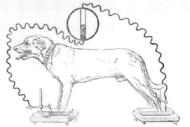

the contraction. One of the most fundamental and certain facts in physiology is that the active state of a living tissue is marked by a fall of electrical level; in other words, an electrical depression is the best, most certain, and most delicate physical sign of physiological action; it proves the fact that living tissue is in excitement just as certainly as a dog's bark proves that a living

Augustus Waller's lecture on electrocardiology. The Wellcome Library

The Purification of Hypertensin. By W. S. PEART (introduced by R. R. PORTER). (*Medical Unit, St Mary's Hospital, W. 2, and National Institute for Medical Research, London, N.W. 7*)

Purification of the pressor principle hypertensin or angiotonin (Braun Menendez, Fasciolo, Leloir & Munoz, 1939; Page & Helmer, 1940) has been successful. It was produced by incubation of the enzyme renin from the rabbit kidney with ox serum in the presence of charcoal, from which it was eluted with glacial acetic acid (Peart, 1955).

Pressor activity at all stages was assayed on the anaesthetized rat (Peart, 1955).

Preliminary evidence that hypertensin was likely to be a peptide was obtained by paper electrophoresis at a wide range of pH, which showed that hypertensin was amphoteric, with an isoelectric range from pH 7·0 to 8·5.

(1) The first step in purification was to extract the NaCl saturated solution of hypertensin at pH 1·0 with n-butanol (Skeggs, Kahn & Shumway, 1952).

(2) Partition chromatography was next carried out on a Hyflo column holding the lower phase of a mixture of n-butanol–acetic acid–water (9:1:10 by vol.), with the top phase mobile.

(3) This activity was next chromatographed on a column of silane-treated Hyflo holding the upper phase of a mixture of n-butanol–0·25 % trichloroacetic acid (1:4 by vol.), with the lower phase mobile. Two peaks of pressor activity were obtained; the faster running peak had 5 % of the total activity.

(4) The main peak was adsorbed on Hyflo and eluted with 0·02 M ammonium formate. Low-pressure distillation of the eluate yielded a white powder, which was 1·5–3·0 times as active wt./wt. as noradrenaline.

Hydrolysis in 6 N-HCl followed by paper chromatography revealed leucine, phenylalanine, valine, tyrosine, proline, aspartic acid, arginine and histidine, with a trace of alanine. Spectrophotometry showed no evidence of tryptophan.

(5) The peptide thus obtained was tested for homogeneity by paper electrophoresis; hydrolysis of the active fractions showed the same pattern of amino acids, suggesting that the material was homogeneous.

Recent reports of purification of hypertensin from different species indicate pressor activity associated with larger numbers of amino acids on hydrolysis (Skeggs, Kahn & Shumway, 1954; Bumpus & Page, 1954; Kuether & Haney, 1955).

REFERENCES

Braun Menendez, E., Fasciolo, J. C., Leloir, L. F. & Munoz, J. M. (1939). *Rev. Soc. argent. Biol.* **15**, 420.
Bumpus, F. M. & Page, I. H. (1954). *Science*, **119**, 849.
Kuether, C. A. & Haney, M. E. (1955). *Science*, **121**, 65.
Page, I. H. & Helmer, O. M. (1940). *J. exp. Med.* **71**, 29.
Peart, W. S. (1955). *Biochem. J.* **59**, 300.
Skeggs, L. T., Kahn, J. R. & Shumway, N. P. (1952). *J. exp. Med.* **95**, 241.
Skeggs, L. T., Kahn, J. R. & Shumway, N. P. (1954). *J. exp. Med.* **99**, 275.

genetic transmission. They maintained that his classification assumed that one was either diseased or healthy. In the early 1950s they showed that the hypothesis was unsustainable. Comparing the relations of hypertensive and other out-patients, they found that at every age the blood pressure of relatives of hypertensives was higher than that of the other two groups, suggesting a genetic component; but the difference was so small ("expressed by a regression coefficient of a little more than 0.2") that the gene was not a dominant one and environmental causes were more significant. Moreover, the distribution curves showed that the difference between normal and high blood pressure was quantitative, not qualitative. As people aged, their blood pressure tended to rise. Essential hypertension was an artifact, not an entity, and referred to "that section of the population in which arterial pressure exceeds an arbitrary value and in which no other disease is found to account for the arterial pressures observed. According to where we draw the line, so we can make essential hypertension as common or as rare as we wish." One might as well speak of essential tallness.

Platt maintained in reply that there were two distinct groups in the general population: those whose pressures rose steeply with age, and those whose pressures were little affected. He admitted that the proposition would require a twenty-year study for proof.[35] The two continued to disagree about how to read the evidence, with Platt waving charts that he described as bimodal and Pickering described as Gaussian – that is, as showing two and one populations respectively.

Pickering's theory was confirmed by a twenty-year study of a small Massachusetts town of 28,000 people. When the American Public Health Service began the Framingham study in 1948, so little was known about heart disease that smoking was not at first included as a risk factor. New variables were added, and, by its end, the Framingham study did identify the major risk factors.[36] You couldn't do this sort of long-term study in "restless" Paddington, but you could do it in the countryside. Researchers including W.E. Miall, a Mary's graduate, confirmed Pickering's position by taking the blood pressure of thousands of people in two Welsh villages over several years. They found some genetic links but also a variation of 36 per cent to 67 per cent due to environment.[37]

By the mid-1970s the graduated distribution of high blood pressure had become a foundational notion of medical epidemiology. In 1976 the classic textbook *Epidemiology in Medical Practice* began its discussion of health surveys with the example of hypertension. The authors, D.J.P. Barker and Geoffrey Rose, asserted that clinical knowledge alone could never suffice to define disease, because it was an artifact "of the selective processes governing hospital admission." To prove the argument, they illustrated the distribution of diastolic blood pressure in middle-aged men graphically, pointing out, "The curve is continuous and unimodal, having only one peak. 'Normotension' merges imperceptibly into 'hypertension', and any definition of an upper level of normal is clearly arbitrary." In most diseases, the question was "not so much 'Has he got it?' as 'How much of it has he got?'"[38] Hypertension, from this perspective, became the model for understanding disease more generally. The concept of graduated blood pressure and the field of medical epidemiology mutually and simultaneously established one another.

Geoffrey Rose, like Miall, was a graduate of St Mary's and had been Pickering's registrar. He became one of the leading epidemiologists in Britain, with appointments at St Mary's and the London School of Hygiene and Tropical Medicine. The epidemiology he helped to establish was frankly imperialistic: unlike existing specialties such as venereology or orthopaedics, it made general theoretical claims. It cited statistics to undermine non-statistical clinical judgment. Barker and Rose showed that clinicians couldn't agree on the presence or absence of ankle pulses in most patients, while cardiologists couldn't agree that a given ECG tracing revealed ischaemia. "Opinions ranged from that of the sanguine Dr. N, who thought that only 5 per cent were abnormal, to that of gloomy Dr. F, who saw evidence of ischaemia in no less than 58 percent. One can imagine the confusion that would result if Dr. N and Dr. F were to conduct surveys on the frequency of heart disease in two different populations."[39] This was the old debate between objective and subjective methods, between the sphygmograph and the educated finger, in new form. The epidemiologists produced an objective calculus of subjectivity, and then reduced that subjectivity by the minuteness of their instructions. Where Platt and Pickering had argued about the reliability of blood pressures taken by nurses, Rose framed rules so detailed that anyone could perform them and get the same results.

Minutely structured observations created finely differentiated clinical findings. Aided by Miall and Rose, Stanley Peart chaired a working party for a large MRC-funded clinical trial into the treatment of mild hypertension. In 17,354 patients with mild hypertension, some received a beta-blocker, some a diuretic, and some a placebo. The drugs did not prevent heart attacks and had only a limited effect overall on the incidence of stroke. But when the diuretic was given to older men in higher risk categories, it did significantly reduce the likelihood of stroke and coronary thrombosis.[40] By surveying enormous numbers of patients and by correlating the variables on a computer, the working party was able to devise clinical indications beyond the scope of a single practitioner or even a single consultant.

The new epidemiology also began to scrutinize healthy people with all the intensity it had previously reserved for the sick. Health is a second-order

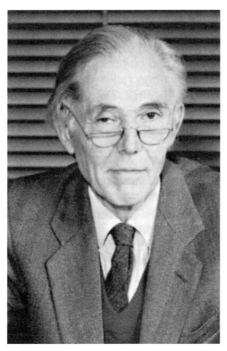

Geoffrey Rose.
St Mary's Hospital NHS Trust Archives

concept, dependent on the study of ill-health, which itself had to be finely tuned. One could not know the prognosis of high blood pressure until one had distinguished it from ordinary blood pressure, and unless one could know the prognosis of high blood pressure, there was no point in throwing all the resources of pharmacology at it. That had never really worried anyone in the past. Traditionally, doctors built up clienteles by giving patients what they wanted – namely, drugs. Patients and hospital governors footed the bill, and neither were in a position to dispute the clinician's judgment, except by seeking a second opinion. But under a state system of medicine, the government had both the grounds and the authority to question and undermine existing therapeutic regimes. It had the grounds because, under the new centralized regime, small adjustments could bring enormous savings. It had the authority by grace of the new medical statistics.

If illness were only a quantitative deviation from health, as researchers like Pickering and Rose argued, then it would be susceptible to audit, to rational calculus. This was the other side of the breakdown of clinical judgment into measurable, formalizable minutiae. It was not merely disease that was quantitative: the very act of reasoning itself became mere addition and subtraction, multiplication and division. Medical judgment could by this token be subjected to political judgment. The state could wield an authority over the doctors that the hospital governors had never attained.

Politicians had reason to encourage medical epidemiology as a discipline. But it would be wrong to suggest that clinical epidemiology checked medical costs. Epidemiology moved the goal posts of health, so that more and more of life seemed essentially unhealthy. This can be illustrated by another line of research that emerged from the Pickering-Peart medical unit: the Kenya hypertension survey, undertaken during the late 1970s.

During the 1970s researchers grew interested in the rapid increase in so-called western diseases such as cancer and hypertension in non-western countries. If, as the clinical epidemiologists suggested, hypertension was a disease of environment and lifestyle, then its pathogenesis might be better understood by comparing societies as well as individuals. With Peart's support, workers at St Mary's collaborated with researchers in Kenya to study the effects of migration on blood pressure. They found a group, the Luo tribe in Kenya, who had low blood pressures that did not rise with age. Then they shifted their focus to Nairobi, Kenya's capital, and measured the blood pressure of Luo immigrants. Over three hundred new immigrants were followed for up to two years, but it was evident that even at one month blood pressures were higher. The Luo migrants were eating more salt, and the investigators hypothesized that the stress of migration made them less able to excrete it.[41] The study suggested that modern urban society was itself pathogenic. The model of stress-induced disease could be applied to Britain, and it suggested rising demand for NHS services.

The Kenya study was developed in the new department of clinical pharmacology, headed by Peter Sever who came to St Mary's as a student in 1965. If Pickering was the first generation of medical academics at St Mary's, and Peart was the second generation, Sever was the third. His father was an international rugby player and friendly with Tommy Kemp, who suggested that young Peter might be happy at St Mary's, as indeed he was.[42] Sever received an education informed by both traditional and academic standards. He recalls Jack Litchfield as "one of Mary's finest clinicians of the old school … He was extremely widely read, and was able to give an informed opinion on virtually any medical case that he came into contact with. That just doesn't happen today. We are all so super-specialised that if we see anything that's remotely outside our field, you know, we tend to call in somebody else. That just didn't happen thirty years ago. Physicians covered virtually everything. And he really was a fantastic diagnostician and he was also entirely up-to-date with the latest treatments. He was a very sympathetic man. He had an incredible rapport with his patients. And again, that's something that you often don't see today. He wasn't a scientist, but then he never professed to be, and he never wanted to be." Stanley Peart, by contrast, "approached everything as a scientist would do. He would question everything. And if you made a statement about a patient, he would always ask why. And if you said, well, you'd read it in a book, he'd say, 'No, that's not the answer I want. I want the scientific answer.'"

Sever asked Peart for advice about a career in research. He recalls that Peart replied, "Well, you've got to go and be a scientist before you can do medical research ... You must have some training in basic scientific methods." Peart sent Sever to the biochemistry department where, under Professor Tecwyn Williams, he completed a doctorate in drug metabolism, studying how amphetamines affected the body. The amphetamines he studied behaved like adrenaline and noradrenaline. In the medical unit, a visiting Australian, Austin Doyle, was trying to show a link between those two hormones and hypertension. Sever was intrigued and, on finishing his PhD, he moved to the unit. The team produced a controlled study of young people with hypertension, showing excessive sympathetic activity.

In 1980 St Mary's created a department of clinical pharmacology and named Sever to the chair. It was becoming clear that the action of drugs needed more careful study: until the thalidomide disaster of the early 1960s, there was almost no drug regulation at all in Britain. Medical students had to be taught what drugs to combine and what to keep apart. The new department was tiny – "One man and a dog. Didn't even have a dog!" – but would become one of the school's largest, with a staff of fifty. Drug companies now provide much of the research funds, though Sever is careful to ensure that the research remains independent and scientific. He continues to study hypertension, but his interests have moved on from hormones to the cell structure of the vessel wall and – using imaging equipment developed in the nuclear fuels industry – the patterns of blood flow in the arteries.

Clinical pharmacology, clinical epidemiology, and angiotensin were all offshoots of the research program that Pickering introduced to St Mary's and that his students carried on. There were other offshoots as well. Peart and four workers – J.J. Brown, D.L. Davies, A.F. Lever, and J.I.S. Robertson – continued to investigate the renin-angiotensin system and especially the role of ionized calcium and sodium in stimulating renin release.[43] The laboratory work on the neurohumoral mechanisms enabled Sever and his group to explain why migrating Luo experienced raised blood pressure on moving to Nairobi. Stress caused an increased sympathetic outflow, primarily to the heart and kidneys, that overrode "the negative feedback inhibition of renal sympathetic nerve activity which would normally be expected with sodium loading." The normal homeostatic relationships were imbalanced.

Lever, Brown, and Robertson moved to Glasgow and created a research institute of their own. Peart continued to study renin and other pressor substances at St Mary's. Dogs and rugby players made fine research subjects for many of these experiments. From time to time there were mishaps, and Francis Diggins recalled being at the receiving end of one of these. When being prepared for injection with a new hormone that raised blood pressure in animals, Diggins "began to shake and shiver, and feel hot and cold, and feel bloody ill, and they had to whip the infusion out. My temperature went up to 105, and they put me up in the ward, and my wife threatened to murder Stan Peart!"[44] The giving set probably contained pyrogens.

The Surgical Unit and Its Offshoots

The medical unit also helped the surgical unit to develop vascular surgery. The foundation of this work was laid by Felix Eastcott, one of Moran's rugger scholars. Eastcott was born in Canada but raised in the West Country, where two of his uncles were medical men. Coming from a soccer school, he played only third-string rugby at St Mary's, but he enjoyed the student life tremendously. While still an undergraduate, on the advice of the physiology lecturer, he took his Primary FRCS, along with a few other students, "the ones who were getting reasonable marks, and didn't mind holding back our clinical work for three months." When the war began, he was evacuated to the Hammersmith Hospital, where the postgraduate atmosphere was enquiring rather than didactic, "just the opposite of Mary's." A stint as surgical registrar at Harefield provoked an interest in thoracic surgery.

At the end of the war, Porritt proposed Eastcott for a registrar exchange with the Peter Bent Brigham Hospital in Boston. The PBB was a world-class centre for surgical research, and by associating with it, St Mary's joined the vanguard of vascular surgery. Eastcott was assigned to the laboratory of a biochemist-physiologist. Eastcott recalls, "And after about a week, he said, 'Well, how are you getting on with your preliminary reading?' I said, 'Well, it's ... frankly, it's double Dutch to me!' 'Oh,' he said, 'I wondered about that!' So he said, 'Well, look,' he said, 'There's a guy over in the dog lab, who's taking out arteries and freezing them and putting them back in again. Do you think that would be ...' I said, 'That sounds absolutely up my street. I would like to do that.' He said, 'Right. Let's go over and have a look.'"[45] Thus was Felix Eastcott introduced to Charles Hufnagel and David Hume, two great pioneers in transplantation surgery. By the end of the year, Eastcott had done a hundred major grafting operations.

Eastcott returned to St Mary's as assistant director of the surgical unit in 1950–51. Charles Rob had already come from St Thomas's to replace Pannett in the chair of surgery in 1950. The unit was, jointly with the physiology department (for it had no lab of its own), investigating tendon grafts in rabbits and using arterial grafts to bridge gaps in a divided ureter.[46] However, few British surgeons were performing vascular surgery, and the field was wide open. Under Rob and Eastcott, St Mary's became an internationally famous centre for vascular surgery.

One success was the thromboendarectomy of the carotid artery performed in 1954.[47] The case was a sixty-six-year-old housewife who had suffered dozens of transient left-sided cerebral and retinal ischaemic attacks. For about twenty to thirty minutes she would find herself unable to move her right limbs or left eye, or speak, or swallow. David Sutton, the hospital radiographer, performed the new procedure of a carotid arteriogram and showed that the vessel was almost completely occluded by an atheromatous lesion, which was, Sutton, Rob, Eastcott, and Pickering decided, sending bits of atheroma "flying off into the brain." The only solution seemed to be to replace the occluded artery, but the patient would die if the blood supply to the brain was cut off for more than fifteen minutes.

When Pickering warned that a terminal stroke was imminent, Eastcott agreed to operate. The team cooled the woman's body temperature to 28°C, opened up the carotid artery, and performed a direct anastomosis between the common and internal carotid arteries. The entire procedure took twenty-eight minutes.

This was not, in fact, the first thromboendarectomy: one had been done in Texas a few months earlier. However, when Eastcott wrote up his account, his operation was the one that became internationally famous and widely imitated. His first inkling of this came several years later when he went to a conference and found himself staring at his own slides.[48]

The thromboendarectomy has become a routine measure to prevent stroke, but it was less successful at curing stroke, which was what the surgical unit then tried to do with it. There were other firsts, including some of the first operations to replace an artery with a vein, leaving the saphenous vein in situ, performed by a visiting Dane, Karl Hall.[49]

The surgical unit was an early pioneer of a more drastic treatment for renal failure: kidney transplantation. Ken Porter, a pathologist, put the idea forward, enlisting the support of the medical unit, including Peart and James Mowbray, who in turn enlisted the support of surgical colleagues Ken Owen and J.R. Kenyon. Once again there was American influence upon the work: Mowbray spent a year in Peter Brent Brigham learning peritoneal dialysis. Porter did the pathology for one of the leading American transplant units in Denver and mediated between that team and St Mary's. The procedures evolved with experience. Initially, live donors were used, and the patients were irradiated to prevent rejection. Cherry Wise and Elizabeth Carless, two newly qualified nurses at St Mary's in the early 1960s, remember nursing an early case in a private room which they scrubbed from top to bottom. The patient, a man who had gone into total renal failure, received a new kidney from his wife. The wife told Cherry Wise that "she'd given him her kidney, not so much for his sake, because I think she realised that he was very likely to die, but for the sake of all those who had kidney failure in the future."[50] The patient did indeed die: the irradiation reduced his immune response, but it also made him vulnerable to fungal organisms that hadn't been entirely eradicated. The nurses were invited to attend the post-mortem meeting on the case and shown slides of the monilia fungus that had invaded his arteries and bronchia.

In 1959 the team at St Mary's began to work with cadaveric kidneys taken from healthy young people who had had died unexpectedly. About the same time, Ken Porter brought Roy Calne, the man who had established cadaveric renal transplants, to St Mary's. Calne had attended a lecture by immunologists Peter Medawar, Rupert Billingham, and Leslie Brent in the mid-1950s when the three announced they had transplanted organs in mice by inducing tolerance when the mice were immunologically immature. Because no such tolerance could be induced in mature animals, Medawar told the audience that the work had no clinical implications. Still, Calne was excited, and he began trying transplants using irradiation. With Porter, he tried an anti-leukemia drug said to arrest antibody production in rabbits. By 1960, the two men had some success with dogs, with some transplants still functioning at one month. Calne then moved to the Peter Brent Brigham, where they were still irradiating, and brought azathioprine with him.

At St Mary's, while Ken Porter's lab flourished, the surgery was stalled. Bill Irvine, who had replaced Rob as professor of surgery in 1961, offered Calne a registrarship. He was invited, Calne speculated in an interview, to do the kidney transplantation, "I think to take away from the other surgeons who were doing it and had one hundred per cent fatality with irradiation. They didn't want to change, no one ever does want to change, but when it was pointed out to them by Stan Peart, who was professor of medicine, that their results weren't very good – in fact, they couldn't be worse – there was reluctant agreement to change to immunosuppression and we started to get some better results."[51] Soon afterwards, Calne moved to the Westminster Hospital.

By the mid-1960s St Mary's had a flourishing transplant team with survival statistics better than the average. Of the thirty-eight patients given cadaveric transplants before July 1965, only five were still alive in 1968. Between July 1965 and June 1968 another seventy-six transplants were performed on sixty-five patients, and half were still alive in 1969.[52] That year Porter parlayed the transplantation work into a new experimental pathology wing, funded privately and by the University of London.

Ancillary Sciences: Two Examples

One research department spawned another. Metabolic studies and radiology grew from and supported the surgical work. Surgery, no less than medicine, requires a precise knowledge of the action of chemicals, hormones, and fluids in health and disease. Trauma, including surgical trauma, can cause many different metabolic disturbances, such as excess hydration leading to swelling and oedema. When lost fluids are restored, they must be the right fluids, with carefully measured proportions of such chemicals as potassium and nitrogen. This is pathological chemistry, but at St Mary's pathological chemistry was done by forensic toxicologists. They were very good at locating and measuring arsenic, the poison of choice for English murderers, but they were not au fait with other developments in the field. Without precise measurements, the consultants were hard pressed to diagnose

Victor Wynn. St Mary's Hospital NHS Trust Archives and the Royal College of Surgeons of England

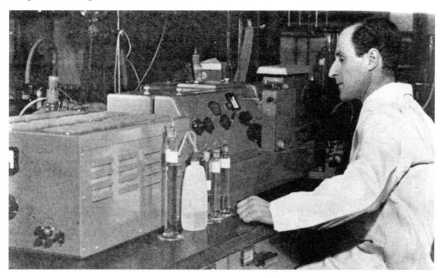

and manage their patients. Hence, Peter Sanderson built a flame photometer in the medical unit, and Victor Wynn built one in the surgical unit. Under Wynn, precise measurement of human metabolism became a far-reaching program of research, leading to his appointment as the first professor of metabolic studies in England.

Victor Wynn came to St Mary's from Australia in 1950 with a Nuffield postdoctoral fellowship. He found St Mary's "Dickensian," if no worse than labs elsewhere in Britain. Though qualified as a physician, he was appointed to the surgical unit by Charles Rob, and he soon took over the unit labs, which were standing idle. There, he developed and perfected a series of techniques for measuring metabolic activity such as osmotic exchange among body cells, water intoxication, and pH balances, which became standard in the field.[53] Without Wynn's measurements, the surgical unit could never have developed as it did. His studies of fluid retention and excretion were crucial to the development of the kidney work at St Mary's.[54]

Subsequently, Wynn turned to anabolic steroids, which were developed during the 1950s. These acted on protein metabolism, enabling muscles to store protein and therefore to bulk up. Suddenly they were being prescribed for all manner of complaints, but no one knew anything of their long-term effects. Wynn discovered that the steroids had serious side effects, and the use of anabolic steroids for therapeutic purposes was rapidly reduced. He was also one of the first to study the long-term effects of the contraceptive pill and to link it to thrombosis.[55] At the end of the 1960s, he created a public furore when he announced on television that the pill in its current form was dangerous. Subsequently, high-oestrogen contraceptives were replaced by contraceptives with a low oestrogen content.

Wynn had an ambivalent relationship with the rest of the medical school. When he came in 1950, he was almost alone in applying a quantitative approach to clinical medicine. The traditional consultants had little use for his work, but happily that meant he could follow his own research agenda. Obtaining the school's approval was easy, obtaining money and beds less so. He created space in Clarence Wing by displacing the domestic staff. His lab was built in the Mint Stables, a spectacular multi-storey building erected in the late nineteenth century for the horses that carried the goods transported up by rail to Paddington station. Convincing British Rail to sell the disused property proved easier than convincing St Mary's to buy; but with money from the university, the Nuffield Foundation, and with a friendly construction company working for free, the lab was finally opened.

Like Almroth Wright, Victor Wynn attracted a lucrative, international consulting and private practice, and he invested the receipts in the labora-

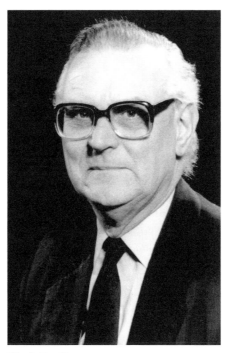

Hugh Dudley.
St Mary's Hospital NHS Trust Archives

tory. He also attracted enormous grants from the American National Institutes of Health. By the time he retired in 1986, he was attracting approximately £80 in soft money for every pound he was paid by the medical school. He used these funds to establish a new research clinic, the Cavendish Clinic, funded by the Heart Disease and Diabetes Research Trust, which he had set up in 1980.[56]

Radiology was another line of work that developed with the surgical unit. Ernest Rohan Williams, who was head of radiology at St Mary's until 1963, had done house jobs in both the medical and surgical units in the 1920s. Though he concentrated on gynaecology and ultrasound, he brought in David Sutton, a specialist in vascular and cardiac work who ensured that St Mary's led the country in that field. Sutton produced dozens of papers and monographs, including a standard textbook, and by the time of his retirement in 1983, ten of the twelve London teaching hospitals had a consultant radiologist who had trained at St Mary's.[57] The radiologists laboured to import the latest technologies including, most recently, a magnetic resonance scanner, permitting the surgeon to scan and operate simultaneously. Oscar Craig, who filled Rohan Williams's position in 1963 (and, like Williams, became a president of the Royal College of Radiologists), specialized in the radiology of the gut, another focus of the surgical unit.

Gastric Surgery

Gastric surgery has always been a focus of research and practice in the St Mary's surgical unit, beginning with Charles Pannett, continuing with Bill Irvine and Hugh Dudley in the 1960s and 1970s, and maintained into the twenty-first century by Ara Darzi. While the NHS consultants developed the vascular work, the Academic Board determined to maintain the gastric work in the unit. Irvine was appointed as a gastric surgeon but decided to take on some of the vascular work. Unfortunately, under the strain of trying to undertake this new and difficult field, he had something of a breakdown and in 1973 was removed from his post. When his successor, Hugh Dudley, came, the surgical unit was in the doldrums: "Morale was at a low ebb and the research was desultory."[58]

Dudley soon changed all of that. Born in Dublin and trained in Edinburgh, at the end of the 1950s he studied surgical metabolism at the Peter Bent Brigham. He held appointments in Edinburgh and Aberdeen, then held a chair in Monash University in Melbourne, and developed an expertise in trauma by serving in Viet Nam. When he came to St Mary's, he brought considerable energy to the task of building up the unit. He was a prolific researcher and writer, producing many elegantly written papers and several monographs, on a wide range of subjects. He reinvigorated the Surgical Research Society of Great Britain as much as he did his own department. With an assistant director, Peter Fielding, he developed the large bowel cancer project, a large-scale audit of surgical results, at a time when many surgeons still shied away from publicizing their negative results. He castigated reticence as harmful to patients and the progress of surgery, a viewpoint gradually coming to prevail. His surgical innovations ranged from technical improvements to instruments to the practice of colonic lavage in emergency bowel surgery. At his retirement in 1988, surgeons from around the world gathered to testify to his influence on the development of their profession.

Dudley's successor was Pierre Guillou, who trained in Leeds and specialized in the treatment of tumours, but after four years, he returned to Leeds, to take up a chair. With Guillou's departure, the surgical unit fell back into the hands of the vascular surgeons, as NHS consultant Averil Mansfield became the acting chair. She had joined St Mary's in 1982 as Felix Eastcott's replacement and on Guillou's departure was given a personal chair, becoming the first female professor of surgery in Britain. The press remarked at the time that her achievements in this very macho world were the more remarkable for her distinctly unmacho, gentle, and genial manner. Mansfield and her colleagues have carried on the vascular work at St Mary's with

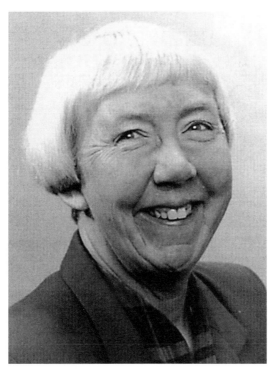

Averil Mansfield.
St Mary's Hospital NHS Trust Archives

great success. Cardiac surgery is a boom industry, and the department remains one of the leading centres. It takes referrals from across the country, performs some of the most drastic operations, and has trained leading vascular surgeons.

While the vascular surgery remained a very strong line of work at St Mary's, direction of the academic surgical unit passed back to the gut surgeons with the appointment of Ara Darzi in 1998. Darzi, who trained in Dublin, specializes in laparoscopic or keyhole surgery, using miniaturized cameras that permit him to make very small incisions. Related technologies developed within the department in partnership with industry, include retroperitoneal balloon-dissection, endoscopic surface guided repair of inguineal hernia, and video rigid sigmoidoscopy. Darzi is also involved in the development of robotic techniques and has, further, patented a computer program that teaches and assesses surgical skill. Watching him lecture, one has the sense of a powerful force being unleashed.

Ara Darzi is fully representative of the old and the new in surgery. While he is every inch the consultant surgeon, with faultless elegance of manner, speech, and dress, his academic profile is untraditional; he publishes extensively and is at the forefront of the mechanization of surgery. In his hands, surgery merges with both science and technology. His appointment signals

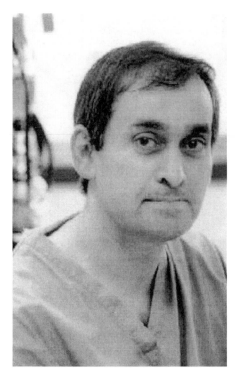

Ara Darzi.
St Mary's Hospital NHS Trust Archives

a new era for surgery, which has remained largely wedded to its craft traditions. (Darzi himself denounces the current academic pressures on surgery and points out that verbosity and skill are not the same thing.[59]) Under Darzi, the surgical unit continues to be a centripetal influence. He integrates St Mary's and the institution with which it has become enmeshed: Imperial College of Science and Technology. Because surgery was moving that way, he was appointed; now that he is appointed, surgery will move further that way.

Other Academic Units

Clinical science sprang up in new academic units as beds became available. Paediatric beds were plentiful after 1948 when two local children's hospitals joined the St Mary's teaching group, and thus in January 1949 an academic unit was formed in paediatrics, under a part-time director, Reginald Lightwood, who doubled as an NHS consultant. The unit had no labs of its own until 1951, so much of the work centred on the treatment of children in the community. There was also a program of research into neonatal respiration, while Lightwood himself specialized in renal acidosis of newborns.

Aleck Bourne's dream of an academic unit in obstetrics and gynaecology had been long frustrated by the lack of beds and the objections of colleagues who were reluctant to see this mainstay of general practice become too academic. In 1960 these obstacles were finally overcome, and Ian Mac-Gillivray was named professor. His research interest in blood pressure and fluid and electrolyte balance in normal pregnancy and in pre-eclampsia converged with those of the other professors. Still, much of the obstetrical and gynaecological work remained and remains in the hands of distinguished NHS consultants. Sir George Pinker served as president of the Royal College of Obstetricians and Gynaecologists and consultant to the royal family, including the queen from 1973. It was Pinker who insisted that the children of the prince and princess of Wales be born in the Lindo Wing, the first royal heirs to be born in hospital. Pinker initiated a successful project when he observed to James Mowbray, then a lecturer in the medical unit, that he often saw healthy young women who suffered repeated miscarriages for no apparent reason. Drawing on observations made in Boston, Mowbray developed a treatment with purified paternal lymphocytes, resulting in over 1,500 live births over the next fifteen years.

Lack of beds hampered the expansion of clinical departments at St Mary's. As other schools specialized, St Mary's was left behind. The school's annual report for 1960–61 struck a note of desperation: "The Medical School Council and Academic Board feel it is absolutely essential that building of the new Hospital should commence in 1966." The rebuilding project remained mired in the politics of health rationing for two more decades, and the clinical professoriat remained small. By 1970 St Mary's had nineteen professors, most of them either in or offshoots of the preclinical departments. Pharmacology, for example, developed from the physiology department, while the chair in metabolism grew out of the chemical pathology department. These departments had only a few beds at best. Others chairs were funded with private donations or research money. A rearrangement of beds in the hospital district enabled the school to create an academic department of psychiatry in 1973. Geoffrey Rose, named professor of epidemiology in 1971, used an out-patient clinic rather than beds. The next clinical chair to be created was that of Peter Sever in clinical pharmacology in 1980.

When the number of beds was finally increased at the Praed Street site, the University of London had no spare money for new chairs. But at the end of the 1980s, money for new appointments was found in NHS funds, and the clinical professoriat expanded at last. By the early 1990s the school counted six professors of basic science, seven professors of pathological science, and twenty-seven professors of clinical science (including three shared with other schools) spread across ten departments: obstetrics and gynaecology, anaesthetics, clinical pharmacology, medicine, paediatrics, general practice, radiology/radiotherapy/oncology, psychiatry, and public health.

The history of St Mary's Hospital and Medical School after 1945 reflects the explosive growth of science but also the braking effect of limited resources. When Moran brought in George Pickering, he ensured that the school would be at the forefront of clinical research for the foreseeable future. Pickering's own research interests were only the initial spark to the development of a wide-ranging program. His outstanding teaching skills attracted highly able young men and women to the medical unit, and his wide network of friends and alliances enabled him to find research positions for these young men and women.

At first the government's support for the expansion of the medical schools seemed almost unlimited. So long as a dean could argue convincingly that a new appointment would advance science and provide better clinical care, he was likely to get it. In 1982 Denis Brinton, dean from 1946 to 1952, recalled those days wistfully in a private letter: "But those were the days for Deans! 'Spend all you can, old chap,' the authorities said."[60] In those early years, the obstacles to expansion were local: the lack of beds and the conservatism of the consultant staff. To understand how these obstacles were overcome, it is necessary to stand back from the development of the academic units and survey the increasing scientization of the medical school as a whole, as the next two chapters undertake to do. The following section then raises the matter of political support, or lack thereof, for the expansion of the hospital.

❦ 11

The School Scientized

THE SECOND WORLD war marked a turning point in British science. As historian Dominique Pestre remarks, it was a "scientific and technological war" that "mobilized and trained a large number of scientists, engineers, and technicians, and has never ended."[1] Until the war, government funding for science was fairly small.[2] After the war, science commanded a new influence in Whitehall, and its investment in scientific education and research increased. The Medical Research Council, for example, received less than £150,000 per annum until the mid-1930s, and only rose above £200,000 towards the end of the Second World War. Those MRC funds increased tenfold during the 1950s and a hundredfold during the 1960s.[3] Universities and learned societies received £1.5 million in government research and development funding in 1945–46 and £8.3 million in 1950–51,[4] while total government spending on higher education rose from £26 million in 1937–38 to £90 million in 1954–55.[5]

Demand for science in the medical schools was growing. They already had science departments to teach basic biology, chemistry, and physics, as well as applied medical sciences such as physiology, biochemistry, and pathology. New technologies like the electron microscope, the ultracentrifuge, electrophoresis, and radio-labelling permitted closer study of the molecules involved in the process of disease and might, for example, lead to a new vaccine or a new drug. The age of "biomedicine" was launched.[6]

Scientific research and medical research grew closer in spirit and technique. Hospital consultants still controlled the wards and dominated hospital policy, but they could no longer dominate school policy. Using UGC money, the University of London required the medical schools to hire scientists for the preclinical departments. As more and more scientists were hired, the balance of power shifted. Encouraged by the general atmosphere of science-worship and by the examples of large research institutes scattered around the country, these scientists were very demanding. At St Mary's they formed a powerful coalition of interests, organized around the physical space of the old Inoculation Department. Already by 1950 university inspectors observed of St Mary's that "a spirit of research appears to be active throughout the School."[7]

Previous chapters have neglected the preclinical sciences to focus on the clinicians. This chapter redresses the neglect by sketching out the development of the major preclinical departments over the course of the twentieth century: biochemistry, anatomy, and physiology. It also surveys the postwar fortunes of four pathological sciences: bacteriology, immunology, haematology, and virology. The old Inoculation Department maintained an income from vaccines that sheltered its pathological departments from developments occurring in other scientific fields. Both its income and scientific reputation declined until the end of the 1950s, when the departments were reconstructed.

The early scientific departments at St Mary's were idiosyncratic. One man would run a preclinical department, often single-handedly, for decades. However, once the departments began to grow, from one-man shows into genuine departments with readers, lecturers, research assistants, and graduate students, the population fluctuated. At the junior level in particular, there was a new interchangeability of staff across departments, hospitals, and countries. As science education developed throughout Britain, junior scientists increasingly shared common terms, concepts, and equipment. Often researchers visited other schools for a few weeks or months to learn and transmit new techniques. There was a great deal of travel to and from the United States, home to some of the world's largest research establishments. Individual research projects were increasingly embedded in international research agendas.[8] There was greater standardization of people and concepts. In Kuhnian terms, the community or paradigm with which an individual researcher identified him or herself became an international one.

André Malraux has observed that the world has become a "museum without walls" whereby all forms of art, whatever the intention of the artist, are comparable and classifiable, part of a continuum.[9] So too, science has come to exist in a "laboratory without walls." It has become "science" as well as a congeries of sciences, although disciplines and even laboratories still have their own subcultures. No single event in the history of recent science can be told outside this international context. As the previous chap-

ter has established, an adequate historical account of any one scientific department, or even one line of research within a department, requires a
chapter in itself – a deeply technical chapter and one not confined to any
particular institution.

In the 1790s the Marquis de Condorcet argued that the more facts and
relations between facts that were discovered, the more general and simple
knowledge would become: "In proportion as the understanding embraces
more complicated combinations, a simple mode of announcing these combinations renders them more easy to be treated."[10] The marquis was too
sanguine. The specialization of medical knowledge, a product of the
growth of medical research, led to a fragmentation of the British medical
field.[11] It was a process that the great generalists of the London teaching
hospitals resisted as best they could but that nonetheless finally transformed those same teaching hospitals as they too became fragmented. A
handful of researchers became dozens, then hundreds, pursuing hundreds
of research projects, each with their own language, technique, culture, or
paradigm. Viewed from an institutional perspective, that of the school as a
whole, the effect was intellectual heterogeneity. In short, this chapter bears
the unhappy burden of conveying narrative inadequacy: individual disciplines become alien and incomprehensible to the general reader, and the
"big picture" becomes one of intellectual incoherence.

Postwar science at St Mary's cannot, therefore, be adequately examined
here. But that inadequacy is itself an important point of departure for further analysis. As the science became more unknowable, the consequences
of its being known grew. Claims to specialized and expert knowledge,
knowledge impenetrable to any but specialized experts, are at the core of
the modern medical profession and, indeed, of the whole institutional
structure of modern science within which medical scientists claim standing.
As the threshold between professional and public knowledge shifts, so must
the analytical focus of this book. Previous chapters have asked how medical men knew what they knew. Subsequent chapters will pay greater attention to how knowledge claims were successfully translated into
institutional and political power, and the consequences of this success. This
chapter straddles the two approaches. It begins by recapitulating the processes described in the previous chapter so as to show how rudimentary,
idiosyncratic research was transformed into highly specialized research
programs in one preclinical science department after another, culminating
in the reconstruction of Wright's Institute. It describes the kinds of activities that occupied and occupy most researchers at St Mary's most of the
time. Meanwhile, at the institutional level, it identifies the growing collective strength of these scientists and the ways they advanced their fields,

sometimes in the face of obstruction from the clinicians. *Pace* Haldane, these men proved that state-of-the-art science could be done in an independent medical school. But their very success was to prove the school's undoing. If medicine was, at bottom, really science, then it followed, according to Haldane's late-twentieth-century counterparts, that medicine should be studied and taught in a university.

Two events marked the turning point for St Mary's. One was the end of Moran's long regime. Lord Moran had become a senior statesman of medicine, impatient with the minutiae that occupy the time of a dean. He became an absent autocrat. By the early 1940s although he was re-elected each December, the vote was no longer unanimous. At the end of the war, he was deposed, and Denis Brinton, the neurologist, became the new dean. The coup was substantially the work of the preclinical departments and of Arthur Huggett in particular. Huggett produced countless memos on policy, for example, complaining that St Mary's had the lowest Treasury grant among medical schools in 1945. Fifteen years later, it would have one of the highest, thanks to a series of aggressive deans. Moran had not been conspicuously hostile to science, as his appointment of Huggett and Pickering demonstrated, but it was only after his departure that the school could be substantially reformed.

The second milestone was the 1944 Goodenough report. This was the work of an interdepartmental committee on medical education that included some distinguished clinicians. The report advised the government to invest in medical education so as to put it on a sound scientific footing. In October 1942 St Mary's was invited to give evidence to the Goodenough committee. The MSC drew up a memo entitled "The Development of the Teaching Hospital along University Lines."[12] Two things, as they saw it, were at stake. On the one hand, teachers should be full-time salaried teachers with advanced qualifications. Medical education should resemble university education. But it should not lose its special identity: clinical teaching. Thus, on the other hand, the memo demanded close relations between hospital and school. It even suggested that teaching hospitals should have a common governing body "with that degree of autonomy usually assigned to governing bodies of constituent colleges or departments of the University to which it belongs," and where teachers would predominate.

The teaching staff got most of what it wanted. There was not a common governing body: hospitals came under the NHS and schools under the University of London. But hospital and school policy were closely integrated. One effect of Goodenough was to subordinate hospital to school policy. Teaching hospitals only maintained their autonomy from local authorities so long as they had a school attached. Keeping that school afloat became the number-one priority among hospital governors: their own appointments were at stake. Because Goodenough specified that teaching hospitals should have between seven hundred and a thousand beds, the teaching status of a small hospital like St Mary's seemed precarious, so the governors were all the more anxious to placate the university authorities and the academic staff.

From 1948 both St Mary's school and hospital were state institutions, but they remained substantially autonomous. The school was probably the more closely inspected of the two, by the university and the General Medical Council. But though it relinquished some autonomy, the school was well recompensed. Salary costs rose from roughly £15,000 to above £50,000 in 1947 and above £100,000 two years later. By the early 1960s the figure doubled again. Government grants underwrote the expansion. This dramatic increase in funding transformed the atmosphere of the medical school. Before the war, salaries were largely restricted to those who did not practise medicine: the staff of the preclinical departments (as well as the academic units). Research positions were almost non-existent. A lecturer and a few student demonstrators might make up a department. After the war, professors, supported by readers, lecturers, technicians, and research students, became the norm. Medical school science departments began to resemble university science departments.

The scientists sensed the change of public mood and pressed their advantage, demanding greater support for advanced teaching and research. In October 1943 Huggett the physiologist, Idris Jones the biologist, and George Ellis the chemist sent Moran a memo that argued that the preclinical departments should teach less and have more money and time for research.[13] Individuals should be able "to develop without economic trammels." The workload should be one part teaching to two parts research, and one third of the teaching should be small-group "investigational" teaching – blood counts, titrations, dissections, nerve stimulations – rather than mass lectures. Full chairs should be created in physiology, biochemistry, chemical pathology, and pharmacology, with top salaries at £2,000. As a result of this petition, a larger subcommittee was named, representing all the preclinical departments and chaired by Huggett, which made even bolder demands. It demonstrated that St Mary's had fewer scientific staff than other London teaching hospitals. The average staff in physiology departments, for example, was seven, and St Mary's had only three.[14] A decade earlier, these arguments would have sounded extreme; by the 1940s they seemed self-evident.

Renewing the Older Departments

Take biochemistry. The department was created from the old chemistry department in 1948, with R.T. Williams in the inaugural chair.[15] His predecessor was George Ellis, who came into St Mary's in 1921 with a BSc to teach organic chemistry. Ellis had investigated the recovery of oil from waste during the war, and his research work was in cholesterol and the auto-oxidation of oils, work for which he eventually received a DSc. During the 1920s Ellis supplemented his income by working as a London gas examiner, analysing coal gas to ensure that it conformed to statutory composition and calorific value. One of the other candidates in 1921, George King, was hired as a junior lecturer, and he began to teach ex-servicemen older than himself, according to one appreciation of King, "during those years when the staff had to fail to notice fireworks on feast days and to learn to handle the occasional riot with unobtrusive tact." The post was only part-time, so King also worked as the biochemist to the Margaret Street Hospital. Then, during the 1930s, he took charge of the physics teaching at St Mary's while still maintaining the chemistry. His early work was in fish respiration, but under Ellis he too took up the oxidation of oils and obtained a DSc in 1943, at which point he became a full-time lecturer.[16]

On his retirement Ellis advocated that a chair be created in biochemistry. He, King, and their students had, he argued, already attracted an international reputation. (The students were A.C. Frazer and H. Stewart. Frazer performed important research on fat metabolism, the properties of the oil-water interface, and related questions of nutrition and toxicology. He became an advisor to the WHO and the British government, and obtained a chair in Birmingham. Stewart became professor of pharmacology at St Mary's where he worked on pain and analgesia with Dame Cicely Saunders.) But their research had been done between consulting work and an onerous teaching load, without institutional support. Ellis had had to improvise research apparatus, for example, painting linseed oil on the glass panels of his bookcases in order to get films for oxidation. Sometimes he obtained research grants, as in 1926 when he was granted £20 by the Inoculation Department for apparatus.[17]

It was very different for the new department of biochemistry. R.T. Williams made the department the flagship of basic science research at St Mary's, attracting vast sums of money from companies interested in the physiological effects of chemicals with agricultural or industrial uses. He also came as an established scholar with a reputation for teaching and research. Williams was born and educated as a chemist in Wales, and then went to Liverpool. He began by studying the structure of glucuronic acid, obtained by feeding animals with camphor and borneol. Glucuronic acid was thought to play a role in detoxifying toxic substances by facilitating their excretion from the body.

Thus, unusually for a chemist, Williams was drawn to biological chemistry. He created the field of detoxification, a field that was to become of great importance, arguing that foreign compounds had their own biochemistry, distinct from the biochemistry of natural substances.[18] In 1947 he wrote a classic textbook. He investigated food additives, locust pesticides, abused drugs, and thalidomide. After that drug became front-page news in 1961, Williams's work was in great demand, and funding for drug metabolism studies increased exponentially. He also investigated animal experimentation, identifying metabolic differences between species. His arrival at St Mary's coincided with the development of new techniques of investigation, such as radio-isotope labelling, chromatography, and infrared absorption spectrophotometry. He was able to introduce these techniques into St Mary's quickly because he had strong support from industry and government.

The final line of William's Royal Society obituary remarks, "It is given to few to be an architect of new science; such was the fate of Tecwyn Williams." In effect, Williams created a large research establishment at St Mary's. His publications were legion, and so were his students. In 1958 he had five PhD students; five years later he had ten. Researchers in 1958 included two individuals funded by Salsbury's Laboratory (based in Iowa) studying the detoxication of meat additives in poultry; two others were sponsored by Distillers Company to study the metabolism and toxicity of fungicides used in wrapping paper; another studied insecticides with money from Shell Petroleum. The American Instrument Company donated a spectrophotoflurometer in exchange for a consultation.[19] Williams was also funded by the Colonial Office, the Ministry of Defence, the Agricultural Research Council, and the Medical Research Council. Visiting researchers in a given year came from Ibadan, Ghana, Milan, Michigan, and Iowa. By the time he retired in 1976, nine of his students had been appointed to chairs, and others were senior scholars approaching that rank. Williams became an FRS in 1967; in 1973 he won the CIBA medal of the Biochemical Society; he was awarded a host of honorary doctorates from universities around the world. He also worked hard to transform undergraduate education at St Mary's, establishing a BSc program within the school and serving as deputy dean.

Anatomy and physiology also saw changes. J. Ernest Frazer ran the anatomy department from 1911 to 1940. Born in 1870, he trained at Bart's and pursued a surgical career until a post-mortem infection of the hand

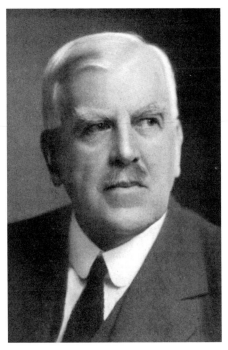

J. Ernest Frazer. Heinemann and
St Mary's Hospital NHS Trust Archives

diverted him to anatomy (though in wartime he took charge of surgical out-patients.) In 1911 he was unanimously elected as the first full-time anatomy lecturer, at £350 per annum. He commanded a demonstrator and a dissection-room attendant (dismissed in December 1915 for seduction and impersonating a student).[20] Operating expenses were £36.5.0. In 1914 Frazer was made professor by the University of London. After the war, on his threatening resignation, his salary was increased to £1,000, and he was allocated an assistant lecturer. Still, until his retirement, the salary costs of the department were well below £2,000. For nearly thirty years, with a shoestring budget and minimal assistance, Frazer ran the anatomy department at St Mary's as one of the leading centres of anatomical teaching and research in London. In a small laboratory overlooking South Wharf Road, he put together his classic, much-reprinted textbook *The Anatomy of the Human Skeleton*. As well, he became a leading embryologist of his day. He invited school alumni to send him embryos and gathered an incomparable collection illustrating normal and abnormal embryonic development.[21] He also attracted brilliant students, such as Ida Mann, who used his collection to write the first English study on the embryology of the eye.

By contrast, Frank Goldby, who held the chair from 1945 to 1970, commanded some of the best resources in the school. Goldby, who trained in Cambridge and King's College, was a comparative anatomist with a special interest in the degeneration of the peripheral nerves. By the time he retired, the department consisted of two professors, one reader, two senior lecturers, four lecturers, and several research assistants and graduate students. This collectivity published more than a dozen articles annually. A BSc program began in 1955. In 1950 the department received MRC funding for freeze-drying equipment, the better to study cytology. It was at the forefront of cell ultrastructure: in 1961–62, Goldby obtained £12,000 from the Wellcome Trust for an electron microscope, used by A.S. Breathnach for his work in epithelial cell anatomy and pigmentation. In 1965 anatomy cost slightly more than biochemistry to run, at £23,400 compared to biochemistry's £23,000; a decade later, the figures were £65,000 and £71,000.

After Waller quit the physiology chair in 1902, the department declined. Dickson Wright, master of the pithy put-down, recalled learning "anatomy under the great Frazer and physiology with the obscure Ellison and Roaf."[22] From 1920 to 1934, B.J. Collingwood ran the department. He had qualified at St Mary's in 1901 and worked with Waller on chloroform, and had been professor of physiology at Dublin before returning to St Mary's. A popular teacher, flamboyant and dogmatic,[23] Collingwood studied coagulation of the blood, and from 1923 marketed an anticoagulant, "protagulin," that brought in a few hundred pounds a year.

Collingwood's successor, Huggett, or "Hugo," was less popular with the students, who behaved badly in his classroom, once setting off pigeons. But when the rugby team spotted him attending a fancy-dress ball as a snowflake, they warmed to him. Huggett quietly turned the physiology department into a first-rate research centre. His own work, which earned him an FRS in 1958, was in foetal and placental physiology, a field that he did much to establish. He would immerse an ewe in a warm bath and maintain the foetus outside of its mother in this solution to study the gaseous and metabolic exchange. He laid the groundwork for research on neonatal development of the human, performed in collaboration with the obstetrics department. Huggett attracted large research grants, including £100,000 from the Wellcome Trust for a new wing with animal houses. (Lab workers recall chasing an errant sheep down Praed Street.)

Huggett trained some distinguished physiologists including his own successor, A.D.M. Greenfield, who came to St Mary's in 1934 as a medical student, and replaced A.C. Frazer as demonstrator in 1941. Like Huggett, Greenfield became an authority on blood flow. During the war he studied the problem of Spitfire pilots blacking out during fast turns. He built an enormous centrifuge, using a Buick back axle as a pivot, with a lead weight at one end and anaesthetized guinea pigs, cats, or monkeys at the other, their arterial, venous, intra-cardiac and intra-thoracic pressures, respiration, and heart-beat measured as they whizzed around in the small space of the physiology laboratory at a speed described as "terrifying to behold." The entire school shook with the force of the centrifuge. Greenfield showed that blackout was due to the breakdown of control by the carotid sinuses and that a water-suit could prevent it, a discovery the RAF soon put into practice.

Greenfield's centrifuge was a wartime casualty after an incendiary bomb fell through a skylight in February 1944. When one researcher exclaimed, "Thank Heavens the E.C.G. is undamaged," Greenfield exploded "Damn your E.C.G., it's only worth a couple of hundred; what about my centrifuge!"[24] Later work into the problem of weightlessness in space travel was funded by the Ministry of Defence. Greenfield went to Belfast, where he succeeded another Mary's man, Henry Barcroft, as professor of physiology, after Barcroft moved to St Thomas's. Greenfield returned to St Mary's as professor in 1964, only to leave in 1968 when he was appointed dean of the medical school in Nottingham.

Thus did the school expand. It had attracted some first-rate scientists before the Second World War, but these men had to cope with a near-complete absence of research facilities. Few were able, as J.E. Frazer was, to parlay their connection with the medical school into a solid research base. After the war more research money was available both internally and externally. Following nationalization, the hospital spent the income from its endowment fund on capital or clinical projects that could not get public funding, and on research. The fund was earmarked for consultants, on the understanding that laboratory scientists could find funds elsewhere.

Funding Research

Enormous funds were becoming available for research, both state-sponsored and private. Research council spending grew from £2.9 million in 1945–46 to £130 million by the early 1970s. About half the pie usually went to the Science Research Council, while the Medical Research Council accounted for less than a quarter. Private funding for medical research also expanded enormously. Some funding agencies sponsored work on particular diseases: the Heart Foundation, or the Imperial Cancer Research Fund, for example. Others were set up by a wealthy benefactor; the Nuffield Foundation was born of Morris Motors, while the Wellcome Trust was the brainchild of Henry Wellcome, a pharmaceutical manufacturer.

Without an exponential increase in research funding, the school could not have grown as it did. In the mid-1950s the total research income of £10,000 per year amounted to one-twentieth of the school's total income. Nearly £4,000 of the £10,000 came from the hospital Endowment Fund and a like amount from government research councils. A decade later, in 1967, research income amounted to £214,000, received from over a hundred donors. By the early 1970s it had doubled again to reach £480,000, almost a third of the school's income. By the early 1980s the research income at St Mary's was £2.29 million, equal to two-thirds of its grant from the UGC. Most of the research grants now came from private foundations (£1,180,000) rather than research councils (£360,000), with further money coming from international organizations (£410,000) and industry (£320,000). Finally, when St Mary's began to negotiate the merger with Imperial College, UGC income and research income were near parity, at £3.7 million and £4.4 million respectively, of a total income of £12.7 million.[25]

An agency that had a particular impact on St Mary's is the Wellcome Trust. A brief account of its development helps to flesh out the context for the school's development. Henry Wellcome was born in 1853, the son of an American lay preacher. He began professional life as a pharmacist and then, in England, with Silas Burroughs, made a fortune selling mass-produced tablets that he patented as "tabloids."[26] He founded a research laboratory in 1894, and Henry Dale worked there from 1904 to 1914, before he moved to the MRC's new National Institute for Medical Research at Hampstead. When Wellcome died in 1936, he left the shares of his pharmaceutical company to the trustees of his will to support medical research and medical history.[27] Henry Dale, now Sir Henry, a Nobel laureate and future president of the Royal Society, became chairman of the five trustees who awarded the grants. The funds were spent on an ad hoc basis, in response to requests. At first the amounts were small, and up to 1957 only £1 million had been awarded. After that the pharmaceutical firm began to flourish, and the income rose to £1 million per annum and increased gradually after that. Initially the funds were mainly used to provide accommodation and equipment. Sir Henry Dale retired in 1960, aged eighty-five, and a new generation of officers began to expand the program. By 1970 the income had risen to £2.5 million and the trust began to fund research programs rather than infrastructure.

One of the energetic new officers was Peter Williams, who served as a scientific secretary and later as director of the trust, charged with administering the grants and liasing with research groups. After graduating from St Mary's in the early 1950s, Williams had published *Careers in Medicine* and had worked for a few years for the MRC as a grants administrator and administrator of their tropical medicine branch, before moving to the Wellcome. St Mary's did well out of the Wellcome Trust, figuring in the top-ten list of its recipients. Between 1957 and 1969 St Mary's received £424,000 (out of £14.2 million); over the next fifteen years the grants amounted to

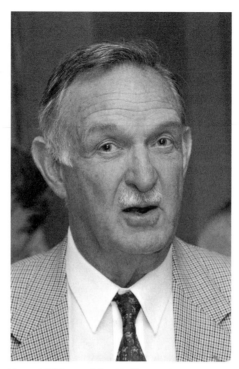

Peter Williams. The Wellcome Trust

nearly £3 million (out of £66 million). This was better than any other London undergraduate teaching hospital, save University College, a much larger institution. St Mary's was becoming a place of serious research.[28] Williams insists that St Mary's did not enjoy any special influence over the trustees. He was not the only link between St Mary's and the Wellcome Trust. Over the years, a number of Mary's graduates and staff have been Wellcome trustees, including Henry Barcroft, Helen Muir, and Stanley Peart. Neurologist Harold Edwards joined the trust's staff in the early 1980s, soon after stepping down as dean at St Mary's to direct a program for Wellcome-funded senior lecturers. In 1983, David Gordon, a senior lecturer on the medical unit, became a program director at the Wellcome while keeping up a clinic at St Mary's. He finally left London to become dean of the medical faculty in Manchester.

The Wellcome Trust helped shape British medical science. It remained a "people place," according to those who worked with it. Time and again the Wellcome funded new projects by young researchers that the MRC would eventually recognize as important centres for state-of-the-art research. In the 1980s and 1990s, the trust sold Wellcome's pharmaceutical company and with the capital received became the largest medical research charity in the world.

Wellcome and other foundations helped build St Mary's. As the school outgrew Moran's buildings, research laboratories had to be put into odd corners like the hospital basement, converted shops on Praed Street, or the old stables of the Post Office. Fortunately Moran had taken a lesson from St Mary's founding governors and had left room for further building as funds permitted. The medical school and the Pathological Institute occupied two wings, forming an L-shape, and there was space to erect two more wings, one to the north on South Wharf Road and another to the east, next to the Nurses Home. But in 1948, with other schools in greater need of rebuilding, the UGC flatly refused the school's request for the funds.[29] Ten years later the school raised £100,000 on its own through a centenary fundraising campaign, and also secured £50,000 from the Shepherd Trust and £70,000 from the Wellcome Trust; the UGC paid for the rest. The Centenary Wing opened in 1961. In 1967 the Wellcome Trust and the Variety Club offered to pay for the final East Wing, contributing £100,000 each. This wing became a centre for experimental pathology. Moran's vision was not entirely fulfilled: instead of a graceful quadrangle with a fountain, an ugly workshop stood in the courtyard.

Research foundations also helped to people the buildings, often with new kinds of scientists. In 1957 Pfizer funded a chair of immunology for ten years at £5,000 per year (the first such chair in the U.K.). In 1962 the Fleming Memorial Fund provided £75,000 for a chair in virology. These negotiations succeeded in part because immunology and virology did not require scarce hospital beds. The immunology professor, Rodney Porter, was not medically qualified and had no patients. In 1961, however, an offer by the Empire Rheumatism Campaign of £25,000 towards a clinical chair of rheumatology was refused. The haematology department, on the other hand, created in December 1960 with MRC money, received four beds.

Renewing the Wright-Fleming Institute

Virology, immunology, and haematology were all housed in the Inoculation Department, which had become a shadow of its former self. Sir Almroth Wright, a frequent visitor in the department almost to the end, died in 1947. Sir Alexander Fleming succeeded him as director of the department, renamed the Wright-Fleming Institute (WFI), legally affiliated with the medical school, but retaining its own governing council. Fleming was by now elderly, and he had none of the fiery charm of his old chief. Most of the old financial backers were dead too, though new ones presented themselves, anxious to show their gratitude to the discoverer of penicillin. The WFI had other sources of income, worth about £60,000 in 1949. It began to charge the hospital for routine bacteriology work after 1948, and it continued to run out-patient clinics for bacterial infections, whooping cough, allergies, and immunization for travellers. Freeman's desensitization allergy clinic was enormously popular, too popular in fact, now that patients expected free service. The Ministry of Health and the school both insisted it be scaled down from 15,000 to 10,000 attendances per year.

In the other clinics, patient numbers were declining. By 1949 patients coming for bacterial vaccines dropped from eighty to eight per week, and for whooping cough vaccine, from sixty-five to ten. Antibiotics killed the demand for Wright's vaccines. This threatened the viability of the entire Wright-Fleming Institute. Service income alone could not support research in the manner to which the WFI was accustomed. Salaries and wages came to £40,000 at the end of the 1940s, paid for primarily by the income from vaccine and pollacine sales of around £35,000. But the institute was still losing thousands of pounds annually. The threat was not immediate, for the institute had a quarter-million pounds banked. However, because Fleming, unlike Wright, had not parlayed his discoveries into a steady source of income, long-term decline loomed. One solution was to branch into other lines of treatment. The institute began to develop diphtheria toxin, which rose from less than 10 per cent to nearer 25 per cent of all therapeutic sales between 1950 and 1951. Quietly, up on the third floor, Himmelweit developed a flu vaccine that went into a large-scale MRC trial in 1951 and into commercial production by the mid-1950s. In 1956, the institute produced more than 500,000 doses of flu vaccine that it sold for £79,741.

Fleming retired as professor of bacteriology in 1949 and as director of the Wright-Fleming Institute in 1955, replaced on both counts by Robert Cruickshank. Cruickshank had made his name in 1937 by introducing into England a test to identify carriers of staphylococcus aureus. At the WFI in the early 1950s, he chaired an MRC working party testing the new antibiotics aureomycin and chloramphenicol; he also investigated the virulence of tuberculosis.

A report describing work in the WFI at the time shows a number of different projects were being undertaken. Fleming and his wife, Voureka, were investigating the effect of antibiotics on bacterial morphology. A.P. Fletcher was testing terramycin on patients and studying proteolytic enzymes. A.C.F. Ogilvie was exposing human blood to immunized rabbit serum. Four bacterial chemists were comparing penicillin to potassium tellurite, using radio-isotope techniques. A staff of eight, including graduate students, ran the bacteriology lab and investigated penicillin, virulence, bacterial genetics, hospital cross-infection and the staphylococci of out-patients. Derek Rowley led a group that investigated bacterial lipopolysaccharides and non-specific resistance to infection. Others refined diagnostic tests or infected inoculated mice with staphylococcus. In the toxin department, an improved diphtheria antitoxin was developed. The vaccine department studied whooping cough.

Cruickshank worked hard to modernize the WFI and its research agenda. He introduced an epidemiological angle that made the research much more relevant to the hospital and reinvigorated the teaching. Yet he was personally unpopular: in 1954 some of the older staff accused him of making "derogatory personal remarks" and failing to ensure that adequate precautions were taken with virulent pathogens. The charges were dismissed, but perhaps they hastened his departure to Edinburgh in 1957.

With Cruickshank gone and both the bacteriology chair and the Wright-Fleming directorship vacant, St Mary's took stock. The school left the chair vacant for three years while it reorganized the troubled institute. What to do with all the old vaccine clinics? A.W. Frankland, who joined the institute at this time, recalled that the bacterial vaccine clinic catered largely to "all these old Paddington ladies, and I don't believe that it worked at all but they loved having it."[30] The ladies and their vaccinators were both dying out; newer staff were less accommodating. When Alan Glynn inherited the boils clinic in the basement of the WFI, he was frankly shocked at what he found:

It really showed you what the Wright-Fleming had come to. I mean, there wasn't much you could do for boils, chronic boils at that stage, you treated acute ones with penicillin, that was no problem. But these people who'd got chronic ones, you know, they'd come with the whole of the back of their neck thickened with craters of old boils and new ones. And what the clinic had been doing for some twenty years, I suppose, was giving them staphylococcal vaccines, which did damn all! And the notes … (on cards about eight by five inches) … [on] the first page, if you could still find it, would say "Boils" or something. And after that would be a list of 0.1, 0.2, 0.3, 0.4 ml of vaccine given, you know, in increasing doses. Very rarely was there ever any comment about whether it did any good or not, or any comment at all, actually! And I thought, "What am I doing here?" They asked me to do some other clinic. And I said, "Well, what's that?" They said, "Well, it's boils, strokes, all the infectious diseases." And I thought, "Christ!"

One of Glynn's earliest patients was a schoolteacher of about fifty who appeared and announced she'd come for her injection.

I said, "What injection?" You know, I had this pile of notes, but, you know … "Ah!" she said, "Well …" Basically, she'd had TB in glands in the neck some twenty or thirty years before and had got better, as they often did. Not necessarily, but they often did. And she'd been treated at St. Mary's for many years, apparently, with injections of something which was called "tubercle powder." And the woman who ran the clinic, who was not a nurse, she was very definitely a lady, produced this bottle, and I looked at it, and it was a little bottle, a brown bottle, with a rubber cap so old that it was perishing, the rubber, with some nasty powder inside. God knows what it was! And it said, "Tubercle powder."… And I thought, "God! What do I do? I can't give her this!" You know, I wouldn't have dared! And I said, "Well, you know, it is some twenty or thirty years since these glands were better, you can probably stop now." "Oh no, no," she said, "If I stop … I can't possibly." So I said, "Okay, we'll give you an injection." And I fiddled around, and I gave her an injection of saline.[31]

One can imagine scenes like these occurring in GP offices across the country. Bacterial vaccine sales dropped by a third between 1955 and 1956, from 910,771 to 632,166. The institute's annual report blamed the decline on the fact that "medical students nowadays receive little or no instruction in the use of therapeutic vaccines," adding defensively, "It may be maintained that there is little scientific support for the efficacy of these vaccines but many experienced doctors have been convinced of their usefulness in chronic or recurrent catarrhal conditions, skin infections, chronic rheumatism, etc."[32] But it was no longer acceptable for a self-proclaimed research institute to defend its activities by appeal to "many experienced doctors" rather than to clinical trials or laboratory research. Nor did respectable research institutes sell a "public school vaccine," made from the sterilized throat organisms of public school boys. The Wright-Fleming Institute, once the focus for scientific activity at St Mary's, was now judged by the medical school to be living on its reputation.[33]

Albert Neuberger, the head of chemical pathology at St Mary's, was made director of the Wright-Fleming Institute with a mandate to shake things up. Neuberger was a "bulky, untidy figure" with a pipe in his mouth, who champed his jaws, worked his lips, and murmured when he was deep in thought.[34] He was often deep in thought and came to Mary's as one of its most distinguished appointments. Born in Bavaria, he obtained an MD in Wurzburg in 1931 and then left Germany for England, obtaining a PhD from University College. During the war he worked in the biochemistry department at Cambridge and served in Delhi. In 1943 he moved to the MRC-funded National Institute of Medical Research at Mill Hill, and became head of its biochemistry division in 1950. He was an editor of the *Bio-*

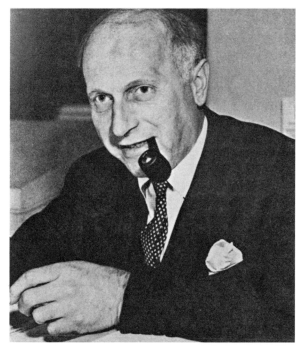

Albert Neuberger. St Mary's Hospital NHS Trust
Archives and the Royal College of Surgeons of England

chemical Journal from 1946 and served on the MRC, the Agricultural Research Council, and the Council of Scientific Policy. In 1955, at a time when St Mary's was still at the fringes of scientific research, he joined the staff with an FRS already after his name, largely so that he could run his own department. The laboratory was in the Clarence Wing of the Hospital. With £20,000 in start-up grants from the Rockefeller Foundation and the Nuffield Trust, and staff brought over from Mill Hill, Neuberger soon built up a small department with a reputation as a forensic authority and very little research tradition into a powerful base for science at St Mary's. He then began to transform the medical school in its image.

Neuberger's appointment marked a turning point at St Mary's. A basic rather than a clinical scientist, he was interested in protein metabolism, and in particular the biosynthesis of porphyrins (the "organic moity of the haem group of haemoglobulin") in humans and other mammals. Using radio-isotopes, he had played an important role in identifying the origins of the carbon and nitrogen atoms of protoporphyrin, and the enzymic steps in biosynthesis. The work earned him an FRS in 1951. At St Mary's he continued the work using photosynthetic bacteria. He took up glycoproteins as well and again performed some important work, examining the linkage between the sugar and the peptide parts of the protein. He also had researchers studying the function of glycoproteins in cells.

By 1970 Neuberger had built up the department so that it had, in addition to himself, four senior lecturers, two lecturers, three research assistants, two graduate students, and two consultants, as well as a further professor and four research workers in its steroid unit. Just as Almroth Wright was a pathologist who wouldn't do the routine hospital pathology, so too Neuberger was a chemical pathologist who wouldn't do the routine chemical pathology. That work was done by a separate team directed by B.J. Houghton: in 1968 a staff of eight was doing 200,000 tests on 45,000 requests per year.[35] Most of these – 75 per cent – were electrolyte estimations, blood sugars, serum proteins and liver function tests.

The chemical pathology department nominally oversaw a steroid unit and also a metabolic unit under Victor Wynn. Wynn was originally based in the surgical unit, but as his research program expanded beyond electrolytes and fluid intoxication to endocrinology and steroid work, he was moved to chemical pathology. In practice, however, Wynn was his own man entirely. The steroid unit, under V.H.T. James, performed routine investigations into endocrine disorders and also undertook research into normal and abnormal steroid excretion, and the effects of steroid administration on the endocrine system. James worked closely with the clinicians. With the surgery professor, William Irvine, James's unit investigated steroids in breast cancers. They found high concentrations of oestrogen hormones and tried to discover whether hormone therapy could affect the disease's course. They also investigated the mechanism of hormone uptake. With the medical unit, they asked whether testosterone could inhibit hirsuitism. James worked out a new method of measuring secretion rates of testosterone. Another area of assay research was the pursuit of a test to identify aldosterone in peripheral human plasma.

Developing assay techniques served both the research and the routine work of the department. As Neuberger remarked, because work was mostly done on micrograms of material, "methodology is of considerable importance and much of the effort is in the direction of improving and assessing the procedures used." Gas-liquid chromatography was permitting ever-finer assays, using picograms of steroids.[36] Important funding agencies for the steroid work were the MRC, the Wellcome Trust, the British Empire Cancer Research Campaign, and the National Institutes of Health.

Having worked in a leading research establishment and having established a flourishing research department in St Mary's Hospital, Neuberger was well equipped to undertake the renovation of the Wright-Fleming. With the institute's chairman, Lord Cohen (named in 1957), he decided to stop all the commercial production. In 1958 the two advised the medical school that, with production at about £35–40,000 per year (worth twice that to Parke Davis, which actually marketed the drugs), the WFI was too small to engage in the "cut-throat business" of commercial production. Himmelweit's flu vaccine typified the problem: the vaccine had been developed with MRC funding, which would be stopped if the institute marketed it commercially. The terms of the grant required Himmelweit to publish his results, enabling larger firms to make and sell the drug more cheaply. If production stopped, then the WFI could "regain its character" and its scientific standing and attract leading microbiologists. The minutes for 2 October 1958 record that after a "very long and detailed discussion in which every member of the Council present took part it was agreed to give up the production of bacteria vaccines and toxoids for commercial purposes." The minutes do not record that the WFI had been rejected by most of the reputable bacteriologists in the country.[37]

In late 1958 the medical school was feeling unusually optimistic about the institute's financial future. That year, three years after Fleming's death, it negotiated an agreement with Howard Florey in Oxford to launch a Fleming memorial appeal. Members confidently expected to raise more than a million pounds with which to endow the Wright-Fleming Institute. Within a few months, however, the optimism dwindled and they tried to resuscitate the agreement with Parke Davis. Parke Davis was having none of it. The drug firm believed it was not getting the best service and insisted on ending the contract on 1 January 1960. So St Mary's turned to Beecham's, which had never before sold vaccines, and formed an agreement for £80,000 worth of vaccines for a year. A year and a half later, in July 1961, production was moved to the Beecham's plant, with the WFI receiving royalty payments of £30,000 rising to £40,000 over seven years. The only link between Sir Almroth Wright's Inoculation Department and the Wright-Fleming Institute now consisted of a few aging staff who could sometimes be persuaded to reminisce about "the old man" in the *Hospital Gazette*.

The Fleming Memorial Fund was never as lucrative as St Mary's hoped it would be. In November 1955 the Duke of Edinburgh (recruited by Arthur Porritt) presided over a meeting with representatives of various universities and learned societies, who gave cautious support, pending Florey's approval. In December, Florey and his colleagues at the Dunn School of Pathology met to discuss their mixed feelings.[38] They opposed the notion of a statue to Fleming and a "Fleming" appeal, though they welcomed a "Penicillin Memorial Research Fund." But, Florey observed, if they refused, Mary's might do their own appeal. "If we can keep the committee in being, I think Mary's will be under control." Sir Henry Dale advised the Dunn workers that the name "Fleming" couldn't be discarded because it was too valuable a catchphrase; but, he reassured them, the St Mary's

crowd "were good fellows." In the event, Florey rebuffed the initial over-
tures, and it was not until 1958 that he agreed to support the fund, with 40
per cent of the first million going to Oxford and 60 per cent to St Mary's.
The fund was constituted, with distinguished representatives from across
the country to manage it. They gave £75,000 to St Mary's to endow a chair
of virology.

The virology department was finally established in 1964. Himmelweit
was deemed too old and the chair went to K.R. Dumbell. Dumbell was
trained at Liverpool and then moved to the MRC common cold unit. He became an expert on smallpox, advising the WHO in its program of eradica-
tion and investigating its relationship to other poxes, comparing DNA
sequences. His team also tried to treat smallpox by blocking an enzyme that
permitted the virus to proliferate. There wasn't much scope for smallpox research in Paddington, but the department did see a lot of cytomegalovirus
and herpes.[39] Cytomegalovirus affects pregnant women and can cause birth
defects; it is also seen in people with compromised immune systems. The
special clinic furnished many interesting questions for the virologists.

The haematology department was established in December 1960. P.L.
Mollison, the first chair of the department, came to St Mary's from the
Hammersmith Post-Graduate Medical School. Mollison brought his MRC
experimental haematology unit with him, thus ensuring that his research
would continue to be supported. He also brought a haematologist to take
charge of the diagnostic work. At first he taught the students how to type
blood for themselves; on reflection, he decided it was safer for them to refer
samples to a haematology lab. He did away with the St Mary's tradition,
which Almroth Wright had introduced, of taking blood samples with a
finger prick and introduced instead venesection. The students, who were
responsible for collecting blood, complained mightily. By 1972 they estimated that they were taking 42,000 blood samples a year.

Mollison had taken up a research career as the result of a chance posting
at the outbreak of World War II. The dean of his medical school, St
Thomas's, sent him to one of the four blood supply depots created in London to cope with the anticipated heavy casualties. These centres were administered by the MRC as the field of blood transfusion was thought likely to
develop rapidly. The ABO system had been discovered at the turn of the century by Karl Landsteiner and others, but the Rhesus groups were only discovered in 1939. Mollison was taken off routine duties and began work on
red cell preservation. With others he showed that acidified citrate solutions
preserved red blood cells well; the solution they recommended, ACD, soon
became the standard solution for preserving blood. Its efficacy was measured by the survival of stored red cells in the circulation after transfusion.[40]

After the war the MRC established a blood transfusion research unit, with Mollison in charge, at the Hammersmith. At first the unit concentrated on haemolytic disease of the newborn, a disease that Mollison was the first in the U.K. to treat with exchange blood transfusion. Much of his later work addressed red cell survival, and particularly the way in which survival was affected by incompatible antibodies. Initially, he studied patterns of destruction of very small amounts of incompatible red cells labelled with radiochromium. Later, with N.C. Hughes-Jones, a member of the MRC unit, he worked on quantitative studies, relating the rate of destruction to the antibody load. Hughes-Jones, who, like Mollison, was later elected an FRS, had trained at St Mary's and played an important part in the unit's relations with the medical school.

When Mollison left the Hammersmith to come to St Mary's, he left Britain's premier research hospital. At the Hammersmith, he said, "there was strong encouragement for clinical investigation, and it was expected that many different laboratories would become involved with any patient with an unusual problem."[41] At St Mary's, by contrast, consultants did not like their patients to be investigated unless a specific invitation had been issued. Several laboratory scientists of that period have said in interviews that the consultants did not seem entirely to appreciate the clinical uses of these sciences. Much of Mollison's research work was performed on healthy volunteers. As well, the haematologists had four beds of their own. Other members of staff at St Mary's engaged in haematological research included Ernst Neumark, a Bavarian, who came to London in 1933 and joined St Mary's in 1946 as "third assistant pathologist," and studied the diagnostic value of biopsying the bone marrow, where blood is formed; in the medical unit J.F. Ackroyd studied platelets and their lysis in sedormid purpura.

Like Mollison, Rodney Porter had an established reputation in a new field when he came to St Mary's in 1960 as the first professor of immunology at St Mary's and in the country. Had haematology and immunology been long-established, university-based disciplines, St Mary's might not have attracted scientists of this calibre. Porter was a biochemist, trained in Liverpool. After a stint with the Royal Engineers he went to Cambridge, then to the National Institute for Medical Research at Mill Hill where he had come to know Neuberger and Stanley Peart. Porter was interested in antibodies, those parts of the body's defence system that Ehrlich had identified in the blood serum. He wanted to identify their structure, applying new techniques in amino-acid sequencing. Antibodies were large molecules, and so he broke them into three fragments and studied those fragments. Two fragments, he discovered, were almost identical, and they both had an

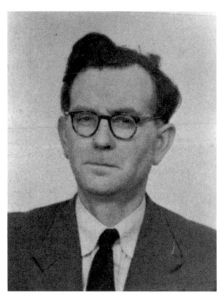

Rodney Porter.
St Mary's Hospital NHS Trust Archives

antigen-binding site; the third could be crystallized and it turned out to contain complement receptor. This work was published in *Nature* in 1959 and paved Porter's way into St Mary's.

Also in 1959, an American named Gerald Edelman showed that a particular type of antibody, y-globulin, was made of three or four peptide chains. At St Mary's, by developing specific antisera against the fragments and assaying them, Porter isolated their four peptide chains in soluble form and with some of their biological activities intact. The four-chain model proved to be applicable to other antibodies, and it laid the foundations of all subsequent immunochemistry. As Porter's successor at St Mary's, Leslie Brent, observed, "It was now possible to study questions such as specificity, affinity, diversity and heterogeneity and the interaction of antibodies with various cell types at a new level of sophistication."[42] In 1964 Porter was made FRS, and in 1972 he shared the Nobel prize with Edelman for the work. Oxford University finally did the expected thing and acquired Porter as a biochemistry professor in 1967, and he also became director of an MRC immunochemistry unit. His subsequent work in complement was cut off abruptly by a fatal road accident in 1985.

Porter was an enthusiastic walker and presided over the Mary's mountaineering club, but in other respects he was somewhat out of place. A very "pure" laboratory scientist, he didn't think much of medicine as a rigorous system of thought. His lectures soared above the heads of the medical students. His obituary described him as "a brilliant scientist who was not always able to communicate his thoughts and ideas at a level intelligible to outsiders." When Leslie Brent was belatedly appointed his successor in 1969, the department was almost defunct, the apparatus covered in dust, and nobody seemed particularly to welcome another onslaught of those indigestible immunology lectures. Brent, who had previously taught in science departments, found the medical students reluctant to exert themselves and persistent in their demands that the material be simplified. In 1969 the *Gazette* printed the complaint of one such student: "Even having thoroughly studied Immunology from other sources since the lectures, I still cannot make sense of my notes which consists of graphs (some even three dimensional) without indices or parameters, mice and other rodents with enormous syringes in their backsides and occasional expressions scattered around like 'lymphocytes; IgG; complement fixation etc.'"[43] It was a fair cop, for Brent had spent much of his career inserting syringes into mice.

Brent was trained as a zoologist rather than an immunologist and was teaching zoology at Southampton at the time of his appointment to St Mary's. His supervisor was Peter Medawar, one of the pioneers of modern immunology. Even before Macfarlane Burnet published his famous argument in 1949 that immunology was concerned with the distinction between self and non-self, Medawar had done work on skin grafts to show that immune response accounted for graft rejection.[44] Ad hoc skin grafts had been performed for many years, with all sorts of competing and incompatible claims for success. It could be difficult to distinguish a failed skin graft and a successful one, though hair growth was one sign of success. Medawar showed conclusively that grafts between different people generally could not succeed. But some could survive – between twins, for example. Medawar and his team spent the next two decades investigating the conditions under which grafts could be made to survive.

Brent had originally enrolled in zoology in the University of Birmingham with the intention of becoming a schoolteacher, but when his charismatic zoology professor invited him to do a PhD, and to follow him to University College London to do it, Brent happily agreed. At Medawar's suggestion, he took up tolerance as the subject of his PhD thesis and with Medawar and Billington showed that tolerance could be induced in foetal or newborn mice. As the three discovered and announced in 1953, very young animals are "immunologically incompetent" and do not react against foreign cells. So, if an antigen is inoculated at an early age, the immune system will not later identify it as "non-self" but will accept it as "self." The reaction is wholly specific, and other antigens will be resisted. This was the first suggestion that tolerance could be artificially created. However, there seemed to Medawar, Billingham, and Brent to be no obvious clinical applications of this discovery.

The three men produced many more studies together. They engaged in a debate as to whether rejection was cellular or humoral. This was reminiscent of the dispute between Erhlich and Metchnikoff as to whether bacteriolysis was primarily cellular or humoral; Almroth Wright had resolved it by arguing that bacteriolysis was *both* cellular and humoral. In the latter-day dispute, once again the truth lay in the middle. Lymphocytes are the major cause of graft or transplant rejection, but antibodies in the blood serum also play a role. In 1969, at one of the Almroth Wright lectures, Sir Peter Medawar explained the principles behind anti-leucocyte serum and its use in transplantation to a crowded and rapt audience at St Mary's.[45] Brent's interest in transplantation made him an obvious choice for St Mary's, where he continued to work on transplantation problems. He showed that small (subcellular) fractions of allogeneic tissue did not provoke immune responses and could be used to promote tolerance and permit skin grafts. He and his team demonstrated that the lack of responsiveness was mediated by suppressor T lymphocytes. In 1974 Brent established a clinical immunology laboratory with a senior lecturer, Helgi Valdimarsson, who later became the first professor of immunology in Iceland.

The immunologists had a natural ally in the old allergy clinic of the Inoculation Department, in so far as an allergic response is an immune response. In the 1950s St Mary's still had the largest allergy clinic in the world, with six thousand patients. Freeman's successor, A.W. Frankland, raised the clinic to new levels of efficiency. Interviewed in 1999 at eighty-seven years of age, Frankland was still a bundle of energy, enthusiasm, and scientific curiosity, his arms showing the prick-marks of recent experiments with allergens. In the past he had given himself near-fatal allergic reactions. Frankland entered St Mary's in 1933 and early on became interested in venereology, mostly because that was the only clinic running in evenings, "so if you'd nothing else to do, you could go into the VD Department, so you were well-trained, or you saw a lot." Joining the services, he took charge of a large VD hospital in Singapore and then spent three and a half years as a prisoner of war. Returning to St Mary's in 1946 as an ex-service registrar, he worked for a time in the VD department and then moved across to the John Freeman's allergy clinic.

Frankland ventured to do what no one there had done before: he organized a double-blind controlled trial of the bacterial vaccines that John Freeman was still using in his clinics. When he proposed the trial to Fleming, Sir Alexander agreed to it, observing, "It must work, mustn't it, Frank? Because he's doing so well with it." What Frankland suspected, and the trial confirmed, was that, as he told Fleming, "It's working only because everyone believes it works, and he believes it works, and the patients believe it works, and you follow up your successes, and you don't do your failures." Frankland and W.H. Hughes (a believer in the vaccines) found that a saline injection worked just as well. Fleming, was, according to Frankland, perfectly happy with the results, though Freeman would never speak of them. More than forty years later, Frankland is still exuberant at having pulled it off, exclaiming with obvious delight, "I didn't lose my job, which was amazing!" Frankland had other scientific successes, such as the demonstration that when people reacted to dust and dry rot, it was as an allergen rather than as a mere irritant. During the late 1940s and early 1950s, he prowled the bombed-out houses of London gathering specimens of dry rot for the project.

Frankland's appointment caused some technical difficulties, for there was no such thing as an NHS allergist. Labelled a bacteriologist, Frankland wrote to the University of London protesting, "I know no bacteriology. I'll have to be something else." Another problem concerned the funding for his position. Frankland had private sponsorship in a wealthy businessman connected to the Anglo-Persian Oil Company with some very interesting allergies. Under the NHS, his position was not entirely regularized and so, when he retired in the mid-1970s, there seemed to be little money either for a replacement or for his pension. He moved to Guy's, where he spent twenty years, and he still sees patients. The allergy clinic was pruned down, and the Pollen Farm, set up on land given by Lord Iveagh at Woking, was closed. When Brent protested the change, he was told that, after all, "allergies were not life-threatening."

Meanwhile, the bacteriology chair was filled in 1960 with the appointment of R.E.O. Williams. Williams qualified at University College in 1940, and after house jobs, went to the Birmingham Accident Hospital with the goal, like that of Fleming in the last war, of studying the bacteriology of industrial wounds and applying the results to the treatment of war wounds. In 1942–43, he worked with Lady Florey applying penicillin locally. He also developed what would be his major area of research: paths of infection by streptococcus and staphylococcus. St Mary's had learned to be curious about paths of infection and had named officers to study the problem and take such measures as installing fly screens in the window of the operating theatre. But with the appointment of R.E.O. Williams, St Mary's acquired a cutting edge researcher who would bring the latest science to the problem.

Williams began to study patterns of cross-infection using bacteriophages – that is, viruses that attack bacteria. His team could identify distinct strains of staphylcoccus and then trace their path from patient to patient. This permitted a far more rigorous and more certain identification of paths and carriers. Alan Glynn wrote on Williams's departure, "Epidemiology to

Robert Williams has always been quantitative. As he says, it is not enough
to know that a particular pathway exists, you also need to know how much
traffic there is on it."[46] One early finding was that the dust floating about
the wards consisted largely of shed skin cells full of staphylococcus. R.R.
Davies and W.C. Noble then studied desquamation, discovering that the
average medical student undressing and dressing in a small cubicle shed approximately 400,000 epithelial squames and 25,000 skin bacteria.[47] On
the wards, brooms and mops were replaced by specialized vacuums.

Older lines of research did not die out entirely. T.D. Brogan investigated
the factors in the serum that enabled phagocytes to engulf wax particles.
These factors, it was thought, might be deficient in people whose phagocytic action was deficient. In other words, Brogan continued Almroth
Wright's line of research into the ways in which blood serum facilitated
phagocytosis, even if he didn't describe the process as "buttering up" the
germs. Two workers, W.B. Brumfitt and A.A. Glynn, studied lysozyme,
which Fleming had discovered just after the First World War. They showed
that lysozyme existed in phagocytes and that they destroyed bacteria after
phagocytosis by cutting the long chains of sugars that form a rigid wall, like
chain-mail, and keep the antibodies at bay. First they studied the process in
the bacteria *Micrococcus lysodeikticus*, which was not pathogenic, and
subsequently Glynn extended his studies to the more important pathogenic bacteria, such as *E. coli*. In that species the lysozyme broke up the wall
only after the antibody and complement had exposed the sugar chains of
the cell wall. Later, Glynn and a research student, Chris Howard, showed
that the strains of *E. coli* resistant to this process were more likely to cause
infection, for example, in the urinary tract.

Alan Glynn had trained at University College, and he sought a career at
the intellectual end of medicine. After registrar posts at St Mary Abbot's in
South Kensington and at the Red Cross Memorial Hospital at Taplow, he
saw a post advertised as joint senior registrar to St Mary's Hospital Medical School and the Wright Fleming Institute. The job seemed ideal, providing access to both labs and wards. Once he got there, however, he found
himself at a loose end. Cruickshank didn't really know what to do with him
and was away himself most of the time on WHO business. Glynn wondered
if coming to Mary's had been a mistake: he wasn't interested in rugby and
didn't approve of the vaccine clinics. Ignoring Cruickshank's suggestions
that he study the epidemiology of chronic bronchitis, he quietly began to
hunt for antibodies to *Haemophilus influenzae*, a common cause of infection in chronic bronchitis. When Cruickshank left, Glynn had a long talk
with Neuberger who invited him to take up full-time lab work, and Glynn
began to settle in happily. Once R.E.O. Williams came in, the place was

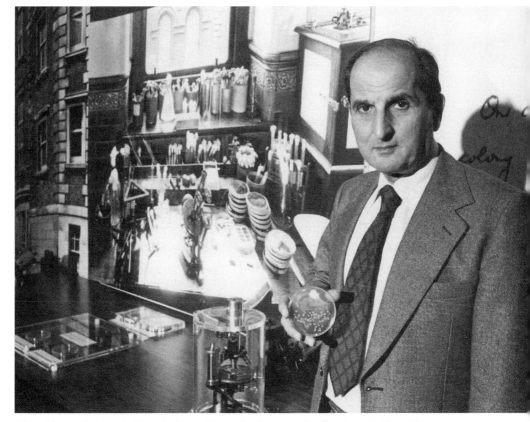

Alan Glynn. St Mary's Hospital NHS Trust Archives and collection of Alyn Glynn.

transformed: "It had come into the modern age and was working properly." After Williams became the director of the Public Health Laboratory
Service in 1973, Glynn rose through the department to succeed him as the
professor of bacteriology at St Mary's. Seven years later, Glynn joined
Williams in the PHLS.

Under Williams and then Glynn, bacteriology became once again a flourishing department. In 1965 it had seven academic staff, plus seven research
students, three of them on MRC funds. Research areas included the inter-
acting antibacterial mechanisms of antibodies, lysozyme, and complement;
anaerobes and gut cancer; antigens in urinary tract infections; virulence and
resistance in gonorrhoea; and work leading to the description of a gene that
controlled resistance to salmonella and some other infections. The diagnostic bacteriology was mechanized. Under Williams and Glynn, as under
their predecessors, bacteriology was firmly rooted in both laboratory and
hospital and helped to infuse science into clinical care.

Williams was a key figure in the "scientization" of the medical school. In 1968, thanks to Huggett's machinations, Williams was elected the first academic dean. Traditionally, the school was run by a very few physicians, sometimes by rival parties of physicians, as in 1920 when Wilfred Harris went up against John Broadbent and William Willcox to get Charles Wilson elected. The surgeons largely stayed out of the internal politics, making their power plays on the larger public or professional arena, in the pursuit of the enormous wealth and titles that leaders in the field could expect. After the Second World War and the retirement of Moran and Hope Gosse, it was a gastroenterologist, Tommy Hunt, who became senior physician and "led the pack." Hunt had come to St Mary's on a scholarship (sports and academic honours both played a part) and by 1929, three years after qualification, was on the out-patient staff. He got on well with Pickering, and the two worked together to obliterate the remaining antagonism between the NHS and academic staff.[48] The way was therefore cleared for the entirely academic triumvirate that dominated the school during the late 1960s and early 1970s and went by the name "Stanley Deanberger." On Friday mornings Peart, Williams, and Neuberger met to drink coffee and plot strategy. Under this regime the academic departments enjoyed unprecedented support for their staffing and teaching policies. Williams was succeeded by Harold Edwards, a consultant neurologist, but academics continued to dominate the important committees.

Between 1945 and 1980, thus, the preclinical departments at St Mary's became full-fledged scientific departments. Some commanded international reputations. They performed "big science," attracting enormous research funds that permitted them to bring in the expensive equipment and the teams of researchers that state-of-the-art scientific research required. They took up more and more of the curriculum. The "investigational teaching" that the preclinical lecturers had demanded in 1943 became firmly entrenched, as did other forms of teaching to encourage independent research. In 1965, for example, the pathologists introduced the "research project" as a compulsory part of the course. The students, gathered in the Almroth Wright lecture theatre, greeted the announcement with an "angry silence." But soon anger had changed to enthusiasm. The students were encouraged to present their projects to the class and were thus exposed to the atmosphere of a research society. One student, David Tunbridge, described his experiences to the *Gazette* in 1967. He had been "outraged" on hearing that so "unglamorous" a group as the pathologists were permitted to encroach so profoundly on his clinical years. He and his fellow students found it impossible to think up suitable topics. Then he clerked a series of renal cases but failed to notice the patients suffered from peripheral neuropathy. Humiliated by his chief, Tunbridge wondered why he hadn't picked it up. He found that very little had been published, which only whetted his appetite further and led him to write up the experience as a research project. He observed that with the introduction of the research project, the library changed from a reading to a reference room and original papers became less authoritative in his eyes: "The amount of double-checked rubbish which is published was brought home, along with the warning that we were probably in the process of contributing to it."[48]

The story of science at St Mary's is not one of unrelieved, linear expansion. In 1968 the first MB courses – basic chemistry, physics, and biology – were terminated, and henceforth the school would only accept students who obtained these prerequisites elsewhere. As a consequence the biophysics department was downgraded from a research to a service department. Sixty years earlier, to offer an incomplete education had seemed to the staff at St Mary's to flirt with disaster and possible closure. By 1968, so great was the pressure for admission to medical schools that the danger had disappeared. It was becoming apparent that medical schools had to be more specialized institutions. They needed proper science departments, but they couldn't maintain them in every preclinical and clinical department. Especially in a small school like St Mary's, it was necessary to be selective: by the 1970s and 1980s, David Gordon observes, "you could not hope to appoint in every area."[50] St Mary's was slow to wake up to that fact, or perhaps the academic board closed its eyes to the full implication of this. If every school could not offer a full education, some sort of division of labour had to be worked out; and once the principle of a rationalized distribution of teaching had been established, there was no telling where it would end.

For all their measurable strengths, the scientific departments at St Mary's were no more secure than in 1910 when faced with the threat of Haldane. In 1979 Margaret Thatcher became prime minister. Her election coincided with a financial crisis in the University of London in which key figures decided that preclinical departments in the London teaching hospitals were too many and too dispersed and should be concentrated. And the preclinical department at St Mary's should be the first to go.

12

Teachers and Students

THE GROWTH OF the sciences in English medical schools was justified primarily by their contribution to teaching. As the University of London inspectors engagingly remarked in 1950, researchers made good teachers because "students benefit by the livelier attitude of mind of the teacher."[1] The development of scientific research exercised a growing influence over teaching as science and its corollaries, including the increase in state funding, introduced a new seriousness and a new sense of public accountability into the student culture.

Administering the New Curriculum

As the scientific departments of the medical school grew in size and in number, the encroachment of science upon the traditional medical curriculum was inexorable. The process of specialization speeded up, in large part because the NHS established clear career patterns, with jobs at the end of them, for the different specialties.[2] Courses became more technical, as scientific explanations of disease began to underwrite the curriculum. New work on metabolism, for example, explained how drugs worked at the cellular or even the sub-cellular level, replacing antiquated theories of humoral balance, counterirritation, and autoinoculation. If they were to prescribe drugs rationally, students had to learn the basic mechanisms of biochemical activity. Mis-prescribing remained a serious concern, especially regarding antibiotics. Licensing and professional bodies like the University of London, the General Medical Council, and the royal colleges took expert advice and upgraded their examinations and diplomas, forcing the medical schools to tailor their courses to the examinations.

Students resisted the scientization and specialization of the curriculum. They complained that preclinical lectures were too frequent, technical, and boring, when they should have been in the clinic. The interwar period was recalled as a golden age for students. As dean, Moran kept lectures to a minimum, having himself been bored by them.[3] His students perpetuated his outlook. At Academic Board meetings, Tom Kemp, a clinical teacher, took the students' part, always demanding that they be given fewer lectures and more responsibility. In 1970 Kemp discussed education in the *Gazette*, quoting Moran's piece on "The Student in Irons" and lamenting that "facts continue to be hurled at students like hand grenades." Teachers, he asserted, should mostly help students learn for themselves: "The real teachers are in the beds."[4]

Everyone knew that there was a problem, that the curriculum was too crowded. All the specialists demanded more time for their discipline.[5] Boards of studies tried to mediate between competing claims. Despite periodic stabs at reform, it was not until 1991 that the GMC finally cried "enough." In a paper entitled "Tomorrow's Doctor," the GMC told the schools to develop a modular method of teaching. They should distinguish between an absolutely minimal core of basic information that every student must know, and the wider field of medical knowledge that students should know how to access without learning it from memory. This program, called "problem-based learning," amounted to a radical reform of the curriculum. It was only possible because over previous decades a new kind of student had been created. The Second World War was a watershed in the construction of this new student.

Moran understood "science" the same way he understood everything else, in its relation to human virtue and to public-school virtues in particular. In 1921 he mused, "To think scientifically – what does it amount to? An end of cant, of prejudice, of irrational emotions; a beginning of sound premises, of logic, of true values." Thought, like rugby, was a form of character purification. Moran's idea of curriculum reform was to encourage students to teach themselves, with very little supervision from on high. He didn't concern himself with the pace of study. Students could dawdle through school so long as finances permitted. For most, finances did permit: in 1938 almost 90 per cent of students at St Mary's were entirely self-supporting.[6]

Life at Moran's Mary's was leisurely. The school commissionaire, "Admiral" Law (as the former naval petty-officer was called), remembered that "students had more money to spend before the war, and drinking, in particular, was on a much more liberal scale ... At the same time, exams did not cause so much worry as they do now." When one student qualified at the end of thirteen years, the others slapped him onto a stretcher and carried him around the hospital to be congratulated.[7] Another student, an old Etonian, played all the games and skipped all the lectures, and declared St Mary's to be the best club in London.[8] Frankland, who came to St Mary's in 1934, recalled that "we were a very happy, happy-go-lucky lot, and not very serious I think. If you wanted to work, you worked hard. And if you didn't want to work, no one seemed to bother you, you just kept on and that was that. You'd have to go in for exams, I suppose, occasionally, be prepared for them, but no one seemed to worry you in those days."[9]

The change began even before Moran's departure. Medical students were excused military service for the duration of their studies. To drag out one's studies was therefore unpatriotic, and the students were the first to demand a crack-down on slackers.[10] But what began as a wartime intervention became routine after the war.[11] Medical schools were told to reserve half their places for ex-service men, by a government anxious to avoid the unemployment of the 1920s. Ex-service students received a grant that they would lose if they failed to pass their exams. The new dean, Denis Brinton, thought it unfair to have two standards, so he required all students to pass their exams or leave the school. As the school secretary, Edgar Stevenson, recalled: "He got things going – one chap had been there twelve years! So [Brinton] went through every record and set a target for each student, and if they didn't reach it they were out."[12] In July 1947 fifteen students were downgraded from the conjoint program to that of the Society of Apothecaries, and nine were dismissed. During Brinton's deanship from 1946 to 1951, 9 per cent of servicemen and 17 per cent of students who came directly from school were dismissed. Not all approved of this cleansing of the Augean stables. In 1949 when John Ambrose, a veteran, boxer, and rugby player, failed his physiology exam for the second time, according to Arthur Dickson Wright, "it took all the efforts of the Rugby Club supporters on the staff to keep him."[13] Their efforts were well rewarded. In 1952 Ambrose captained the rugby team, and his quick thinking won them the cup (he turned a free kick into a try, the legality of which was much debated in the press the next day). Ambrose became, Dickson Wright remarked, "a wonderful and much-loved general practitioner, as so many chronic students are."

Another reason for ruthlessness was a new pressure on places.[14] In 1900–01, 20,000 students were enrolled in British universities; in 1938–39, the figure was 50,000; and by 1954–55 it was 82,000, a figure that tripled during the 1960s. In 1900 only .8 per cent of the public entered a university; in 1939, 1.7 per cent, and in 1954, 3.2 per cent. At St Mary's the intake soared from an average of sixty-six during the 1930s to ninety-seven

in 1947. Admissions then stabilized, but applications rose beyond manage-
able levels. In 1950, statistics on ten London schools showed that only 18
per cent of the 2,394 applicants were accepted.[15] During the 1950s, about
five hundred to six hundred students applied annually to St Mary's, about
60 per cent of whom received interviews.

Compounding the pressure for places was the reintroduction of women
students. In 1947 the University of London compelled all London medical
schools receiving UGC grants to admit women or lose the grant. Immediately the pool of applicants increased. The university specified a minimum of 15
per cent female students, and for many years, 15 per cent remained the maximum proportion of women accepted in most of the London teaching hospitals.[16] Eight of the ninety-seven students admitted to St Mary's in 1947
were women.

Denis Brinton was not entirely pleased by the reintroduction of women.
He entered St Mary's as a student in 1925, the first year that women were
turned away. Relations between the remaining women finishing out their de-
grees and the male students had been bad, and Brinton dreaded seeing it all
happen again. Certainly the feeling at St Mary's opposed admission of women. When the British Medical Students' Association advocated the move,
students from St Mary's were "strongly opposed."[17] Evidence from the women
is mixed. One woman admitted in 1947 complained that male students
made their lives miserable; others describe a good deal of acceptance.

One young student from Girton College in Cambridge, Judith Fitzsimons
as she then was (now Judith Hockaday), came to St Mary's in 1950 on the
advice of her physiology tutor who knew of Brinton's reforms. "St Mary's
was known to be a very friendly place, and many of the staff were very involved in the sporting clubs, the music clubs, whatever. And there was great
friendship, and very few barriers." One barrier was the lack of an equivalent to the men's common room, where students and staff mingled as
equals. The women had a room in the basement: "So we were very separate. But I don't remember it mattering actually. We knew we were a very
few of us, but we knew had every right to be there. I mean, we had no problems or inhibitions in any sense. And in the nature of things, we were a fairly capable, competent group of people, got into Cambridge, and survived
that, so we had that confidence. We knew we were okay, and I think ... for
a woman to be doing medicine then was a great commitment, and you
wouldn't get that far unless you were totally committed and sure of your-
self, in intellectual terms ... I made very good friends. It was a very good
time, actually. And then, after qualifying, there were in-house jobs. That
was tremendous fun. And one was totally part of the community."[18]

In Hockaday's view the teachers were a greater obstacle than the students. They were unable to view young girls as "potentially their equal," in

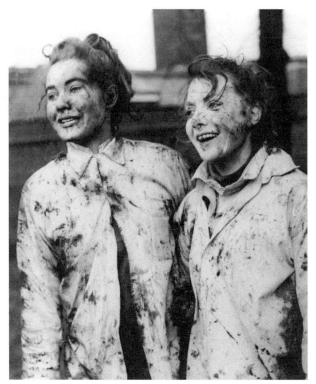

At the rag. Collection of Victoria Cattell

the profession. "I think that is a critical thing, because in a profession, once you're accepted into a profession, you're equal to everyone else in it, even if you're just qualified, compared to the Senior Professor. He's a doctor, you're a doctor, that's a very real professional state." Hockaday did specialist training in Boston and became a consultant in Oxford, specializing in paediatric neurology.

The women adapted well to Brinton's reforms. In 1959 it was found that most of the male students had failed their MBBS exams and most of the female students had passed.[19] Still, not all women students were paragons of sobriety. When the male students behaved riotously, as at the rugby cup match, so did the women. In 1964 male and female students fought a pitched battle with St Thomas's, lobbing plaster, soot, and flour, careening around in souped-up lorries and taking hostages. Victoria Cattell was one who took part. Sent by the team's marshal to secure an iron bar lying on the field, she was captured by opposing forces and rolled in the mud until rescued by a newspaper photographer, who snapped a photograph of her and another female student.[20] Their smiling faces proclaim their sense of belonging.

The postwar deans of St Mary's had an unenviable task. Again and again Mary's students performed poorly on examinations. In 1950 thirteen students failed their first MB so badly that they were dismissed. In 1958 Mary's students did particularly badly in anatomy and physiology.[21] In 1959 one-third failed pharmacology, in 1963, two-thirds. Some argued that the school should dismiss out of hand all who failed their first MBBS exam. Others from both the academic and the rugby factions – Pickering and Kemp – argued that "it would be unfortunate if students felt that the only important thing was the passing of examinations"; other qualities should also be prized.[22] To some extent the lecturers were as much victims of the curriculum as were the students. The University of London and the royal colleges set standards, and the Academic Board, though it might chafe,[23] had to abide by them.

But if the lecturers objected to the restrictions, the increases in salaries muted their criticisms. The students were also subsidized, both indirectly by the Board of Education's grants to the school and directly by the subsistence grants they received from local authorities. The effect was to make the students more, not less, vocal critics of the medical establishment. Aware of the costs of their education, they looked for value for money. They monitored the school with as much energy as the school monitored them.

Students Confront the Curriculum

The old medical school functioned at two levels: the level of governance and that of what might be called "civil society." The lecturers governed, reporting (sometimes) to the hospital governors and occasionally to the Board of Education inspectors. The students studied and occupied themselves with cultural activities, which one student of the 1880s, T.M. King, called "secular studies" – namely, "all those pursuits which though not recognised by examining boards are or will be of use to us as Medical Men and as citizens."[24] Students were no more worried by lax teaching than teachers by lax students. Where teaching was bad, the students responded in a spirit of self-reliance. That there was bad teaching there can be no doubt. J. Ernest Frazer, for example, taught advanced students brilliantly, but when he lectured, his booming voice disappeared into mumbles. Every once in a while a discernible phrase could be detected and quickly became a stock phrase among the students, repeated amidst peals of laughter over a pint at the Fountains Abbey. One student of the 1930s, when asked if they ever thought of complaining, looked blank and responded, "To whom?" Such obstacles became for the students a way of bonding more closely together, relying on one another for advice to get through exams.

The pub was one venue for bemoaning bad teaching; another was the medical society. From time to time the society staged quasi-serious, quasi-entertaining debates on the curriculum. In 1925 one woman asked for less "lordly disdain" and fewer loud laughs from teachers, while Stuart Craddock complained that his medical clerkship was entirely spent carrying specimens to the pathology department.[25] In May 1932 S.A. Mackeith complained that anatomy was too detailed, a remnant of the "days of five-minute amputations when minute knowledge was necessary." Suggestions for reform, however, made Frazer apoplectic.[26] At that the end of the discussion, Sir Ernest Graham Little invited concrete criticisms of the curriculum, and several students responded with letters to the *Gazette*. But on the whole, this sort of criticism was rare before the Second World War.

During and after the war, students became increasingly self-assertive. The war veterans of the late 1940s were self-confident men of independent judgment. W.D.A. Smith was aged twenty-eight when he entered the medical school in 1946. When he failed his second MB, he placed part of the blame upon the school itself. There were too many exams and not enough opportunity for reflection. In pharmacology, experiments and lectures were not coordinated. In organic chemistry, "Early memories are of walking the lab. in search of apparatus and chemicals, at times being uncertain of the colour and state of the contents of the bottle that I was looking for. A lasting memory will be of the far end of the laboratory, where everyone crowded round the blackboard to copy out instructions for several experiments, all of which even the more able and conscientious rarely found time to complete." In biochemistry, only students with access to the notebooks of the previous years' students could identify the carbohydrates in a solution. In physiology, there were no tutors (a problem at the end of the war, when few senior students had taken time out for scientific studies) so one had to learn techniques from books. Again, in the dissecting room, students were "left to get on with it with the aid of their dissecting manual."[27]

Student unions amplified the protests. A union came to St Mary's on the eve of the Second World War in characteristic Marian fashion. Moran called a rugby player into his office, and told him, "'Ah, Graham Jones. Graham Jones. Come and sit down. It's come to my attention that nowadays, one's expected to be, perhaps, more democratic in student life. And so I want you to set up a Union,' he says. 'And I want you to be Secretary, and who do you think should be President?'" This was, John Graham Jones recalls with a hearty laugh, "Democracy at its absolute best!"[28] There already existed a student club that ran the clubhouse and kept the billiards table in working order. This club drew up a constitution for the new union and called general meetings to ratify it in June 1939. The object of the union was to promote recreation, manage the clubs, and further the interests of the students.[29]

Almost at once, however, the union emerged as an independent voice for student autonomy, at loggerheads with the dean. The union sought financial autonomy and independent control of club monies. Worse, from Moran's perspective, it sought to formalize relations within the school and bypass himself. He faced an adversary in union president Alasdair Frazer, the physiology lecturer (and recent graduate of Mary's) who saw a chance to counter the dean's autocratic rule of the school.[30] Moran complained that Frazer was becoming a "second Dean." In 1940 the students played their trump card by investigating the "number of attendances of the Dean at the Medical School during the past year when he would have been available to students" and the number of "unattended complaints." Moran was busy elsewhere with war work. By 1944, to obtain his approval for a tutorial scheme, the president had to approach Lady Moran, who "promised to write to the Dean (at present with the Prime Minister in the Middle East)."[31]

The absence of Moran and other teachers, the overworked state of those remaining, and the dispersal of the students to sector hospitals all worked to increase the importance of the new union. If students in Basingstoke or Hammersmith were overcharged for their board or were not seeing enough midwifery cases to satisfy examiners, they told the union which told the Medical School Committee. Thus during the war union provided an important service.

Nationally student politics ran at a high pitch during the early 1940s. The National Union of Students alienated medical students by associating itself with a motion denouncing the war. At St Mary's, one hundred students attended the next union meeting and rejected these quislingesque sentiments.[32] The London medical students found themselves increasingly at odds with the NUS and with the provincial students who dominated its medical subcommittee, the British Medical Students Association (BMSA). Mary's students called a meeting of London students in a pub and formed an alternative London Medical Committee, but later rejoined a reconstituted BMSA.[33]

Lively debate characterized the union meetings. In 1943 the St Mary's union invited speakers to address the Beveridge Report. It circulated questionnaires that revealed that a "majority of the Medical School thought want should be abolished, that £2 a week was adequate for this purpose and that special provision should be made for the deaf, if not for the halt and the lame. The proposal for a complete State Medical Service was opposed but it was thought that some financial help should be given by the State to the health services."[34] Students from St Mary's denounced the nationalization of hospitals at the BMSA and at the Socialist Medical Association.[35] These students took their cue from the new union president, Arthur Dickson Wright, who denounced the scheme at union meetings. A student member of the union executive and *Gazette* editor was Robin Abel (the son of Dickson Wright's best friend), who agreed that the NHS was "communism at its worst." On the other hand, George Bonney, second secretary of the union, recalled widespread support for the NHS: "All our lives, we'd known nothing but a State service. It was either the Emergency Medical Service or the Armed Forces. And we didn't want to go hanging around the vans, hanging out for a fiver! We wanted to do the work, and get paid a reasonable sum for it."[36]

During the 1950s the union concentrated on selling ties and pints, but during the 1960s the students began to reassert themselves. No longer satisfied to have a union and a *Gazette* to express their concerns, they demanded direct power over school governance. In March 1963 the students obtained representation on the curriculum committees. By the end of that decade they were represented on the Academic Board itself and began to demand representation on the hospital's board of governors. At the same time, sporadic student commentaries on the state of teaching became a sustained campaign. In 1960 "Cobber" wrote amusingly but critically of his introduction to the wards, taking blood specimens and urine samples. He tried to get to know the patients but found that they seemed to "establish a better rapport with the man who sold them their papers and cigarettes, and the woman who wheeled round the book trolley." His surgery attachment was spent chipping ice off the roof. The hospital was too crowded to admit casualty cases, which were diverted to Paddington General, while on Praed Street the seventeen students on the firm saw a few drunks and infected toenails.[37]

A stream of letters seconded Cobber's complaints. Students felt bored and neglected. One surgical student asked rhetorically, "When will the teaching authorities wake up to the fact that the School needs persons on its staff, who will teach and like teaching so that half the student's time spent in the hospital is not entirely eaten away with frustration and sapping of genuine enthusiasm?" Another just wanted someone to talk to: "What every student wants is the *right* to discuss anything he wishes with *some* member of the staff – and the assurance that the matter will not rest there if it is something which concerns everyone."[38] In 1962 the *Gazette*'s editors, Gershy Hepner and David Wilkinson, complained of the "total lack of official communication between students and staff."[39] A few months later at a retreat in Windsor, all the old complaints and some new ones were aired: "the meeting felt that only rarely are students stimulated." Lectures were too scientific. On the wards, "The student in the teaching hospital wanders as a stateless person – rebuffed by sister, turned off the ward, told to take quarter-hourly blood pressures, wasting much time waiting for the chief and so on. All the time he is anxious to get experience and be of some genuine use."[40]

A small scandal erupted in 1963 when a student, Peter Maguire, wrote a report on clinical teaching. He complained that there was no timetable so lectures overlapped, there were too many lectures, pathology appointments came too late to be useful, and so forth. He sent the report into the *Gazette*, but the dean, Mitchell Heggs, stopped publication. The *Gazette* appeared with two blank pages. Discussing the matter in July 1963, the Academic Board agreed to permit publication. Within a few months Maguire was helping to rewrite the clinical curriculum. Thus the school gradually accommodated itself to the new climate of student self-assertion.

Students now demanded to be at the centre of hospital relationships – a radical change to traditional relationships between teacher and student. Students and staff at St Mary's had always lived separate lives. There was understood to be an unbridgeable gap between entrenched authority – by its nature authoritarian and unreasonable, something to be borne – and youthful rebellion that circumvented the rules set by authority. Interwar students practised "tactics," as distinct from "strategies." Tactics have been described as forays upon the enemy carried out within sight of the enemy. Tactics do not keep what they win, and take no hostages. By contrast, strategies elaborate "systems and totalising discourses."[41] Students of the 1960s practised strategy. They forced the educational establishment to remake itself so to conform to their demands. They had a host of new allies ranging from government officials and inspectors to national student unions. Slowly but steadily they carried the day. The students relinquished some self-reliance, but in return the whole creaking structure of the teaching hospital was turned about to become student centred. Blood-taking was assigned to paid staff. Students were given someone to talk to: tutors, councillors, directors of study, and other officials with liaison duties. Course evaluations began to generate critical feedback.

The Student Critique Broadens

Some accused St Mary's of failing to provide a university-standard education. Education was broadly understood to include student culture (or, following the analogy, "civil society"). Did the medical school provide an atmosphere in which human self-development and critical thinking could flourish at all levels, and not just those aspects related to medicine? In

March 1962 a letter by "Freshman" complained that it did not. There seemed no extracurricular life outside rugby, which was a ruffian's pastime. Anti-nuke groups, UN humanist groups, an archaeological society, a functioning art society, even a debating society were all negligible or absent. Without them, "Freshman" charged, St Mary's was more like a polytechnic than a university school.[42] The letter sparked intense debate. One student replied that "although culture at Mary's may not go about in a black shirt, with down on its chin," the school did sustain a lively cultural life. Several pointed out that Freshman's missing clubs were all well represented in the university-wide student union. Ironically, it was just as a university-wide highbrow intellectual life took hold at St Mary's that students who participated in this life grew more critical of the barbarians and philistines around them.

The divide between radical and conservative students, quiescent during the 1950s, resurfaced at the end of the 1960s. When students from the London School of Economics occupied the University of London union building in 1968, St Mary's was polarized. Some cheered on the occupiers, others manhandled them out. The same year also saw an unsuccessful attempt by a group called the "Young Socialists" to gain recognition from the student union at St Mary's.[43] But the real cleavage point was rugby. To anyone reading the *Gazette* in the early 1960s, it would appear that Moran's critics had won the day. Students repeatedly declared themselves anxious that the school live down its reputation as a rugby farm. And rugby did in fact diminish in stature both relatively and absolutely, to Moran's dismay. (It was many years before he forgave Brinton for replacing him, and the "Great Dean" was especially critical of the new selection policies.[44])

Denis Brinton's notion of the ideal student differed significantly from that of Moran. Brinton belonged to a specialty, neurology, seen to occupy the intellectual end of medicine. While not a great academic himself – he published little – he was highly intelligent and cultured, and he sought these qualities in students.[45] Applicants had to write a short essay. Music was a special love of both Brinton and his wife, Joan, who involved herself in school functions, and so musical students were specially encouraged. The strains of Sibelius, Wagner, and Haydn began to waft through the library. Students undertook ambitious musical productions and invited prominent musicians to perform at beautiful mid-summer concerts in Joyce Grove, a mansion in Nettlebed donated to the hospital by the Fleming family. The drama society also went from strength to strength. Music and drama were not new to St Mary's, but were now more formally encouraged, men and women participating in these new societies side by side. Thus Brinton oversaw the development of a culture quite different from the atmosphere of the late 1930s when, according to George Bonney, all the students talked about was rugby, beer, and women.[46]

By 1952 an eclectic culture flourished. The rugby, football, swimming, squash, and cricket clubs all won their respective cups, beating the other medical schools. The athletics club led by Roger Bannister won the cross-country match. There were clubs for boxing, golf, rifle, squash, lawn tennis, and hockey. A sailing club joined the Round the Island race. A motor club had long since replaced the old cycling club. In 1952 fencing and judo clubs were inaugurated. The mountaineering club held several climbs, usually in Wales. The following year, early-morning visits to the river were revived with the boat club.

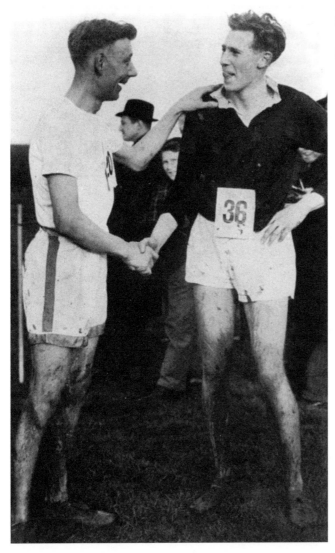

Bannister wins the inter-hospital race, 1952. Collection of Sir Roger Bannister

An arts society organized exhibitions, with paintings by students and celebrated artists. There were also a bridge club, a chess club, a gramophone club, and a photographic society. The Christian Union had weekly reading and prayer meetings and brought in missionaries to speak. The drama society performed *Lady Windermere's Fan*. The musical society heard Solomon play. The film club showed *Battleship Potemkin*. The medical society held debates.

The new culture was reinforced when Brinton revived the ideal of a hall of residence. This was the old Oxbridge ideal of an inward-looking life of the mind set apart from the hurly-burly and sordidness of London and of Paddington boarding houses in particular. As one student remarked in 1953, "We are heartily sick of digs, with their difficult landlords and ladies; the uncertainty of tenure – being expelled in the face of invasion by a foreign horde; the fusty, dowdy rooms whose furnishings vary from heavy, dark, Victorian monsters to dirty, green-painted plywood, all covered with a thick layer of pernicious London dust; and, horror of horrors! – the brownish flowered wallpaper and the 'Monarch of the Glen.'"[47] Brinton moved heaven and earth to obtain land and put up two student residences, Wilson House and Lawley House, using money from the University of London and a benefactor, Edgar Lawley. The student residences soon became the heart of the student community. No other London school could provide such extensive housing.

Amidst so much activity, the rugby team declined as the focus for student culture. There was some good-natured rivalry. In 1952 one spirited group of students, likening themselves to the early Christian fathers, formed a Rugby Anti-Committee which played a few pranks.[48] Biology teacher Alan Fisk recalled another confrontation. "At the first Dramatic Society soirée, I was fetched because a delegation had arrived from the Rugger Club to say that they were going 'to bust up the Library.' As always, they proved kindly and, relying on their alcoholic sentimentality, I pointed out that as I was the only member of the staff present, they would probably get me into trouble; I added that there were plenty of streetlamps in Praed St. They went into solemn conclave and decided to withdraw their attack and march instead on Praed St."[49]

Serious tensions only surfaced when the rugby club performed badly. In 1960 a cup-tie loss led to much finger-pointing, especially at freshmen who would rather attend a lecture than a match. The next year, the once-mighty St Mary's was eliminated by Charing Cross in the second round. Keenness had so declined that the school sometimes couldn't field a complete team, and players were unfit from lack of practice. The claims of rugby versus culture were much aired in the *Gazette*. When sporting types lamented a decline of school spirit, the highbrow editors defiantly responded, "The idea of a strong 'hospital spirit' (the type that has advertised their foolishness on the fence opposite Wilson House) is surely a rather childish concept and belongs to the short trousers decade."[50] The new eclectic life was more to their taste. They cheered an ambitious performance of *The Marriage of Figaro* with the remark, "Gone are the annual pantomime and bacchanalian orgies thinly disguised as Gilbert and Sullivan."[51]

It would be wrong to exaggerate the divide. Rugby players were not *ipso facto* lowbrow philistines, even if they sometimes played the part. Many turned their hands to other sports and activities, often as rowdy as rugby. The swim team was a force to be reckoned with, almost as mighty as the rugby club. Year after year it beat all comers in water polo. Thrashed once too often, the Metropolitan Police took revenge by making the entire forward line of the Polytechnic Swimming Club honorary policemen for one night.[52] Swimming club galas ended with broken bottles and blood in the water. Uproarious cultural activities such as rag week and the annual soirée brought all the students together for a long laugh at themselves. One reviewer observed, "The three Ss, Shop, Sex and Sport, are the stones from which the jewels of its humour must be cut."[53] Rugby was often sent up, as were teachers. Some teachers took part in the soirées, dressing up in wigs and jeans as rock stars, for example. For years, the two men who worked most closely with the students, Harold Edwards, the dean, and Oscar Craig, the director of clinical studies, performed a skit that culminated in one soaking the other with a soda siphon.

But the correspondence in the *Gazette* reveals more than just rivalry between highbrows and lowbrows. "Freshman" wanted the whole person to be represented somewhere at St Mary's. This reflected a broader change in the *Gazette*, one that left the alumni feeling puzzled and alienated. Increasingly the editors included prose and poetry with no relation to St Mary's. They replaced the much-loved Virgin and Child on the cover with non-representational modern art. In September 1962, after complaints against the irrelevant and "mostly mediocre photographs, accompanied by nebulous commentary," as well as papers by outsiders, the editors replied that they wished to broaden the outlook of the student and to try "as far as possible, to get away from pure medicine as a subject for articles."[54] In December 1962, Leonard Ley, a Yarmouth GP who had graduated from St Mary's before the First World War, stopped his subscription in protest against the *Gazette*'s "silly puerilities." In 1968 Welsh GP (and founder of the Royal College of General Practitioners) David Kyle wrote to complain. He had entered St Mary's on a scholarship in 1930 and, succeeding Moran as editor of the *Gazette*, made it once again a lively organ of student culture. The new *Gazette*, he objected, was "everything a hospital magazine should not be," full of medico-literary articles one could find anywhere rather than local news. And as for the cover, "I thought I was holding it upside down."[55]

The paper, like rugby, had always been a bridge between old and new Mary's graduates. Young Mary's men and women had always needed the old, to help them find practices and become established. Now the students were less needy and could be more cavalier. The student editors began to insist that the *Gazette* served only the current students, and "its most positive service lies in showing that medical students do have a life beyond the medical school."[56] Regular features that served to delineate and reinforce the St Mary's community disappeared from the *Gazette* during the 1960s. Obituaries were one casualty. The old men and women like Leonard Ley who read the *Gazette* for news of their friends lost interest. The students did not feel the loss.

This was a significant change in the medical student culture, made in the name of social conscience and an awakening to the claims of the larger community. Many students had long debated matters of social justice and formed clubs such as the missionary society in the name of service. Their work with hospital patients, still "the poor" until 1948, was ostensibly philanthropic. But as the middle classes entered the hospital, caring for the sick no longer satiated student idealism. "The poor" had to be served in other ways. The students began increasingly to think and write about community in a more sociological sense. Photo-essays of impoverished Paddingtonians grounded their often-abstract disquisitions. They became involved with local projects: sponsoring boy's clubs, for example, or painting the houses of pensioners. Vicky Cattell, a student of the 1960s, recalled, "The poor old-age pensioners, they were so terrified! I remember, we went to this flat, and this couple were there, clutching mugs of tea as we marched in. None of us knew anything about paint. We didn't know the difference between gloss paint and emulsion paint. And I remember putting the gloss paint on the wrong thing, and trying to wipe it off with newspaper. I think we left the flats in worse state than we started! I know they were glad to get rid of us!"[57]

During the 1960s "community" became something defined by sociology textbooks rather than an experience shared with one's predecessors. The students of the 1960s who had grown up under the NHS felt little in common with the older alumni scattered about the countryside, and they turned their backs on them. Until the postwar period medical students probably had more in common with qualified practitioners than with other university students. Old and young shared in the shock of the first dissection, the first day on the ward, and the happy memories of such coping mechanisms as the soirée. A common professional identity smoothed out generational differences. During the 1960s this changed as the "generation gap" and youthful rebelliousness pitted old and young against one another.

In 1963 one correspondent complained to the *Gazette* that some students were a "disgrace": "Imagine the apprehension of a patient who is confronted by a long-haired bearded weirdy, who wishes to conduct an examination."[58] The writer, David Dodds, was a current student, the son of a vicar, so this was a dispute among the young, but it provoked a frank attack on the older generation and the dead weight of tradition. In defence of his own beard (grown to hide a spindly neck), D.P. Evans argued hotly, "All medical schools are bogged down by much useless tradition, every member is made to conform as closely as possible to the accepted and stereotyped 'Doctor.' There is hardly an ounce of original thinking in the whole hospital, interest in matters of culture is almost non-existent, and the course leaves most peoples' minds ineffective, immature, and philistine."[59]

By the late 1960s positions had polarized. To some students any communication with the alumni through the *Gazette* seemed a sell-out. In 1969 one idealistic student, Philip Birch, objected to shop-talk – articles about medicine – as reactionary, done to please a reactionary constituency of alumni: "One wonders if the editors are tradition-bound by an image of their postal readers: the bombastic ultra-Tory, the general 'old-boy,' and those nearer home, who don't want to think that 'chaps' at their 'old-hospital' are delving questioningly into the nature of our society (or theirs!)." He demanded that the *Gazette* become an instrument of counter-hegemony: anything less than political debate constituted "quiet approval for the reactionary forces in society, those with power (industrialists, university lecturers, schoolteachers, police, immigration officers, MPs, and journalists)." The editors agreed with Birch, commenting, "It obviously becomes essential that from now on, this publication is used by its readers as a mouthpiece for their moral, social or political convictions. No longer can we afford to be inert in these directions."

A greater contrast with the youthful Moran can hardly be imagined. For Moran's generation (as for the Victorian founders of the hospital) community was a network of relationships occurring outside official purview. Moran distrusted bureaucracy, and his reform of the medical profession – and through the profession, society at large – was to be accomplished by instilling values that would facilitate consensus, and thus concerted action behind the scenes, of the sort that helped him to bring in the NHS. He worked to create a state-within-the-state that would harbour much invisible yet real political power. Doctors would be unacknowledged legislators. From the perspective of half a century later, this state-within-the-state seemed a conspiracy designed to restrict real power to the few (as indeed it was), which should be exposed and stamped out in the name of real democracy, or perhaps even revolution. Any community of equals – if those equals had some power or prestige (as doctors and even medical students undoubtedly did) – that resorted to informal mechanisms of community was *de facto* engaging in a conspiracy to monopolize power. Either one worked to disperse power, or one guarded it; neutrality was impossible, according to the scheme advanced by young Birch and the other student radicals.

The radical tone quieted down over the next decade, and nostalgia and obituaries began to reappear in the *Gazette*. The intergenerational puzzlement, however, remained. Old alumni couldn't understand the politically correct tone that crept into the paper in the 1980s, as students redirected their idealism away from visions of revolution and towards establishing more caring personal relations with patients, relations that were, incomprehensibly to the old guard, mediated by formality and academicism. Late in 1986 the journal published an essay by a mature student at St Mary's, Pat Wright, which had won a BMA journalism prize. Wright recounted the efforts made at St Mary's to broaden the awareness of medical students with sociology lectures on the relationship between class and illness, a community placement in paediatrics, sessions with obstetrics social workers, and three weeks with a GP. At group discussions students were encouraged to reveal something intimate about themselves or to describe their experience with bereavement. As Wright, whose husband had died of brain haemorrhage, "listened to spotty youths recalling the deaths of their pet gerbils," she felt like a rape victim.[60]

Debbie Newton, the *Gazette*'s editor, responded indignantly that Wright had "missed the point." The consciousness of middle-class students had to be raised somehow, so that they could understand the perspective of a single mother in a stinking tenement. In reply M.A. Sparrow took Wright's part and defended the *ancien régime*, when the most important part of education had been informal. "The Mary's I knew used to understand the basics – it didn't matter where you trained or what you knew when you qualified because within two years of doing so you found your own level anyways. Students went to Mary's because they knew they would enjoy themselves (the Welsh because they knew they could find it) and Mary's tried to accept people for whom medicine would be a part of their existence and not a whole. Doctors spend the bulk of their working lives treating people who know nothing of medicine and there has to be other lines of communication." He went on to ask whether St Mary's had "tried to pull its academic socks up so far it is now strangling the life out of the students? Do they believe that the honest toiler who knows 24 of the 25 complications of diseases X, Y and Z is somehow superior to the chap who knows where to look them up?" As for intense personal discussions about masturbation and gerbil death, "What garbage is this? I can think of many in my year who would have quite sensibly repaired to the bar ... The medical profession has always taken itself too seriously. God help us now the students are beginning to do the same." Sparrow denounced the *Gazette* as confused and humourless. Newton replied that Sparrow should humbly admit he might benefit from communication studies. Other letters denounced Sparrow as narrow, palsied, and undiplomatic, and they warned that repairing to the bar encouraged high alcoholism, cirrhosis, and suicide rates among doctors.

For the old guard, human relations were informal. By building up informal mechanisms of sociability among themselves, ranging from sport to humour to music, they enhanced their sociability with others. Inwardness bolstered a sense of common humanity. The new generation rejected this inwardness and looked to sociology to help it relate to the larger world. The old tribal tone was banished forever. From the 1960s students began to spend a great deal of time doing electives in various parts of the world, and the *Gazette* filled its pages with accounts of overseas experiences. The *Gazette* for the final decades of its hundred-year history existed primarily as an organ for students to express their grasp of the world in general, rather than their experiences at St Mary's. Insofar as it represented St Mary's to itself, it did so primarily in the reports of clubs, the obituaries (largely the work of an alumni association, formed in the 1980s), and the regular columns of history by the St Mary's archivist, Kevin Brown, the *Gazette*'s final editor.

Kevin Brown is the history man of St Mary's. Trained as an historian and archivist, he was appointed in the early 1980s at the instigation of the St Mary's alumni association, in an appointment jointly sponsored by the school and the hospital. Brown interprets his task broadly: as well as collecting and caring for the archival records of St Mary's, he has worked hard to tell students, staff, and the wider public about the place's history. He has written prolifically about "tales from the archives," set up the Alexander Fleming Museum, spoken to schools and conferences, and patiently answered questions about who "St Mary" is. Brown's appointment ensured that a good deal of very rich history has been recounted and preserved. At the same time, it relegated reflection on the identity of St Mary's to the province of a propounding expert.

For the first sixty-odd years, writers in the *Gazette* described things that everyone knew, and the attraction was the wit and style of the presentation, and the affectionate recapitulation of favourite truths. The same much-loved stories reappeared every few years for each new generation of students. The old *Gazette* existed primarily to reaffirm membership in a circle

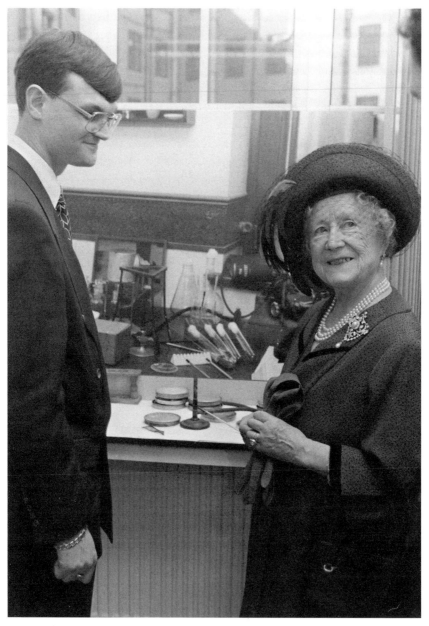

Archivist Kevin Brown welcomes Queen Elizabeth the Queen Mother,
patron of St Mary's Hospital Medical School, to the Fleming museum.
St Mary's Hospital NHS Trust Archives

that enjoyed a special, shared knowledge. By contrast, in the last thirty-odd years of the *Gazette*, student articles tended to be expository: writers claimed some special knowledge of the world that they passed on, such as the experience of doing an elective in Tobago. Often these electives were done in countries with appalling medical conditions. Students treated cases not seen in Paddington for a century: rheumatic children with "hearts the size of buckets" or women who had been in labour a week, to cite two examples from the early 1970s. In writing up their experiences, the students were implicitly or explicitly situating themselves on the political spectrum, finding for themselves an answer to the perpetual question of the relationship between medicine and justice. They seemed to feel an individual responsibility for good behaviour and moral integrity which, in the old days of "honorary" consultants, had been thrown on the profession as a collectivity. As the collective self-righteousness of the profession diminished, individual members needed to find a moral high ground for themselves.

But the written level is only the most overt level of student organization. Student culture is like an iceberg, with nine-tenths of it submerged away from the probing eyes of authorities. Tom Kemp, in arguing for a rugby spirit in 1973, asserted, "Whatever claims may be made for the intellect, our lives will continue to be dominated by what William James has called 'the dumb regions of the heart.'"[61] Rituals of initiation continue to thrive in medical schools, catering to these dumb regions. Off the field the rugby club continues to flout ordinary morality with obscure rites of passage involving gigantic amounts of alcohol and such paraphernalia as funnels, lacy underpants, and head-to-foot plaster bandages in which rival players are encased. Though Kemp insisted that rugby was a democratizing force, the students cock a snoot at this ideal by filing into the stands with bottles of port in their hands. Why port? "Because it is a gentleman's drink," one slightly swaying student explained. Other students do not lag behind in their own rituals, some of them alcohol-drenched, others sober and contemplative. The Christian Society still flourishes. Rag week nets tens of thousands of pounds for charity each year. And student facilities improved immeasurably during the 1980s when a recreation centre was built behind Wilson House, finally freeing the library from the risks of raucous performances.

The St Mary's rugby team remained a power in the land to the end, garnering victories up until it merged with the teams from Westminster and Charing Cross in 1997. The new team of Imperial Medicals has won every cup final since its formation. Into the new millennium the opposing team, especially the "old enemy, Guy's" (actually Guy's-King's-Thomas's) could still be heard heartily consigning "Mary's" rather than "Imperial Medics" to unpleasant places. But though the old traditions and taunts persist, the

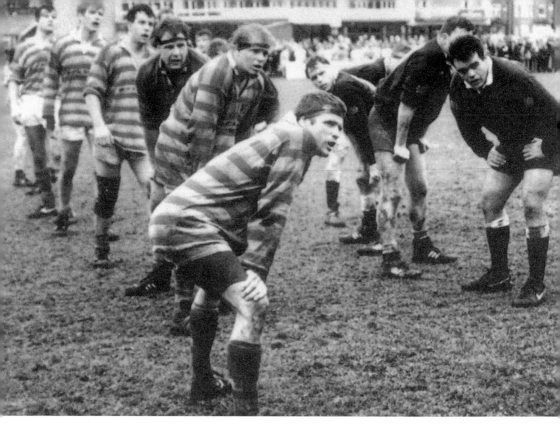

Rugby football thrives.
St Mary's Hospital
NHS Trust Archives

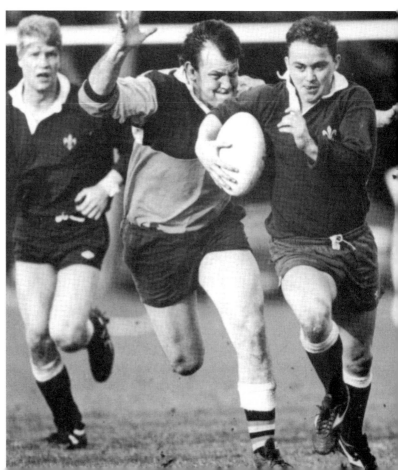

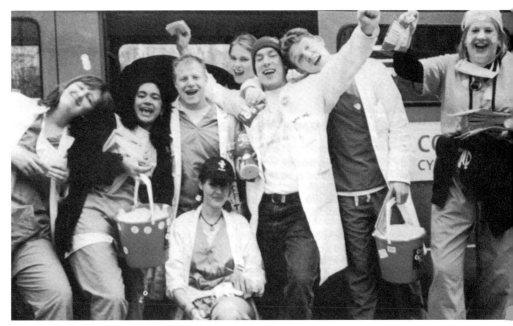

Students collecting for rag week. St Mary's Hospital NHS Trust Archives

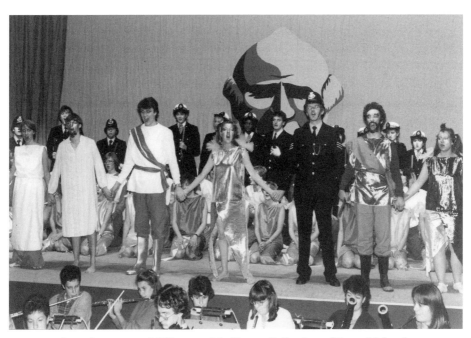

A performance of Gilbert and Sullivan. Collection of Peter Richards

new rugby team is a powerful force for friendship and amalgamation in the new Imperial College Faculty of Medicine. And, assured of academic respect, the team can openly pursue top players by offering a rugby scholarship, the "Cockburn Rugby Scholarship," named for the St Mary's captain and medical superintendent, Cocky Cockburn.

Still, the place of rugby in the medical schools has changed. The schools can no longer compete with the now-professional teams like the Barbarians or Wasps as they once could. Moreover, rugby is no longer, as it was for Moran, a macrocosm of studentship or of the profession. Rugby has been sidelined by the materialist theory of social organization that informed Birch's argument. This theory has found purchase in intellectual politics and university governance. Its influence is most visible in changes to the process of student selection, which is now governed by the principle of social justice.

Student Selection

Formerly, a dean could admit whomever he liked, as Lord Moran, interviewed on his 90th birthday, recalled: "What I instigated was that I picked 'em and there was no exam at all, I just picked 'em; it was an arbitrary process; I didn't consult any committee, I just did it myself, you see. That's a very dangerous method, of course. It depends upon the dean being a very good judge of character. If he isn't, of course, it would be disastrous."[62] By contrast, the modern dean must be *fair*. It is now an accepted principle that all actions that set people closer to or further from a medical qualification are, *de facto*, actions that structure the distribution of power, money, and authority in society. As a consequence, the process of admission has become more standardized and more objective. St Mary's provides a very good example of this change. On the one hand, it became the most popular medical school in the country, fielding the greatest number of applicants for every place. On the other hand, Peter Richards, dean from 1979 to 1995, propelled St Mary's to the heart of the debate over student identity and student selection.

Richards had trained at St George's before serving in Peart's medical unit in the late 1960s. When, in the late 1970s, the staff cast about for a new dean, Peart thought of his erstwhile lecturer, who was one of the most organized men he had known. Richards agreed to come to St Mary's as the first full-time dean when he was offered a personal chair in medicine and access to patients. Once in office, he shifted his research interests from the laboratory to the problem of student selection. Until Richards's arrival, the process followed informal lines that Moran would have recognized. A cen-

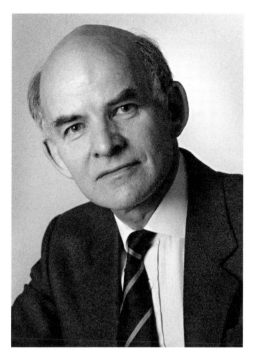

Peter Richards.
Collection of Peter Richards

tral clearing system had been introduced, so the students submitted only one application, listing the schools in order of preference. The school secretary would read over the applications, draw up a short list, and pass this on to the dean for interview. Matthews had done the work for Moran; Edgar Stevenson took it on from 1947 to 1977, and then Keith Lockyer inherited the task. Most applicants were turned away before they made it as far as a medical referee. Richards took over this work himself and did the initial selection of students for interviews. In the fall of 1980, 1,478 applied to St Mary's, of a total 10,810 applicants, and 49,328 applications for all medical schools. Nearly one-quarter of all applicants to London medical schools listed Mary's as one of their five choices, and about 12 per cent of all applicants to British medical schools did so.[63] By 1986, 24 per cent of students applying to medical school in Britain listed St Mary's as one of their choices.

Where Moran felt supremely confident of his ability to select good students, what Richards felt on surveying the stacks of applications was not so much confidence as curiosity. What sort of people were chosen and why? In 1968 a Royal Commission on Medical Education had studied candidates, identifying their class and educational background, among other things. Richards wondered if anything had changed, and whether St Mary's followed the normal pattern. Together with Chris McManus, a psychology lecturer at St Mary's, he set about finding out. They sent out a question-naire to all St Mary's applicants with U.K. postal addresses, 1,361 in total. Of these, 1,151 replied. Interviewed candidates answered another question-naire. Applicants were asked about their social, educational, and family background and their reasons for entering medicine. They were invited to voice their own opinions on selection ("many doing so with great feeling"). The second questionnaire examined personality types, with psychological tests and questions about cultural and sporting interests and ethical, polit-ical, and social attitudes. The results indicated that working-class students were not penalized over middle-class students, but they were less likely to have applied in the first place. Having a medical practitioner in the family did help applicants, as did the date of the application (the earlier the bet-ter) and grades (the higher the better). While Oxbridge students achieved higher grades, "There were no differences between St Mary's, other Lon-don, and non-London schools." Psychologically, applicants were more ex-travert, less neurotic, and less psychotic than their peers.

McManus and Richards also probed the interview procedure. They found that schools that interviewed students, like St Mary's, accepted can-didates with lower academic qualifications but higher ratings of interests. In other words, St Mary's was still prepared to favour character. The rea-sons for doing so were not entirely those of Lord Moran. Richards argued that no examination could test for "humanity, perception, perseverance and good judgement."[64] Brightness alone, moreover, wouldn't always see students through the course. Richards explained, "Medicine is tough, so we look for determination. It helps to survive if you have other talents, so we look for excellence in any other field, from butterfly collecting to music or rugby."[65] Other members of staff at St Mary's privileged rugby in particu-lar. "Rugby players make the best casualty doctors" is a phrase still to be heard in the western end of the hospital.

When Richards and McManus extended their survey of applicants and students to the years 1981 and 1986, they found that, despite protestations to the contrary, medical schools preferred students who ranked them first. The two men also recirculated the applicants round the same referees to see if opinions varied from person to person, and found only small differences. Still other follow-up studies focused on the learning experience. One iden-tified learning styles. Another showed that students who entered in the 1990s gained less clinical experience than those of the 1980s. Another sur-veyed drop-out rates, showing these to be small. The Mary's group also studied the ethnic make-up of candidates to St Mary's and other medical schools. They found that, once grades and other factors had been allowed for, white students were more likely to be accepted than those from ethnic minorities. (Another study using 1990 students showed that ethnic minorities faced discrimination in twelve of twenty-eight medical schools.)

The studies drew attention in influential quarters, such as the UCCA, to some serious questions surrounding selection. Far more public was Richards's decision to invite the BBC in to film the process of selecting and training medical students. BBC editors decided it would be interesting to follow medical students through school and subsequent careers, and they chose St Mary's because Richards had written about medical education and because the school had old-fashioned rugby traditions, yet half the intake was female. The series promised to combine the interest of serious social commentary with the hijinks of *Doctor in the House* or the *Carry On* films (supposedly modelled on a Mary's surgeon). The Academic Board was markedly unenthusiastic, the student union likewise. They agreed to let incoming students decide whether they wanted to be filmed. Richards himself was enthusiastic from the beginning and determined to push the project through. He commented to one journal, "It seemed to be an area of real public interest; we had a duty to lay open the process, and ourselves, to public scrutiny ... I hoped that the imperfections visible to the world would be those involved in the system, and that the pleasures would be special features of St. Mary's."[66] He reserved the right to cut any segments that might harm students' careers, but no cuts were made.

The cameras rolled into St Mary's in 1984 to begin filming interviews. The first episode in the series, showing the interviews, seized the public's attention. Everyone could sympathize with the hopeful young applicants; everyone had an opinion about who should have been accepted. The *Health Service Journal* noticed that a young girl in the Duke of Edinburgh's awards scheme who liked to read obtained unanimous support from a selection panel, while an older man who denounced nuclear weapons was turned away. The *BMJ* saw class prejudice at work when a Welsh boy from a comprehensive school was turned down after he hesitated over questions concerning miners' diseases, whereas when a "sweet girl from a private school in Bolton admits she has no idea what causes people to become tramps, the Dean falls over himself to offer her a place."[67] Richards recalls ruefully that there was almost a revolt over that personable young Welsh boy, who was accepted to the medical school of his choice in Wales.

Reviewers marvelled at the ignorance students revealed. One reviewer exclaimed, "I defy anyone who is committed to the doctor-as-god view not to be shocked to see these godlings stammer out nervous answers to a bunch of unsurprising questions." With its display of eighteen-year-olds learning to draw blood and distinguish the gluteus maximus from the elbow, actually behaving like boisterous eighteen-year-olds, *Doctors to Be*

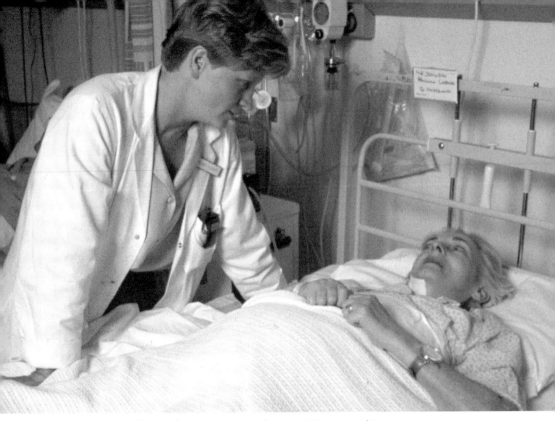

Sarah Holdsworth, in *Doctors to Be*. BBC Picture Archives

John Shepherd, in *Doctors to Be*.
BBC Picture Archives

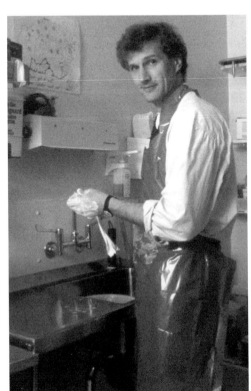

was "set fair to set back the carefully acquired authority of the medical profession 100 years."[68] The BMJ also found the students remarkably ignorant, even after they had passed their early exams and began to see patients. It described a moving exchange between Ese Oshivere, a student of Nigerian ancestry, and a patient with myeloma. Ese giggled nervously on hearing the man describe his condition, and she told him, "I'm only a medical student – I don't know what that is." Her face fell when the patient explained that it was cancer. Another student, Will Liddell, was appalled to discover, after two years, that he couldn't think of the cause of a cough, and remarked woefully, "The depth of my ignorance is astonishing."

The cameras continued to roll as Will, Ese, Sarah, Nick, Fay, Dong, Jane, Mark, David, and John learned to keep their fingernails clean and avoid a ragging from the consultant, to draw blood, to examine patients, and to talk to them. They laughed and cavorted at the soirée and sweated over examinations, which not all of them passed. For their electives, Ese went to Jamaica and treated endless knife wounds in the casualty department, Nick Hollings went to Borneo as a last chance to see people in their home environment before taking up specialized surgical studies, and Dong Chiu, a Chinese Malaysian student, went to Sarawak.

During the early 1990s the series ran again, updating the students' activities and showing them as junior doctors. Sarah had her first house job in the orthopaedics department at St Mary's, where she found herself single-handedly in charge and, within minutes, dealing with a broken pelvis. She and the others were working more than eighty hours per week and suffering from lack of sleep, a diet of junk food, and low pay. They were exhausted and fed up with the work. Their frank statements were haunting. Will confessed that sometimes, preparing for a late-night admission of an elderly patient, "I've felt ... you know, I just wish the patient would die before they get here, because then I won't have to go through the rigmarole of doing an ECG, taking the blood ..." Another of the keen young applicants of 1984 had in his exhaustion committed a mistake in prescribing, and he took himself out of medicine to rethink things. In a newspaper article, Richards compared the experiences of this group to that of his generation: his own cohort had worked even longer hours, but with patient turnovers much lower, there was not the same pressure, and the work was more pastoral.

Since the program was broadcast in the early 1990s, conditions for junior doctors have improved, largely the result of EEC directives. The program itself helped to generate sympathy for the young doctors and support for a change of policy. The series is still ongoing; what will happen to these people next is not yet a matter of history. What is certain is that the lives

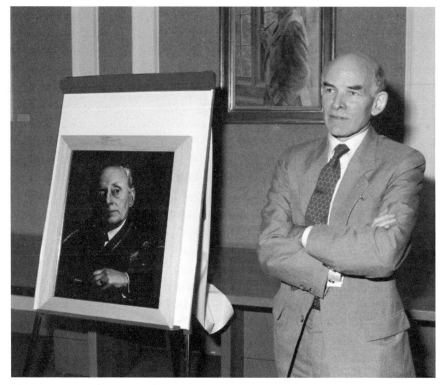

The two "great deans." Collection of Peter Richards

of students on Praed Street will be very different in future, as a consequence of the school's merger with Imperial College.

During the half century that separated Moran and Richards, the students' experience changed considerably, but one very important element of continuity remained. Richards, like Moran, believed deeply in a student-centred school. He insisted that students, not teachers, set the atmosphere for a medical school and that, so long as students are given responsibility and an atmosphere that encourages them to grow spiritually and socially as well as to develop academically, their keenness, energy, curiosity, and idealism will keep the NHS in good shape and patients well cared for. A society that wants its patients treated as fully human beings rather than as passive objects for medical intervention must treat its medical students as fully human beings rather than as glorified technicians. Because people are at their weakest and most vulnerable when they are ill, those treating them must be at their most sympathetic, scrupulously careful of the rights, privileges, and needs of their patients. Medicine cuts straight to the heart of the values of a civilization. Therefore, a medical school must be something like

Plato's republic, an idealized community. It must recognize and nurture the highest values of the civilization that sustains it. These values must permeate from the bottom up, rather than being imposed from the top down.

Both Richards and Moran, in their own fashion, bolstered a student-centred culture at the school, which helped to forge a strong sense of self-confidence among the students and a strong corporate identity. St Mary's supports an alumni association of two thousand members, which maintains scholarships for current students. In forging this identity, Richards and Moran took their cue from the traditions of and culture within St Mary's. Richards even took up the soda siphon that Harold Edwards relinquished with the deanship. Despite such countervailing forces as specialization and liberal guilt, informal mechanisms of culture have persisted in ensuring that students of St Mary's would meet not, in T.S. Eliot's phrase, as "committee members," but as people sharing a wealth of tacit knowledge and values. It remains to be seen whether the new Imperial College School of Medicine with its annual intake of three hundred students can sustain this shared culture, or, indeed, whether it wishes to.

St Mary's
at the Century's End

The Changed Hospital 1
The Big Picture

AFTER 1948 ST MARY'S exercised dominion over a sprawling fiefdom of "constituent" hospitals spread across West London and itself owed fealty to the Ministry of Health, which paid the bills. The money was good at first, though not quite as good as the governors had hoped. In subsequent years the government became less liberal and demanded proof of value for money. The state and the medical profession engaged in a long dialogue about the purpose and efficiency of the NHS, with hospitals at the centre of the dispute. This chapter shows how the hospital authorities learned to integrate these local and larger perspectives. It outlines the state's campaign to subject St Mary's to centralized discipline in the name of efficiency. Social and economic pressures behind the campaign are exemplified by conditions in the district, which was still "mournful Paddington ... a place of transit and transience."[1] Concerns over the relationship between health and poverty continued to shape medical politics in the 1950s as they had done in the 1850s.

Accounts of the NHS, like accounts of mid-Victorian medicine, have tended to focus on politics, and in particular on the wrangling between the state and professional organizations like the BMA. These accounts are not well integrated with discussions of medical knowledge and practice. But medical expertise was at the heart of the confrontation between state and profession. The medical profession based its claims to power and money on science – that is, on the knowledge revolution that had transformed medicine. Politicians could only impose their will on the profession if they could challenge its authority with alternative standards of authority. In response, doctors learned to incorporate politics into their clinical research programs, so as to beat the politicians at their own game. If there was a political logic to the repeated reorganization of medicine, there was also a medical logic to the profession's response. It was a logic informed by political considerations, but equally informed by the clinic, by the limits of what could be known about and done to people's bodies.

Politics and the View from Praed Street

During the run-up to the designated day for the initiation of the NHS in June 1948, the always-precarious finances of the hospital collapsed entirely. Its overdraft had tripled during the economic crisis of the early 1930s, rising from £20,000 to £60,000 between 1932 and 1935, and by 1939 hovering around £75,000. Wartime payments from the government, which reserved 295 beds, reduced the overdraft by one-third within a year. But by the end of the war, with public ownership looming, subscriptions and donations dried up while costs spiralled upwards. The overdraft rose above £140,000 until the Ministry of Health pegged it at £136,000, instructing the governors to sell off securities to keep it below that figure. Thus, on entering the NHS, the hospital *looked* broke, but in fact this crisis was largely an artifact of the NHS legislation. The governors were so optimistic about the long-term economic future that in the mid-1940s visitors were shown a scale model of a projected new hospital.

The Ministry of Health had other priorities. In July 1948 it inherited a badly run-down network of hospitals. As the chief medical officer, George Godber, observed, even those not damaged in the Blitz (as most of the London teaching hospitals had been) were "largely old and defective in structure." But they would have to do: the first new district hospital was not begun until 1957.[2] St Mary's was old but relatively sound by postwar London standards. The project of rebuilding, so dear to the governors' hearts, was postponed until the 1980s. Income for capital projects at St Mary's during the first few years of the NHS hovered between about £30,000 and £60,000 and paid for only dire necessities. By the late 1950s, as economic conditions improved, so too did the grants: that to St Mary's rose to £150,000 per annum, and in the early 1960s a new out-patient wing was built.

On 24 June 1948, when the new board of governors of St Mary's met for the first time, many of the old board of managers attended, including Anthony de Rothschild, who took the chair, Edgar Lawley, and clinicians including Fleming, Cope, and Porritt. But now there were also socialists present. Richard Doll, one of the few London consultants to support the introduction of the NHS, was named to the board by the ministry. Sir Richard

Doll recalls, "I was very surprised when I was put on it, for I held very left wing views at that time. But everyone was very polite to me."[3] Doll had a clinical position and research base elsewhere (though he did use patients from St Mary's along with other hospitals when he and Bradford Hill showed in 1951 that smoking caused lung cancer[4]). As well, Esther Rickards represented the local authority. The real centre of power at St Mary's, according to Doll, was the medical committee, which is to say the consultants. The lay governors largely followed the advice of the medical staff. And, whatever their differences at lower levels, "they were all very careful, the consultants on the Board, never to disagree with each other." St Mary's clung to the principle, voiced by the old board of managers in April 1943, that "the present practice in Voluntary Hospitals, of control of medical affairs by a Medical Committee, should be maintained."[5] There was considerable old wine in the new skin of the state hospital.

Relations between the ministry and the board of governors were, on the whole, cordial and fruitful. The governors continually complained of lack of money, as demand for NHS services among the British public soared far beyond planners' expectations. Only occasionally did political and clinical interests clash spectacularly. One such clash, over the rationalization of hospital services, pitted St Mary's and local political authorities against one another, leaving the Ministry of Health in the difficult position of arbitrator. The sprawling fiefdom of constituent hospitals was unwieldy and often redundant, but proposals for rationalization were controversial.

In 1948 St Mary's had 476 beds on Praed Street, while the Samaritan Hospital for Women provided another eighty-eight beds, the Western Ophthalmic Hospital thirty-five, and Paddington Green Children's Hospital fifty-two. On Harrow Road the old London Lock Hospital with sixty-four beds had been closed down; next door, the Paddington General Hospital with 668 beds was the busiest in the borough, serving the poor and crowded north part of Paddington. In the western part of the parish there was "St Luke's Hospital for the Dying," renamed "St Luke's Hospital, Bayswater," and later changed to the wholly innocuous "Hereford Lodge." Beyond the parish boundary in North Kensington, two further hospitals would also enter the St Mary's empire: Princess Louise Hospital and St Charles Hospital, formerly the Marylebone Workhouse Infirmary. Integration of clinical services throughout the group proceeded slowly and painfully. Gynaecology was transferred from St Mary's to the Samaritan Hospital and ophthalmic out-patient clinics to the Western Ophthalmic Hospital. Relocating obstetrics, on the other hand, proved far more difficult. St Mary's badly needed more obstetric beds, both to meet increasing demand from parturient women and to establish an sixty-bedded academic unit.

But St Mary's Hospital had no spare beds. Ambulance cases were turned away three times out of four in the fall of 1952 and two times of three in 1955.[6] Bed occupancy was at 94.9 per cent for the whole hospital. The consequence was overworked staff and cross-infection. Waiting lists increased substantially during this period. But while adult beds at St Mary's were running at 100 per cent occupancy, children's cots had much lower rates: 75 per cent at Paddington Green Children's Hospital, 66 per cent at Princess Louise Hospital in Kensington, and 79 per cent in the Lewis Carroll Ward at St Mary's in 1952. Children were less sick less often and, increasingly, much of their treatment was done in out-patient departments. St Mary's was a pioneer in providing home care for sick children. A pilot scheme worked out by Freddie Brimblecombe in the 1950s – deemed too experimental to receive Exchequer funding and paid for by the Endowment Fund – provided medical and nursing supervision for children at home. The project was a great success and was finally taken up by the public authorities. But even had the demand for paediatric beds not declined, the St Mary's group would still have been overstocked with two paediatric hospitals. The obvious solution was to "disclaim" one of these and convert it to maternity or much-needed geriatric beds. In November 1952, the Ministry of Health approved the conversion.

This solution was obvious but impolitic. Paddington Green, which began life in 1862 as the North-West London Free Dispensary for Sick Children, had always enjoyed support and subscriptions from local labourers. The door was always open to worried mothers. Paddington Green was the workhorse of paediatric care, while the Lewis Carroll Ward on Praed Street catered to a middle-class clientele. According to Tom Oppé, long the professor of paediatrics at St Mary's, Paddington Green was a bastion of left-wing politics and values, quite different from the "rarefied atmosphere" of St Mary's.[7] Thus when St Mary's began in 1949 to contemplate converting Paddington Green, it quickly learned of the political cost. In October 1949, following correspondence from the North and South Paddington Labour parties, the Middlesex Local Medical Committee, the Paddington Trades Council, the Institute of Psychoanalysis, the University of London Institute of Education, the vicar of Holy Trinity Church, the National Association of Mental Health, the Paddington Conservative Club, and the Paddington Deanery, the board of governors at St Mary's promised to maintain paediatric services at Paddington Green.

Princess Louise in Kensington made an easier target. Endocrinologist S.L. Simpson vainly appealed to the board, arguing that "it would be a blot on the history of St. Mary's if the Board should agree to the destruction of Princess Louise Hospital, which had sought the protection and guidance of St. Mary's in the safeguarding of the objects for which it was founded,

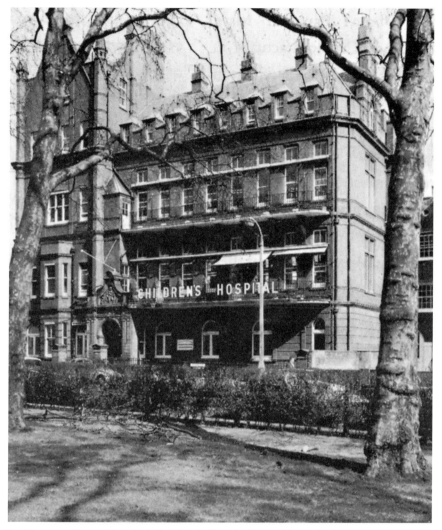

Paddington Green Hospital. St Mary's Hospital NHS Trust Archives

namely the care of sick children in the area in which it stands." Would that they had never applied to join, Simpson lamented.[8] The governors were unmoved. Increasing financial stringency would force the closure of the group hospitals, one by one. At the end of the 1990s only the Western Ophthalmic Hospital remained open. But the governors probably anticipated this outcome all along. In June 1958 board members commented that once St Mary's was rebuilt, "the present Constituent Hospital buildings would no longer be required by St. Mary's and would thus be disclaimed to the Minister."

The minister of Health still hesitated to close Princess Louise Hospital. Peers, municipal councillors, and local organizations had denounced the scheme. There were also legal impediments: the covenant conveying the land specified that it should be reserved for a hospital for mothers and children. To get around the covenant, St Mary's decided to site the new obstetrics unit at Princess Louise, converting the ground-floor wards for the purpose. In December 1960, at long last, Ian MacGillivray was named professor of obstetrics, and in November 1961 the new unit began admitting patients. Soon afterwards, the minister of Health (the fifth since 1955 when the change was first proposed) belatedly approved the introduction of maternity beds at Princess Louise. At the end of the decade, however obstetrics was moved back to Praed Street at the insistence of the obstetricians. Obstetrics had become a high-tech, high-intervention field and needed the support of the general hospital. The bed shortages on Praed Street were eased in 1968 when the Regional Hospital Board relinquished Paddington General Hospital, handing it over to the board of governors for full integration into the teaching group. With two large obstetric wards on Praed Street and Harrow Road, the governors could empty the obstetric beds at Princess Louise. Early in 1969 the minister gave cautious approval to filling them with geriatric patients.

The situation was tragically complicated by a mishap at Paddington General. It had occurred in July 1967, before the governors of St Mary's took charge, but it came back to haunt them in 1969. A seven-year-old boy named David Tomlinson was misdiagnosed with appendicitis and died of a viral infection. The parents complained to the Regional Hospital Board, which found that there had been no malpractice but inadequate care. Only one house surgeon had been on duty that weekend, with no paediatric services, and the nurses were students, too inexperienced to notice the boy's deterioration. The tribunal recommended that the ward be closed or upgraded "as a matter of urgency." The Tomlinsons took their story to the newspapers, while the Department of Health published the report in December 1969. The governors of St Mary's found themselves at the centre of a highly charged medical scandal and under pressure from the Department of Health (now the Department of Health and Social Services) to close the ward permanently.

The board of governors quickly added another house officer and fifty more nurses, bringing the total to three hundred. But they refused to bow to political pressure and close the ward permanently. Paddington General had the busiest obstetrics ward and casualty department in the borough, with more than 50,000 emergency cases seen annually. Inevitably, sick children would come to the hospital, and some sort of paediatric cover was needed. Governors, politicians, and consultants staged a very public row. Defenders of Princess Louise made much of the scandal. Lady Petrie, an alderwoman on the Kensington and Chelsea Council, exclaimed to a journalist, "What fools they are! Putting their children in a derelict hospital when they have a purpose-built children's hospital in their own group less than a mile away." The headline on the next week's *Paddington Mercury* read, "Hospital Chief Hits Back at Lady P."[9] The DHSS finally agreed to permit geriatric patients in two of the four wards, so long as the board also provided for mentally handicapped children in the others. There would also be thirty-four psychiatric beds at Harrow Road, soon to rise to sixty, to service a new academic unit in psychiatry.

Prior to the NHS geriatric and psychiatric cases had been dumped in massive, two-thousand-bed institutions. Under the NHS there was a concerted effort to create smaller, more thoroughly medical institutions, closer to the homes and families of those institutionalized. New psychiatric drugs like chlorpromazine, introduced in 1952, facilitated the change. As well, the medical curriculum was broadened to include these special subjects. But the reforms required more beds than St Mary's could muster. Hence, St Mary's had asked for and received access to the beds at Paddington General Hospital in 1948 and hence, two decades later, it seemed natural to transfer the hospital to the teaching group. In return the governors of St Mary's agreed to assume "district responsibility." Rather than allocating beds according to teaching needs, they would have to consider the district's needs, filling quotas set down by the Ministry of Health. St Mary's was not responsible to the Regional Hospital Board, but the two institutions had representatives on one another's boards, and they worked together, referring patients to one another in time of bed shortages. In November 1960 the two boards discussed responsibility for geriatric beds, with the RHB keen to integrate geriatric cases in general wards and St Mary's keen to keep them out.[10] The RHB argued that students should study such cases, St Mary's, that there was little to learn from them. Only from 1968 did St Mary's seriously take up geriatrics.

Political Pressures

One reason why St Mary's was eager to assume district responsibilities was the erosion of the special status of teaching hospitals. In 1948 teaching hospitals were given special autonomy and funding. By the 1960s, however, it had become clear that this policy tended to reinforce the inequalities in health-care provision that had, for socialists like Bevan, been the point of the NHS in the first place. A study published in 1964 showed that the

North-West Thames Region – home to St Mary's – had the most consultants per capita, 22.8 per 100,000, while Sheffield had nearly half that amount, and the gap had grown by 15 per cent since 1948.[11] The NHS seemed to cause more, not less inequality. This was politically unacceptable.

From the 1960s successive ministers of Health began to look for ways to redistribute health care. This long-term project took many forms over the years, but above all it consisted of an assault on the London teaching hospitals. The special autonomy of the teaching hospitals was removed in 1974 when the boards of governors were abolished and the hospitals placed under new Area Health Authorities (AHAs). Next, other regions began to receive more funding at the expense of London. Finally, the Department of Health tried to pass the extra cost of teaching on to the Department of Education. These initiatives were formalized by the Resources Allocation Working Party (RAWP) established in 1975, but they began to inform department policy from about 1970.

Much of the reorganization was set in motion by the Labour secretary of state for the new Department of Health and Social Services (DHSS) from 1968 to 1970, Richard Crossman. Crossman represented Birmingham, which was near the bottom of the table for health-care provision. As the new merged department's title suggested, health was now to be more thoroughly integrated with social services. Crossman produced a Green Paper in 1970 that aimed at redistributing health care according to objective needs measured statistically, with an emphasis on community services.[12] Before his plan could be integrated, a Conservative government took office and produced its own plan of reform in a White Paper of 1972. The Conservatives did not abolish the regional boards, but they added a layer of Area Health Authorities, largely filled by political nominees chosen for their "management abilities." These AHAs would manage and integrate hospital and community medical services, including the teaching hospitals. Returned to office in 1974, Labour tempered this centralist schema by strengthening local representation (to compose one-third of AHA members).

The reorganizations of the 1970s and 1980s were aimed at disciplining the medical profession in general and the teaching hospitals in particular. The DHSS was in much the same position that the old hospital governors had been a century before. If the St Mary's consultants had demanded a certain treatment or diet be provided, the governors could not refuse on any but economic grounds. Rather than trying to impose financial discipline upon individual clinical decisions, Victorian-era governors chose the far easier path of limiting the number of patients admitted. Comparatively few applicants were admitted into St Mary's but, once patients *were* admitted, nothing was refused them. The rest of the population had to fall back on the scantier provision at the infirmary. However, if all people had to be admitted to a hospital somewhere in the NHS, this form of rationing could not apply. Political authorities had to find a new way to impose financial discipline upon clinical decisions. On the one hand, if hospitals were placed under local authorities, they would be competing for resources with other medical lobbies, such as general practitioners. On the other hand, expert managers, trained to balance books and manage "human resources," could prioritize competing demands with more authority than the amateur governors could command. Both these approaches were adopted.

After 1974, recalls George Bonney, who was on the board of governors that year, the hospital officials "had to start arguing the toss" at the AHA in competition with the Westminster Hospital, the Middlesex, and general practitioners. This was a shock to their pride and independence. Hardest hit was the house governor, Alan Powditch. Under the new regime he became one of a district management team, along with a medical officer, a finance officer, chief nursing officer, and the dean of the medical school. Powditch found that his channels of influence dried up, and he retired in 1977. By that time St Mary's was well and truly dilapidated. Every new minister of Health was shown around Praed Street, and departed, ashen-faced, promising a new building. But there was nowhere to build. Powditch proposed to fill in the canal basin and build atop it, but the public revolted against the idea. Powditch's successor, Terry Hunt, solved the problem by sacrificing Harrow Road. The closure of Paddington General would pay for the rebuilding of St Mary's, and he obtained land from British Waterways by trading off a chunk of the Harrow Road site. Paddington General Children's Hospital would also be closed. The scheme was approved, and rebuilding began in the early 1980s.

Concentration made sense to the NHS planners because the population of Paddington was shrinking as people moved to the suburbs. But residents in Kilburn and Harrow Road objected to losing their local hospital, seeing the rebuilding at Praed Street as "at best irrelevant and at worst a boost to the medical school at the expense of the community." The loss of the hospital would hasten inner-city decay in impoverished North Paddington. Hospitals were seen to provide "a definite but ill defined social role" in deprived communities that no other welfare service could fill.[13] The scheme was opposed by the Community Health Council, trade unions, and residents who formed a "Save Paddington Hospitals" campaign. A Health Council referendum found that residents would accept the hospital closure, if they were given community health services at Harrow Road. A new community hospital was therefore opened in 1985, but later cuts led to the closure and sale of the Harrow Road site.

The reorganizations of the 1970s did integrate the teaching hospitals, however. In the case of St Mary's, integration had the result of increasing rather than decreasing the hospital's share of community resources. If the AHAs had been designed to shrink the teaching hospitals, they were failing in their objective. Instead they amplified the hospitals' demands. The response of Margaret Thatcher's Conservative government was to abolish the AHAs. It also reduced local and professional representation on the District Health Authorities which now managed hospitals, making them more directly the instruments of the central government. In 1983 Thatcher inaugurated a "managerial revolution" within the NHS, adding professional managers at every level. Historian Rudolf Klein argues that while all governments worried about efficiency in the NHS, this concern dominated government policy under Thatcher.[14] Her vision of society, he continues, was of a strong, central state and strong, individualistic consumers, with weak intermediary bodies such as local authorities, trade unions, or professional associations. During the 1980s she delegated executive responsibility for local management of the NHS to the periphery, all the while maintaining legislative and financial control.

During the 1970s and 1980s, then, hospitals like St Mary's found themselves under assault both politically and financially. Political and financial factors were now priorities, trumping the clinical and pedagogical arguments by doctors. But the medical profession has always been politically astute, and it adapted to the new atmosphere. Finding their clinical arguments overturned by sociological arguments relating to distributive justice, doctors quickly mastered and assimilated these arguments. Paddington provided fertile ground for the new, socially conscious medicine. To understand the change, it is necessary to take a step backwards to consider the place of health and of medicine in society and in social policy more generally. Richard Crossman, for example, had come to the Department of Health and Social Services from the Department of Housing, which was, when he took office in 1964, at the centre of a new kind of debate about poverty and justice in modern Britain. Conditions in Paddington were at the centre of these debates. During the early 1960s, Paddington was wracked by social conflicts as serious as any in its history. While these conflicts specifically addressed standards of living, they established a new consensus about the function of the welfare state and framed future debates about health.

Social Pressures

Postwar Britain prided itself on its campaign to abolish poverty, and officials and social scientists believed that they were achieving the goal.[15] This consensus was shattered by the "rediscovery" of poverty.[16] People were no longer starving, but some were leading lives of terrible deprivation. In bombed-out London, housing shortages had enabled unscrupulous landlords to prey on families desperate to find shelter. In Paddington thousands were on waiting lists for council housing. At three hundred people to an acre in some neighbourhoods, it had become one of the most densely populated regions in England. The *Paddington Mercury* was filled with complaints. The Romualds, a family of four living on Shirland Road, inhabited a room ten by twelve feet, with one bed, a shared cooker on the landing, and no bathroom in the house. On Edenham Road a family of nine lived in six rooms, two of them too damp to use, and again there was no bathroom. In the slums on Clarendon Road, water dripped through the ceiling onto children lying in their beds, floors crumbled when stamped on, and drainage was blocked.

The Anglican Church still owned much of Paddington: six hundred acres with five thousand houses. In 1940 ground rents produced £84,000, which was paid into a central church fund.[17] This was a great deal of money to siphon out of a poor, inner-city area. Worse, the church stood accused of making the money on the backs of "enslaved" women: The Ecclesiastical Commissioners, who took over the property from the bishop of London, were landlords to one of London's largest communities of prostitutes. In 1942 a resident of Sussex Gardens, Dr Thomas Stowell, began a campaign of letters to the *Times* to complain that men and even children were accosted in broad daylight by "unhappy women, who are driven on all the time by panders, pimps and bullies on the watch at street corners." The industry was "highly capitalised and highly remunerative and highly organised," with the average bawdy house producing £2,000 in six weeks. The Ecclesiastical Commissioners tried to defend themselves as businessmen, unconcerned with morality, but in 1948 they took action. Rather than trying to house the poor themselves, they sold some ninety acres to Paddington and London County Councils for council housing and began to develop luxury and high-rise apartment blocks on the remaining land. By the early 1960s they insisted that they no longer owned slums or brothels. Their building projects drove up rents and rates, making life harder for the poor families they refused to house.

Many of the poorest were immigrants. Between 1948, when British colonials were invested with British citizenship, and 1962, when commonwealth immigration was again restricted, 300,000 people immigrated to Britain from the West Indies.[18] Nearly half settled in London, especially the poorer areas: Hackney, Brixton, North Kensington, and Paddington. These immigrants brought a colourful culture with them, but they also brought new medical and social problems. Sickle-cell anaemia earned a mention as a rare disease at St Mary's in 1940 when a "half breed negress"

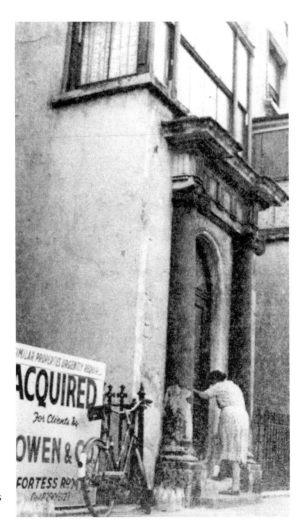

Postwar Paddington.
St Mary's Hospital NHS
Trust Archives and the
Royal College of Surgeons
of England

was diagnosed with it: "The patient submitted with fortitude to the en-
raptured gaze of unnumbered clinicians; and her case is to be written
up."[19] Within a few years, the rarity had become a staple of the haematology clinic. Another problem was syphilis. Bereft of their families, immigrants turned to strangers. By 1965 immigrants constituted 55 per cent
of the caseload in the special clinic at St Mary's.[20]

Immigrants faced discrimination from employers and landlords, so they
were more likely to be poor, unemployed, and badly housed.[22] They were
also blamed for social problems. In 1963 the Paddington and Marylebone
Employment Committee, which had the longest queue in London, asked
for a ban on immigrants until unemployment figures were down. All that
spring, angry letters filled the local press, denouncing or defending immigrants, while violence flared on the streets. In early June two dozen leather
and denim clad teenagers forced their way into the West African Student

Hostel on Warrington Crescent. City councillors warned of a "racially explosive" situation in Paddington. People feared a replay of the Notting Hill riots of 1958 when white thugs went on a rampage.

Matters came to ahead in July 1963 during the Profumo affair. The secretary of state for War had, it turned out, shared a mistress with the most rapacious landlord in West London, a Polish immigrant named Peter Rachman who had died in 1962.[22] Rachman made a fortune by charging exorbitant rents to prostitutes and immigrants, whom no one else would house. Disobliging tenants were beaten or found their gas or power cut off, or even their roof removed.[23] Journalists found lurid copy for their papers: stories of, for example, twenty people sharing one toilet and a single cold tap. Rachman's empire spanned Hammersmith and Notting Hill as well as Kensington, but the enterprising Labour MP for North Paddington, Ben Parkin, ensured that public attention focused on Paddington when he described it in the Commons as "the biggest brothel in Europe." At the town hall, demonstrators demanding housing reform (and, often, nuclear disarmament) crowded into meetings, shouted down council members, and were carried out by the police. The Rachman affair helped to bring down the Conservative government in 1964 and to secure housing reforms under the new Labour minister, Richard Crossman. The British public was shocked to learn that such poverty and squalor persisted in Britain. The incident paved the way to a much larger debate on the nature and incidence of poverty.

The Rachman scandal signalled a shift in the left-wing political agenda. The traditional Labour constituency, the working class, no longer suffered from joblessness or homelessness as it once had. Unemployment figures remained below interwar standards until the 1970s, while home ownership rose from 10 per cent in 1910 to 42 per cent in 1962.[24] Statistical measures of poverty showed a tenfold decrease, from one-third to a mere 3 per cent.[25] As a consequence, traditional Labour party voters began to favour tax cuts over social services. The demands of the poor and of labour unions had coincided in Britain; now they bifurcated, with ethnicity marking a cleavage point.

A new definition of poverty was being framed by a group of left-wing academics at the London School of Economics. They replaced the old objective measure with a relative measure of poverty: the poor were those who were least well off in any society. Poverty was no longer something that could be eradicated. The poverty that was rediscovered in the 1950s and 1960s was "essentially a statistical concept. The poor did not make themselves visible; they were discovered at the bottom of income tables by social scientists."[26] There was some dispute as to where to set the poverty line (the LSE found 14 per cent were poor, the Labour party only 3.8 per cent).

The rediscovery of poverty was accomplished by Richard Titmuss, the first professor of social administration at the LSE, and his protégés Peter Townsend and Brian Abel-Smith (who succeeded him to the LSE chair). Titmuss was not trained in a university but had worked in an insurance office, writing books in his spare time, before being commissioned to write the official war history of social policy.[27] He had received MRC money to study social medicine, and in 1941 he had joined a Committee for the Study of Social Medicine, chaired by the physiology professor at St Mary's, Arthur Huggett. From 1951 to 1955 Titmuss was on the board of governors of the Hammersmith Hospital, and from 1953 to 1955 he was on the North-West Thames Regional Hospital Board, which encompassed Paddington. Sociology was infiltrating the NHS.

Ten years on from 1948, Titmuss saw threats to the hospital service from growing impersonality and bureaucratization.[28] These problems could be solved by putting sociologists in charge of hospitals and sociology in the curriculum, to provide students with "a greater understanding of the dynamics of human relationships ... The task of the future is to make medicine more 'social,' in its application without losing in the process the benefits of science and specialized knowledge."[29] This was an explosive new way of defining medicine. Hitherto, impersonality had seemed a consequence of the scientization and quantification of medicine. Conservative clinicians had fought it by arguing that in its application to the patient – who was not a statistic, and whose body was not a laboratory reagent – medicine was an applied art that could only be learned at the bedside. The concept of "medicine as art" tempered the concept of "medicine as science." Now, however, the language of patient "individuality" was submerged within a new language of the patient as a "whole" person. Sociologists claimed to provide the best way of encapsulating the "whole" patient as a social being.

Social Medicine

Titmuss was not simply lobbing a new concept, grenade-like, into medicine. He had been deeply influenced by John Ryle, who took up the first appointment as professor of social medicine at Cambridge in 1943. In an inaugural address, Ryle drew on Titmuss's early work on poverty when he defined social medicine: it studied groups and it sought to reduce disparities in death and morbidity between those groups.[30] The idea of social medicine reinvigorated a stalled public health movement. Hygienists like R.C. Wofinden, who qualified at St Mary's in the 1930s before becoming a medical officer of health and professor of public health in Bristol, welcomed the advent of social and state medicine together in the 1940s.[31] Public health had been marginal in his own medical training: "If I remember rightly the title was 'Hygiene' and it was badly taught through a brief series of boring lectures which most students avoided." The exam was still modelled on Chadwickian notions of hygiene. Wofinden embarked upon a career in public health because, he said, though he won prizes and distinctions in the medical course, he hadn't enough money to become a consultant, and the junior post in the medical unit was semi-permanently occupied by a New Zealander the rugby team was reluctant to lose. For Wofinden the choice was either public health or general practice. When he discussed the choices with a fellow student of his year, John Crawford Adams (later consultant orthopaedic surgeon to St Mary's), Adams was horrified: "You can't waste your life messing about with drains and sewers," he cried.[32]

In 1950, responding to the new atmosphere, Denis Brinton attached students to the hospital almoners to visit patients in their homes and introduced field trips to industrial centres and general practices. Conservative clinicians such as W.D.W. Brooks objected to even this much innovation, and into the 1960s public health remained marginal at St Mary's.[33] One student who entered St Mary's in this period and became an epidemiologist recalled that, "even if you could spell epidemiology, you didn't want to." His cohort heard two lectures from Geoffrey Rose (hired in 1962 as a part-time lecturer shared with the London School of Hygiene) but remained otherwise untutored in the Titmuss tradition of statistical investigation. As for the practice of social medicine at St Mary's, this remained largely in the hands of the almoners. The chief almoner was Dorothy Manchée, a prominent spokeswoman for the expansion of social services. After her retirement in 1953, the almoners became hospital social workers.

The DHSS began to impose its own brand of social medicine on the teaching hospitals from the 1960s. Sociologists, though institutionally weak themselves, provided the DHSS with a means to discipline the powerful profession of medicine. As Dorothy Porter points out, sociologists relinquished their radical slant,[34] and by way of reward, at least twenty chairs of sociology were created in Britain between 1962 and 1967.[35] The new sociological slant to DHSS policy took two forms. On the one hand, community medicine was strengthened. In 1968 two committees of inquiry (Seebohm and Todd) advanced a "new vision" of community medicine, with expanded responsibilities for hygienists and general practitioners.[36] In 1972 another report described the community physician as a crucial intermediary in the reformed NHS. That year, the Faculty of Community Medicine was established. The MOH lost ground during the austere years of the 1970s, but in the 1980s regional public health directors were introduced across the country. Public health had a new role to play in preventive medicine, in campaigning against diseases of environment and lifestyle – social causes – such as cancer and coronary heart disease.[37] GPs also benefited from the investment into community programs.

Simultaneously the DHSS tried to redistribute resources more equitably across the NHS as a whole. The instrument for this was RAWP, the Resource Allocation Working Party, set up in 1975 to refine the purely geographical redistribution strategies of the early 1970s. RAWP weighed the population of Britain by age and mortality as well as by region. It found London to be heavily over-provided with NHS resources. RAWP offered a seemingly objective, quantitative measure of this disparity and of the necessary redressment. As Rudolph Klein has remarked of RAWP, "The development of new analytical methodologies thus gave new salience to the issue of distribution within the NHS: conceptually they solved the puzzle about which criteria should be used to decide who got what, but politically they intensified it."[38] Crossman had planned to channel more funds towards the poorer regions, without subtracting it from the wealthier ones, arguing, "I can only equalise on an expanding budget."[39] However, recession in the 1970s meant that wealthier regions would be equalized downwards, above all by the closure of hospital beds. Demographic statistics justified the closures. The population of inner London fell from 4.8 million in 1931 to 2.3 million in 1977, as people moved to the suburbs. Beds in inner London, it was argued, might well be reduced by between 20 and 25 per cent.[40] This was the conclusion of the London Health Planning Consortium, formed in 1977 to facilitate planning between the four London Regional Health Boards, the DHSS, the University of London, and the UGC. Hospital beds in inner London, the consortium argued, should be moved to the suburbs. As a result the number of beds was reduced across England by 21 per cent between 1982 and 1993; in London it was reduced by more than 30 per cent.[41]

Through the 1970s and 1980s, the London teaching hospitals bowed to growing pressures for relocation. The Westminster Hospital (airily described by some as a local VD clinic for MPs) was, despite pressure from many MPs, disbanded. Its hospital facilities were relocated to the Chelsea Hospital, and its medical school to Charing Cross, which itself moved to Fulham. St George's Hospital moved to Tooting when its lease expired. The Royal Free moved to Hampstead in North London; King's College Hospital had already moved from the Strand to Denmark Hill in South London. Everyone knew that still more radical closures loomed on the horizon, as soon as the government could summon up the political will to enact them. There was no need of three teaching hospitals in North-West London (St Mary's, the Middlesex, and University College), nor of two in Southwark

(Guy's and St Thomas's) nor even of one in Smithfield (St Bartholomew's). Nor could the teaching hospitals expect the University of London to back them against the DHSS: Senate House was trying to rationalize the teaching. The hospitals desperately sought ways of staving off the blow. St Mary's couldn't draw on Great Historical Tradition, as could Bart's and Guy's. It had some influential patrons, but the older hospitals had armies of them. St Mary's was, as it had always been, one of the newest, smallest, and poorest of the hospitals. But it had two strengths to fall back on: its staff and its patients.

Almost overnight, St Mary's became an important base for social medicine, and this line of work provided hospital administrators with a powerful weapon against politically inspired assaults. Above all, St Mary's had to prove that it was an indispensable *community* institution. This was not difficult. As ever, it was in the middle of one of the poorest areas in London. The railway station and canal prevented the gentrification seen in other once-deprived areas like Islington. Many inhabitants were elderly or newcomers, the poorest of the poor. Illnesses of poverty ranging from tuberculosis to drug addiction were rife. Moreover, the population of the North-West Thames region as a whole was growing. There was thus an argument to be made for continuing and even expanding the provision of medical services in Paddington.

However, the North-West Thames had more hospitals and more consultants per capita than any other region in Britain. The RAWP figures provided a clear argument for reducing services. Any argument to defend Paddington's beds would require a formula that was more sensitive to morbidity than the mortality-based statistics of the RAWP. Precisely such a formula was developed by Brian Jarman, a St Mary's lecturer. While he was primarily concerned with the conditions of general practice, his findings had implications for medical services more generally. The story of Brian Jarman, now Professor Sir Brian Jarman, illustrates the politics and gritty reality of inner London medical practice. It also shows that the unorthodox methods of student selection at St Mary's could have far-reaching results.

The Jarman Index

Brian Jarman came to medicine late.[42] His father was an engineer and his mother worked in a post office. Jarman studied science and mathematics in Cambridge; then, after a stint in the Royal Artillery (where he was asked to develop a nuclear defence plan for Western Europe), he spent the late 1950s at Imperial College studying geophysics. After three years in the field, he was having a medical examination when the examiner mentioned that his

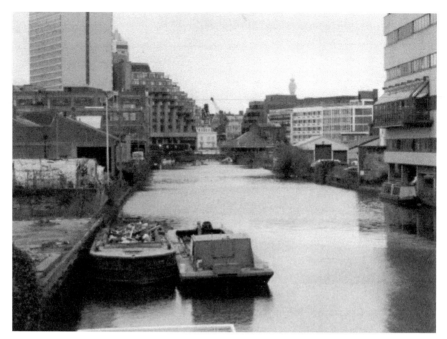

The new wing of St Mary's Hospital (right), overlooking the canal basin.
Photo: Mike Stevens

school, St Mary's, accepted mature students. Jarman applied, passed the IQ test with flying colours, and entered St Mary's at the age of thirty-one. His first impressions filled him with dismay: the lecture hall was full of young men with their feet on the desk, all reading the *Daily Telegraph*. Yet Jarman did well as a student, winning prizes and an exchange to Harvard University. His knowledge of physics and mathematics led him to laboratory research on Doppler flow through the aorta, and he seemed destined for a hospital post. But he wanted to work with people. A chance encounter with a friend in a run-down practice at Lisson Grove, the poor end of Marylebone, captivated him, and he became a locum, then a partner in the practice, to the disappointment of his sponsors at St Mary's.

Jarman's experiences in the practice propelled him towards medical politics. One day a woman came asking to be registered as a patient, saying that she had been turned away by almost every other practitioner in the neighbourhood. This seemed extraordinary to Jarman, for Marylebone was not short of practitioners. Not understanding the nature of the problem, he called a meeting of local practitioners to address it. He was warned to drop the idea quietly. Some local practitioners who relied on private practice did not want to be put under pressure to take NHS patients. These people formed a powerful interest group. Like the hero of Cronin's *The Citadel*, Jarman found himself under investigation by the GMC for fifteen months on the patently ridiculous charge of refusing vitamins to a patient who was not suffering from avitaminosis but rather from paranoid schizophrenia.

Jarman had come to medicine young enough to be an idealist, yet old enough to trust his own judgment rather than become disillusioned by the ways of the world. He concluded that these practitioners had responded to their circumstances. Most inner-city GPs were aging, single-handed, badly housed, and badly paid. The NHS made no distinctions between practices and no allowances for difficult conditions. GPs were reimbursed at a standard rate per patient, and they alone, of all NHS workers, received no London weighting in their salaries. Inner London GPs paid more for their premises and saw clienteles with morbidity and call-out rates above the average, yet they received no special recompense. Sociologists examining inner-city problems invariably studied the East End, with its high rates of industrial illness. In Lisson Grove, Jarman saw quite a different set of problems, characteristic of the West End: high rates of mobility, immigration, and broken homes. The government would, for example, place single mothers on welfare all together in a high-rise building, creating a very local and particular set of problems. Jarman determined to find a way of registering these problems and their impact on demands for GP services so that inner-city practitioners would be properly recompensed.

Jarman's index of underprivilege was developed in three stages. Identifying areas of deprivation wasn't difficult: his final map looked very much like that of Charles Booth, done nearly a century earlier. Even a simple map of population density showed much the same pattern. The difficulty was to find an objective measure of deprivation that would please everybody. Any measure of deprivation and compensation based on such simple criteria as population density would be vetoed by practitioners outside London whose own resources would diminish. Jarman's early proposals were, thus, rejected by the parent body of GPs. At the same time, he became involved in an inquiry sponsored by the London Health Planning Consortium. The consortium commissioned Donald Acheson to inquire into the conditions of general practice in London, and Acheson invited Jarman to join him. The committee invited comments from 4,000 GPs and organizations and developed a list of factors determining workloads, including hazardous occupations, the transience of the population, and psychosocial problems like addiction, marital instability, lack of health education, and high morbidity. The Acheson Committee did identify underprivileged areas in London, but again it foundered on the problem of convincing practitioners from across the country, most of them in leafy areas.

With the help of a statistician at St Mary's, Jarman drew up a question-naire based on the findings of the Acheson Committee, asking how much these factors increased workloads. He sent this to 10 per cent of practi-tioners nationwide.[43] Once scores were assigned to different weightings, the index provided a measure of "underprivilege" that the RAWP had not. On this scale, inner London was shown to have a high degree of underprivilege. Paddington and North Kensington together constituted the fourth most de-prived district in the country. Jarman took this new model to the GP coun-cil. This time, rather than rejecting it outright, the council proposed a test be done to measure the index's objectivity. Four areas would be selected, ranging from Bradford to Norfolk, and both Jarman and the council would then apply the index and see if they had the same results.

The maps were almost identical. When the index was then put to a gen-eral vote, not a single hand was raised against it. In later years, as the Jar-man index became an important instrument of policy, criticisms began to be heard. It was now thought to be slanted towards London, with poor northern districts failing to register high scores.[44] These areas, while not al-ways as socially deprived as some inner London boroughs, often have worse medical services. The index has thus been revised to include some of these factors.

The Jarman index was aimed at redressing imbalances between GP serv-ices, but from 1987 some argued for applying it to hospitals as well. GP services and hospitals are intimately connected. Poor GP services can be compensated for by the local hospital, and overworked GPs sometimes re-duce their workloads by referring patients to hospitals. Moreover, Jarman himself made the leap from practices to hospitals. In July 1994 he gave a controversial university lecture entitled "The Crisis in London Medicine: How Many Hospital Beds Does the Capital Need?" which attacked the bed closings and the demographic and morbidity projections underlying them. Likewise, administrators, academics, and consultants at St Mary's took up the Jarman index to defend themselves against the rationalizers in govern-ment. They also emphasized the place of general practice within both hos-pital and school.

Jarman's appointment to St Mary's a few years earlier reflected a change in thinking. Under duress from the UGC, in 1962 the school hired a part-time lecturer in epidemiology and preventive medicine, former student Geoffrey Rose. Mary's could only afford to pay £500 of Rose's salary, with the London School of Hygiene and Tropical Medicine paying the rest, £2,200. Rose received substantial research funding from the DHSS, £158,083 in 1970. Using these funds, and funds from the Lawley Founda-tion, he brought in a general practitioner to teach the students. First the school named an Essex-based GP, Marshall Marinker, but then Rose convinced his colleagues to create a teaching practice in the vicinity. After heated debates the board of studies gave cautious approval and appointed Jarman as a part-time lecturer.

Jarman built up a thriving department. New lecturers were added, and visiting researchers came. In 1978 the department moved into a health centre, an initiative jointly funded by the DHSS, the Area Health Authority, and the UGC. During the early 1980s St Mary's became the first medical school to integrate an attachment in general practice with the pre-registration house jobs in medicine and surgery. Students spent four months on each attachment. Thus, under pedagogical and political pressure, St Mary's integrated a social perspective into the school curriculum and hospital practice. Jarman was only one arrow in the quiver of St Mary's. Geoffrey Rose was another. The epidemiologist became the leading proponent of preventive medicine of his day. Helped by a series of able graduate students, he developed research projects that showed that the incidence of coronary heart disease was particularly high in western countries due to an unhealthy diet rich in animal fats. Rose became an influential figure in the state-sponsored campaign to reduce hospitalization by educating the public to better health. Epidemiology mediated between the laboratory and the clinic, as well as between politics and medicine, lending intellectual authority to the former and political relevance to the latter.

AIDS at St Mary's

Venereology also knitted together the lab and the clinic and placed both in the centre of politics. Renamed the "Special Clinic," later the Praed Street Clinic, and still later the Jefferiss Wing for Genito-Urinary Medicine, the clinic was one of the most flourishing services of the hospital. Under G.M. McElligott, assisted by R.R. Willcox and F.J.G. Jefferiss, the clinic became the largest in the land, with a commanding influence over both public policy and the development of venereological knowledge. As venereal advisor to the new Department of Health, McElligott was an important intermediary. His assistants were remarkable venereologists in their own right. Both were Mary's students drawn to the clinic because it offered a salary. Both became full-fledged venereologists during the Second World War, when experts in this neglected field were badly needed. RAF hospitals were full of venereal cases and McElligott, as advisor to the RAF, took Jefferiss away from examining recruits to treat these cases. Willcox ran the clinic until his own call-up papers arrived, when he was posted first to the Lock Hospital, then to the forces in West Africa, where he found a "veritable cornucopia of venereal disease." After the war, both men returned to St Mary's, though they retained advisory posts, Willcox at the War Office, and Jefferiss at the RAF.

After the war Jefferiss became a leading venereologist with a special interest in homosexual cases, while Willcox became the most prominent venereologist of his day. Jefferiss built up his practice and his profile locally, catering to a West End clientele, while Willcox flitted around the world, usually on business for the World Health Organization. The two were very different men, Jefferiss quiet, discreet, and subtle, Willcox florid and flamboyant. Willcox probably saw more cases and wrote more articles and books (nearly eight hundred titles) than any other venereologist, perhaps any other physician. A colleague recalled that, if you had a difficult case, you would show it to Willcox because he had probably seen it somewhere, had probably written it up. One of his early successes was to identify an endemic disease in West Africa as non-venereal syphilis. Jefferiss stayed home and ran the clinic with quiet efficiency. The two men competed for patients, and they divided the hospital over their rival bids to succeed McElligott as the clinic's director in 1958. Unfortunately, while venereal disease was on the increase in 1958, the DHSS, looking to earlier statistics showing a decline, cut back on venereological appointments and abolished the directorship.

Jefferiss and Willcox retired at the end of the 1970s. Willie Harris, who had trained in Belfast, came from King's College to take charge of the Praed Street clinic. Thanks to the DHSS cuts, venereologists were in short supply, and a man like Harris was turning down job offers from across the country.[45] He came to Mary's because of its reputation and its large patient base. He and his colleagues expanded the work, pioneering investigations into male infertility. But inevitably, the disease with which the St Mary's Clinic became most famously associated was acquired immuno-deficiency syndrome: AIDS.

Even before the first case of AIDS was diagnosed in Britain, St Mary's prepared for it. In 1981 Harris attended an American conference where he heard about a strange new disease that appeared to strike gay men. St Mary's had an enormous gay clientele who came in for treatment of sexually transmitted infections including syphilis, gonorrhoea, and, more recently, hepatitis. The consultants decided to prepare for an epidemic. They would test the prevalent theory of causation – amyl nitrates – and they would investigate the damage to the immune system. The medical school had just appointed a new immunologist with a special interest in immune disorders. Anthony Pinching was still working at the Hammersmith, due to take up his appointment at St Mary's shortly, when Harris rang to invite him to join the study. If an epidemic did occur, the team reasoned, it would be valuable to trace it from the beginning; if it didn't occur, then that too was interesting.

Harris and Pinching put together a proposal for a cohort study: a statistical study of a population that would be observed over several years. The clinical work was done by registrar Jonathan Weber, whose task was to keep track of the patients' lifestyles and habits, while Pinching would follow their immunological profiles. Half the men were drawn from the clinic's clientele, half responded to an advertisement in the gay press. Rather than a static, retrospective portrait of a population, this study would identify and account for changes as they occurred. This was the first time anyone had applied such a proposal to a sexually transmitted disease.

The scheme was too radical for the MRC, which turned it down. The MRC had a reputation for funding only established figures – which none of these young men were – and conservative, laboratory-based projects. Moreover, the MRC saw no reason to study a disease not actually in Britain.[46] The team then approached the Wellcome Trust, which provided £43,000 for the study. Within weeks the first AIDS patients began to appear at the clinic. Even without a specific diagnostic test for HIV (human immunodeficiency virus), Weber could see that a major epidemic was occurring, because many of the men showed swollen glands, exhaustion, and other signs of seroconversion. When a diagnostic test finally became available in 1984, Pinching went back and tested the original blood samples, all of which had been taken from symptom-free men, only to find that half of them contained the HIV virus.

From the beginning the study marked a new relationship between doctors and patients. There was no shortage of volunteers, for the gay community in London was well aware of developments in the United States. As the epidemic developed, the partners of patients who acquired AIDS and other patients were added to the study. In the interests of finding the relevant variables, these volunteers were fully cooperative, willing to describe their most intimate practices and to submit to medical procedures done for scientific rather than therapeutic purposes. Pinching reflects of the population study that "we were characterising them to the degree as we would expect a laboratory reagent to be characterised. If you get sodium chloride off the shelf, you'd know it was well-characterised sodium chloride, it wasn't anything else. Well, here, we had a sort of a complex mix, but we knew what we were dealing with, and that was, I think, a very important tool of our research, and actually made it quite strong over the years."[47] Almroth Wright had sworn that only the laboratory could produce certain and fully scientific information. Pinching obtained social information, thanks to collaboration between clinic and lab and the cooperation of patients.

By cooperating, AIDS patients could influence their treatment. American AIDS scientists found that if gay patients distrusted the clinical trials they enrolled for, they might swap drugs with other patients so as to avoid the placebos, or they might secretly enter several trials at once. Collectively these patients demanded that treatment regimens put their interests first, above the demands of science. These were, as a group, the most informed and politicized patients that the medical establishment has ever had to deal with, and, by enforcing their demands on doctors, they made medicine far more responsive to the patient's perspective.[48]

Another consequence of this type of study was that the clinicians became deeply concerned with the public health aspect of AIDS. Watching healthy young men sicken and die was traumatic. Even the politicians began to wake up to the disease, responding, Rudolph Klein remarks, "perhaps less to the number of deaths (which were few) than to the number of column inches in the press (which were many)."[49] The disease couldn't be cured, only prevented, by means of public education. The chief medical officer, Sir Donald Acheson, himself a public health specialist, supported this approach. In December 1985 the government allocated £6.3 million to combat AIDS, most of the money going towards treatment and education, with small sums for research and for a counselling scheme for health professionals modelled on the program developed at St Mary's. Pinching threw himself vigorously into the public campaign, warning against unsafe sexual practices, defending innocuous social contact, and labouring to destigmatize the disease. In September 1985 he drove to a school in Hampshire to reassure parents that an HIV-positive haemophiliac boy posed no real threat to their own children. Pinching also served on government and MRC advisory committees concerning AIDS. He brought the campaign into St Mary's by presenting a patient at the weekly grand rounds.

AIDS brought St Mary's a great deal of money and publicity and political influence. These were the fruit of a very real collaboration between the laboratory, the clinic, and epidemiology. The Jefferiss Wing continues to pioneer new programs to bring science, social science, and patients into closer communion. For example, male and female prostitutes each have their own clinics, where they can be sure of getting appropriate counselling and treatment. A nurse who works at the men's clinic is writing a doctoral thesis that fuses clinical and social science: he talks to patients to learn the relationship between their lives and their diseases, so he can advise them on prevention and formulate policy suggestions.

Paediatrics

Social medicine also found a home in the paediatrics department. A foundation was laid by Reginald Lightwood, who qualified at King's in 1921 and worked as a general practitioner before taking up hospital appointments. He came to St Mary's in 1939, when Frederick Langmead retired and medicine and paediatrics were separated for the first time. A mediocre

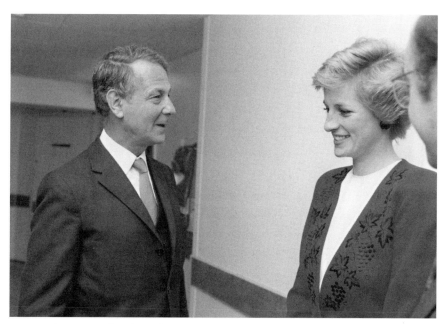

Immunologists Anthony Pinching (right) and Leslie Brent welcome Diana, Princess of Wales, to the opening of the AIDS wards. St Mary's Hospital NHS Trust Archives and collection of Leslie Brent

teacher, Lightwood instead built up the new department as a place of research. He developed an exchange program with Boston, designed an academic unit, and became part-time director. In 1945 he established a course on "The Social Aspects of Child Health and Welfare."[50] Students heard lectures on the use of the almoner and other referral agencies, and visited day nurseries, welfare centres, schools, and special schools for defective or tubercular children, as well as courts and probation officers.

In 1963 Lightwood retired, and Tom Oppé replaced him. Oppé had done some research with Ken Cross at St Mary's in 1950, putting babies into plethysmograph boxes. Ten years later, after working at his own school, Guy's, at Great Ormond Street, and in Bristol, he returned as assistant director to the unit, becoming director in 1963. Oppé had first become interested in the relationship between lifestyle and health while serving in the navy, and this was confirmed by a stint as a tuberculosis officer, then as a sanatorium patient himself. His many publications ranged from studies of metabolism, respiratory function, haemoglobin, and other physiological characteristics of the newborn child to "the medical problems of coloured immigrant children in Britain" to psychosomatic disorders. A close relationship with Freudian psychoanalyst Donald Winnicott at Paddington

Green Children's Hospital led to an interest in psychiatric disorders. Oppé built upon the work of Lightwood and Brimblecombe, continuing and expanding the Home Care Scheme and the teaching of social medicine. In 1967 he helped Geoffrey Rose plan GP attachments and visits to clinics. Oppé also appointed a lecturer, Roma Chamberlain, to teach "community paediatrics" and direct a perinatal mortality survey. All these initiatives put the St Mary's group and North-West Thames region at the forefront of social paediatrics.

Social Medicine Entrenched

Social medicine has found a home in St Mary's. Of course, public health officials think that more could be done. To John H. James, the chief executive of the Kensington & Chelsea and Westminster Health Authority, St Mary's remains inward-looking and elitist. As the consultants freely admit, most teaching is done and most medicine practised at the bedside. On the other hand, James finds both hospital and medical school responsive when he urges them to consider the community in making their appointments. The AHAs have a veto power over hospital appointments, which they use to enjoin their perspective. Social medicine is represented at the highest levels of the hospital and school, articulated by academics and clinicians from within and by political authorities from without.

The hospital and the Health Authority collaborate on some projects. The Kensington & Chelsea and Westminster Health Authority maintains a department of research and development. Senior members include – as well as John H. James himself and Dorothy Wedderburn, professor of management at Imperial College – Professor Brian Hurwitz of the department of primary health care and general practice, and Professor Paul Elliott of the department of epidemiology and public health, both of them based at St Mary's. The Research and Development Committee is funded through the Health Authority and external funding agencies (especially NHS research funds), and it investigates questions relating to the integration of social and clinical perspectives. In 1999 research projects included asking why acute mental health admission figures were rising; investigating whether patients in a GP-run ward at St Charles had better outcomes (they didn't, but they were more satisfied with their treatment); and looking for ethnic and class differentials in the outcome of heart-failure cases.[51]

Not all approve of this paradigm shift. James Le Fanu, a columnist for the conservative *Daily Telegraph*, recently wrote a diatribe against "the social theory" in medicine. He was positively splenetic in his attack on the arguments by Geoffrey Rose and Sir Richard Doll that diet and lifestyle can cause heart disease and cancer. (Their solemn faces peer at the reader from a spread of photographs under the headline "Seduced by The Social Theory.") Le Fanu is no more tolerant of the argument that poverty causes serious illness in Britain. He dismisses the general tenor of sociological arguments of the last forty years with the observation: "Absolute poverty in the form of an inadequate diet, overcrowding, poor hygiene and the lack of protection from the elements can harm the human organization and cause disease. Relative poverty cannot."[52] Absolute poverty, he believes, is too scarce to account for the mortality that has been attributed to it by such commentators as Sir Douglas Black, who produced a report on inequality in health care in 1980.[53] This report was thought so explosive at the time that the Thatcher government tried to bury it. From Le Fanu's perspective, social medicine is too influential; from that of left-wing commentators, it is not influential enough.

If medicine has been sociologized by political pressures, it is no less true that politics has been medicalized by sociological pressures. Medicine became a focus for left-wing lobbying in the early twentieth century because it revealed profound social inequalities. It provided a measure of deprivation and a powerful argument for intervention. In the late twentieth century the situation was reversed. The NHS, viewed as a way of addressing deprivation without redressing social inequality, is a cheap way to quiet the left and buy social harmony. At the end of the century, spending on medicine is rising faster than other government spending, and it dominates budget announcements. The thinking behind this spending is not so very different from the thinking behind the creation of St Mary's, in the 1840s.

Social medicine has been a source of political strength to St Mary's, and it has rooted the hospital thoroughly in the life of the community, breaking down some of the barriers between acute and community care. It has perpetuated the life of the hospital in the face of economic and political pressures for rationalization. Above all, the development of social medicine prepared St Mary's for the new battles of the 1990s. This included the *Report of the Inquiry into London's Health Service, Medical Education, and Research*, the work of a committee chaired by Sir Bernard Tomlinson.[54] The Tomlinson Report signified Judgment Day for the London hospitals. It advocated sweeping changes across medical London: a wholesale re-allocation of hospital resources towards community medicine and general practice. (It was to combat Tomlinson's figures on bed use that Jarman gave his University of London lecture in 1994.) St Bartholomew's and Guy's were to be closed, others were to be amalgamated, and beds generally to be reduced. St Mary's, Tomlinson decided, was in a strong position because most of its patients were local residents, and the hospital was well used. However, neither the school nor the hospital emerged from the report unscathed.

Tomlinson also supported a more far-reaching reform that the DHSS had recently adopted for the NHS as a whole, namely, the development of self-governing hospital trusts. After one administrative reform after another had failed to contain NHS costs, and after suffering one too many bruising encounters with the medical profession, Margaret Thatcher sponsored a review of the NHS. For the first time, advice from the medical profession was ignored. When the review recommended that competitive, commercial incentives be introduced into the NHS, the medical profession which had howled outrage at their abolition in 1948 now howled outrage at their reintroduction. According to the new policy, the NHS was divided into health care purchasers and health care providers. Hospitals, as providers, sell their services to GPs and to district health authorities. On them lies the onus of generating an income through services and balancing their books. The reform required that hospital governance be separated from regional administration and primary care (general practice). Hospitals could apply to become self-governing trusts, run by a handful of political appointees with solid business credentials. St Mary's quickly applied for and obtained trust status. Once again the hospital became largely self-governing. There have been some financial ups and downs, and the hospital was for some years criticized for having a large deficit, but corrections to the faulty funding formula promise to change that.

Tomlinson also made another recommendation that affected St Mary's, namely, a shake-up and merger of the teaching and research institutions in West London. In coping with these proposals, St Mary's drew heavily on its relationship with the local community. The formulae worked out by academics in defence of the hospital now were brandished in defence of the medical school. Changes on a scale not seen since the introduction of the NHS would occur, and, as in 1948, it would be the school's political savvy, its claims to leadership in research, and the value of its community service that would determine whether St Mary's would emerge stronger or weaker.

Science and Strategy
The Merger with Imperial College

FOR GOOD OR EVIL, London's medical landscape was being kneaded like dough.[1] We have seen that there were pressures to concentrate and rationalize medical care in London. There were equally strong pressures to do the same for medical education. Twelve schools were too many. There were equally good and far cheaper facilities elsewhere. London still trained one-third of British medical students, and because most graduates either emigrated or practised within a few miles of their school, other regions remained chronically underserviced.

The problem of London medical education had niggled during the 1950s and '60s, leading the government to appoint a royal commission that recommended concentration. The economic crisis of the 1970s made the matter more acute. Severe cutbacks were imposed, distributed across the schools, which became more and more stretched. No one wanted to grasp the nettle of whole-institution closure. At the end of the 1970s the political will to impose radical solutions was found with the election of Margaret Thatcher's Conservative regime. Government and universities were soon at loggerheads. The structure of university funding was recast: the UGC was closed down as being too representative of the universities rather than political interests, and a new formula was devised to favour institutions with strong research records.

The arguments for concentration were not all political. Since Goodenough, medical schools had flourished as places of science, accommodating scientists like Rodney Porter or R.T. Williams who had little interest in the clinical applications of their research. But research required resources beyond the capacity of individual medical schools. Granting institutions began to favour large-scale research centres. The United States set the pace for the development of big science, and it tallied up discoveries at breakneck pace.[2] Other countries scrambled to keep up.

Political values, economic necessity, the changing structure of research, and demographic changes made a major shake-up of medical education inevitable. That much everyone knew. It only remained to see which schools would survive. The more savvy began their defensive campaigns long before the threat materialized. St Mary's was not among the more savvy schools, and it was shocked to discover one day in March 1981 that it was first in line for the axe. This chapter identifies the interplay of political and scientific forces reshaping the London medical schools at the end of the twentieth century. As with the confrontation between the DHSS and the hospitals, this was not simply a confrontation between power and knowledge but required a redefinition of knowledge, the better to serve power. Once again, St Mary's was in the thick of the struggle.

Reorganizing the University of London

The story begins with the Royal Commission on Medical Education that reported in 1968: the Todd Report.[3] Todd concluded that London medical schools should be "twinned." Neighbouring schools should combine their facilities and, eventually, their infrastructure, including St Thomas's with Guy's, the London with St Bartholomew's, and St Mary's with the Middlesex. The schools hated the idea. They did form joint policy committees, and some even made joint appointments or developed shared courses, but serious change was staved off. Mergers would require new buildings, and there was no money for new buildings. At St Mary's the feeling against amalgamation was "almost unanimous." The paltriest of negotiations continued to the end of the 1970s. One Middlesex man recalled, "It was an agreed hidden agenda, that we met and did nothing. And this happened everywhere."[4]

Meanwhile, things got worse. Funding plummeted: in 1976 alone the University of London's grant was cut by 6 per cent. The schools moved into deficit. That of St Mary's was £20,000 in 1973; a decade later, it had risen tenfold. Clinical commitments made it difficult to impose cuts. Meanwhile, the cost of medical education rose inexorably. The medical schools absorbed 30.5 per cent of University of London funds in 1969–70, and 35.5 per cent in 1978-79.[5] Doubly squeezed, the other faculties demanded drastic action. The university named a working party on medical teaching resources headed by Lord Flowers, the rector of Imperial College; it warned that "financial support for medical teaching in London has been so reduced that a stage may be reached when all the total revenue available will be insufficient to enable all the existing Medical and Dental Schools and Postgraduate Institutes to continue as viable units."[6]

In June 1979 the new dean of St Mary's, Peter Richards, put together a submission that described the school as a place of good morale and serious science, situated in a populous and deprived region with sufficient patients to train all its clinical student intake of one hundred. The argument was a compelling one, as Noel Annan, the vice-chancellor of the university, cautiously indicated when he visited St Mary's on 5 December 1979. When Flowers reported, St Mary's was declared viable as a stand-alone school, though he recommended that the school recoup beds lost on Harrow Road by affiliating with the Central Middlesex Hospital. The district general hospital had a first-rate research record, developed over a forty-year affiliation with the Middlesex, which was deeply dismayed to lose it in the rearrangement.[7] Flowers also recommended that St Mary's form an academic link with the Royal Post-Graduate Medical School (RPMS) in Hammersmith, the leading clinical research institution in the country. Without such an affiliation, both institutions were vulnerable – St Mary's because the "academic strength" of this small school would be uncompetitive, and RPMS because of recent fee hikes imposed on foreign students. Both affiliations, therefore, would reinforce the existing strengths at St Mary's, as would closer research links with Imperial College. All in all, Mary's could celebrate the Flowers report.

Other schools had less to celebrate. Flowers recommended that the Westminster Medical School should be closed down, that the Middlesex, the Royal Free, and University College hospital medical schools should merge around University College, that those at St Bartholomew's and the Royal London should combine, and that King's College Hospital Medical School should close its preclinical departments, merge physically with Guy's, and then combine administratively with St Thomas's to form one large school. Specialist institutions were also recast.

The threatened schools mobilized to court public opinion and political influence in their favour. Accusations and insults flew. St George's and Charing Cross, both left intact, were seen to be over-represented on the working party. Schools touted their own qualities and attacked their rivals: the Westminster, for example, pointed to better results on the MBBS than St Mary's. The Westminster couldn't be saved, because the Westminster hospital was to be closed and rebuilt in Chelsea, so its school finally moved to Charing Cross, recently rebuilt in Fulham. On the other hand, the campaign to save King's College preclinical school was successful, as the university senate overturned Flowers's recommendation. The university had to start again, finding a more vulnerable target for closure. Perhaps the best target would be a stand-alone school, one without the multi-faculty, collegiate status that King's College had used to defend itself, one that hadn't been rebuilt at great expense recently, as St George's had at Tooting and the Royal Free at Hampstead, and one that didn't command much influence in the university.

Even before the senate had rejected Flowers, the report was out of date. Flowers assumed that student numbers would rise, but by early 1981 the university was told to cut student intake. It was also told to prepare for an immediate cutback of 10 to 20 per cent. Flowers was no longer drastic enough: only complete closure of a school would suffice. Moreover, Flowers hadn't carried out any costings. His working party decided that financial considerations shouldn't be determinative, so it didn't bother to compare the savings of closing one school against closing another. However, as the political arguments against closing any one school mounted, the university sought a solution based on financial logic. Acting on the directions of the Joint Planning Committee – the major policy committee of the University of London – in November 1980 the Joint Medical Advisory Committee (JMAC) set up another working party, this one led by Professor L.P. Le Quesne, the deputy vice-chancellor, dean of the Faculty of Medicine, and a Middlesex man. By March 1981 the report was complete, and the JMAC gathered at Senate House to discuss it.

Seeing the writing on the wall, Bart's and the London, Guy's and Thomas's rushed into merger talks so they couldn't be closed. St George's, Charing Cross, and the Royal Free, newly rehoused in state-of-the-art accommodation, were safe. The college schools were unassailable. That left only the Middlesex and St Mary's. Faced with the ghastly prospect of a direct vote between the two schools, Le Quesne suggested a compromise: that University College, the Middlesex, and St Mary's all combine to form one school, with the Middlesex relinquishing its undergraduate clinical school and St Mary's its preclinical school. The other proposals before the JMAC required action on closing one school or other and were rejected; this one, requiring only investigation, was unanimously passed.

Le Quesne's proposal was greeted with disbelief and dismay on Praed Street. It would reduce St Mary's to the status of a district general hospital. St Mary's would provide the Middlesex and UCH with teaching beds but have no serious laboratory research on its own on site. Worse still, the University of London began to behave as though it were a *fait accompli*. The vice-chancellor, Noel Annan, launched a "dawn raid" on St Mary's. Annan was a man of considerable distinction and authority. In the new proposal he saw an opportunity to effect a closure in all but name, whilst placating university lobby groups more powerful than any St Mary's could muster. A decisive man, he acted decisively.

Annan offered to come to St Mary's to explain the university's thinking – ominously, St Mary's was the only school he visited. The meeting was fixed for 23 March, two days before the University of London Senate (on which St Mary's had no representative) was to meet. The lecture theatre at St Mary's was packed with anxious students and staff when Annan, a tall, commanding figure, strode in. He began by telling the audience of his "great love of St Mary's": "Not many of you will know, but I would have been born at St. Mary's, had I not been born in a taxi on the way here. But, having said that, we're still going to close you down."[8] Two days later he announced in the senate that the JMAC had more or less agreed to the Le Quesne proposals, which only needed some fine tuning. On 27 March he published a letter in the *Times* suggesting much the same.

Already, however, Annan was fighting a rearguard action. The speed and ferocity of the strike was unexpected, but the threat to St Mary's had not materialized out of nowhere. Peter Richards had been marshalling forces. All through the winter of 1980–81 the medical press had debated the pros and cons of closing one or the other schools. *Pulse*, for example, couldn't make up its mind. On 7 March it predicted that Mary's would fall because the clinicians were all too busy with private practice to build up a research profile, while St Bartholomew's was so old that "Winkling it out would be a tough job." On 23 March it turned about to argue that Paddington was "deprived enough without losing its major acute hospital," while Bart's had a local catchment of only three hundred residents. In this atmosphere of thrust and counterthrust, school officials assiduously cultivated their press contacts, wrote angry letters, and hired a public relations firm to leak information, raise questions in Parliament, and advise on tactics. On 24 March, Richards called a press conference, and the next day, the day that the University Senate met, angry headlines denounced the plan to close St Mary's. *The Times* called the scheme "vandalism," the *New Standard* "academically and financially disastrous," while the *Guardian* defended St Mary's as one of the most efficient schools in the university. The feisty *Paddington Mercury* told Annan, "Your proposals have been cobbled together in an atmosphere of panic."

The school mustered enough indignation and sympathy to give the University Senate pause. It named two more working parties, one to study East London, the other to study the Mary's-Middlesex-UCH proposal. All three schools were represented on the latter committee, chaired by Sir Richard Way. This group lost no time in declaring the tripartite scheme unworkable. It would weaken either or both St Mary's and the Middlesex so severely that even the mighty University College would be endangering itself to take them on. University College authorities wrote to Richards to say that, notwithstanding their esteem for his school, they didn't want it. The Middlesex was another matter. Dating back to the Todd report, there had been talk of twinning the Middlesex and University College. Geographically, a merger of the two schools made sense. The two institutions were only nine hundred yards apart, and their patients came from north and central London, while St Mary's looked westward.

All the while that he was enthusiastically supporting a merger between the Middlesex and University College, Richards built the case for St Mary's, drawing on clinical and pedagogical arguments. The new hospital wing was about to be built, and the UGC had promised to pay £2 million of the total bill of £12 million to house the clinical science departments. Richards drew on Brian Jarman's work to show that Paddington badly needed better services. The rebuilding had been delayed too long already, and if the UGC pulled out, the result would be more delay and cost. The UGC might save some money, but the taxpayers would gain nothing. But, Richards further argued, the UGC wouldn't save much money by closing St Mary's. Because the school had never (since Graham Little) cultivated a high profile in the University of London, it relied on other resources. Despite low costs per student, the school obtained academic results as good as any other and a research profile better than average. Moreover, St Mary's had already inflicted upon itself such severe cuts that it had all but achieved the ratio of staff to students (1:7) which the university had set out as the target for 1990. As other schools still had lower ratios, further cuts to St Mary's would be unfair; indeed, if the other schools could only achieve ratios already obtained at St Mary's, no one would have to be closed down.

St Mary's laboriously amassed statistics to prove these points. The cost per student of preclinical education at St Mary's was £3,909, compared with £5,894 at the Middlesex, and well below St George's, the Royal Free, University College, Charing Cross, and St Thomas's. The preclinical school had the fourth-highest level of research grants, worth £40,000 per full-time-equivalent member of staff between 1975 and 1980, and it had more publications per staff member than any other: 8.7 compared to 7.3 at University College, and less than four everywhere else. The clinical departments scored even better, with £75,000 per person in research grants over those five years. For every pound the school received from the UGC, it earned another 56 pence in research grants, amounting to £1.5 million in 1979–80. Any statistic that could be quoted to save St Mary's was fired off to the press and the university, and then they were all packaged together in a glossy little pamphlet which, Richards recalls with a laugh, fellow deans described as "outrageous" even as they asked his advice on how to produce one for themselves.⁹

St Mary's waged a very public battle for opinion and a more discreet political battle. That summer Peter Richards, Stanley Peart, and Tom Oppé were added to the University Senate and Richards was soon presiding over the JMAC. Influence was exerted in other quarters. Queen Elizabeth, the Queen Mother, patron of the school, interested herself in the events, as did the newly appointed president, Evelyn de Rothschild, chairman since 1976 of the family banking firm, N.M. Rothschild.¹⁰ Rothschild called on Lord Annan, and as the school officials looked on, these two men of enormous power and influence eyed one another. The school president made it clear that his power, influence, and wealth would be engaged to save St Mary's.

Gradually in the course of 1981 the tide turned. University College and the Middlesex came to terms. St Mary's was confirmed as an independent medical school. Everything looked good. The new wing, named for Queen Elizabeth, the Queen Mother, was finally being built, and student applications had never been higher. Yet Richards and the staff knew that there could be no peace of mind. As Thatcher found her stride in the mid-1980s, cuts to hospitals and universities reached new levels.¹¹ UGC funding for the University of London dropped by 2 per cent each year. Between 1980 and 1986, UGC funding for St Mary's fell by 15 per cent. Thanks to tight economies, fund-raising, and a canny finance officer named Philip Blissett, St Mary's managed to reduce rather than increase its debt, even developing a surplus. But talks among the East London schools had broken down, and if that merger failed, the university might seek a new victim. Moreover, the structure of university financing was changing in a way that seemed ominous for the future of a school like St Mary's.

Reorganizing Medical Research

Since 1908, when St Mary's successfully appealed to the Board of Education, the Exchequer had been funding medical schools. The grant had come to seem an entitlement, but in the 1980s that sense was destroyed. Rather than a grant, the Exchequer money was to be used to purchase services – teaching and research – in a market where schools competed against one another. As the UGC chair wrote to explain, the government would "use the power which that situation gives it to press for higher quality and greater efficiency, just as Marks & Spencer (for example) does in similar circumstances."¹² He hastened to add that the government did not simply wish to buy cheap goods, but it did demand quality goods. It would introduce a research assessment exercise (RAE) to discriminate between strong and weak departments.

To outsiders St Mary's looked small and isolated. Both Le Quesne and Flowers had argued that the school's academic strength could not survive in the world of big science. By the mid-1980s prospects seemed even dimmer. New technologies including new generations of mass spectrometers, electron microscopes, and monoclonal antibodies opened up a new, molecular approach to the study of biological matter. In the 1970s, leading cancer research was virological; during the 1980s, it became genetic. This shift had two general consequences. It put medicine at the cutting edge of scientific modernity and consequently raised the economic stakes.

St Mary's jumped aboard the molecular bandwagon early on. In 1973 the departure of R.E.O. Williams, followed shortly afterwards by Albert Neuberger and R.T. Williams, permitted the Academic Board to recast its biochemical sciences. The new chair of biochemistry was Bob Williamson, who came with a team of ten workers and MRC funding worth £150,000. Trained at UCL and Glasgow, Williamson studied the genetics of cystic fibrosis, a disease that damages the lungs of young people. Sponsored by the Cystic Fibrosis Research Trust, his team began with Duchenne muscular dystrophy as a model to identify the damaged chromosome. As one member of the team, Kay Davies, recalls, they decided to purify the chromosome and "make a library" of it.[13] The purification sorting process was done by shining a laser through chromosomes stained with ethidium bromide. St Mary's didn't have a suitable laser, so the team made regular trips to Glasgow, working overnight in shifts and returning to London with 150 nanogrammes of DNA for experimentation. Once they had a test-tube full of chromosome fragments, they would "pick them out at random" and find those that co-segregated with the disease. When the faulty chromosome was identified, the team would construct "restriction fragment length polymorphisms," (RFLPs) to repair the fault. The new genetic information could then be introduced into the faulty gene by means of a virus. By the end of the 1980s Williamson's team was ready to apply his gene therapy to humans, introducing the genetic information through the lungs with an aerosol. This was the dawn of gene therapy in Britain. It was big science with a vengeance, and Williamson began to attract enormous funds for his work, averaging more than £1 million annually.

His was not the only line of research into gene therapy at St Mary's. Neuberger's department was reconfigured as Pharmacology and Toxicology, headed by R.L Smith. One day NHL consultant Richard Lancaster told Smith that some of his patients were reacting oddly to debrisoquine, an anti-hypertensive drug. Smith and his colleagues injected themselves with the drug, and for the rest of the day Smith was ill. As toxicologist John Caldwell remarked, Smith was known to respond abnormally to some

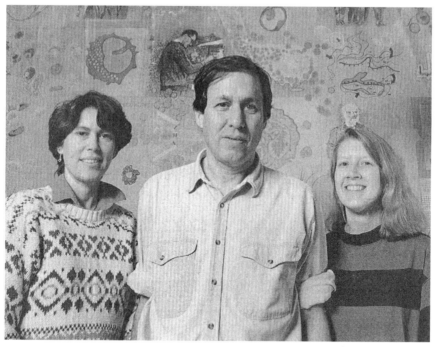

Bob Williamson and his team pioneer gene therapy in Britain. *Daily Telegraph*

drugs: "We knew he was funny, we didn't know why he was funny."[14] They set about looking for other people who were also "funny," and the eighty-fifth person screened showed the same response. The team discovered that 7 per cent of the population had a genetic polymorphism of oxidation – an "inborn error of drug metabolism," as they called it. By the mid-1980s St Mary's had identified several more polymorphisms which they linked with adverse reactions to drugs. Smoking, for example, was more likely to cause lung cancer in people with the polymorphism.[15] At one stroke the mechanistic approach of the lifestyle aetiology was made more amenable to laboratory investigation. This was the dawn of pharmaco-genetics, now an enormous and thriving field of investigation.

Sir Stanley Peart retired in the mid-1980s. His replacement was Howard Thomas, a specialist in liver virology then working with Sheila Sherlock, a renowned liver specialist, at the Royal Free. Thomas wanted to build up a liver transplantation unit, and St Mary's, with its kidney unit, supported this interest. Paradoxically, it was only possible to get NHS approval as a specialist transplant unit if you already had a good track record in the field, and so Thomas had to raise private funds to bring in a surgeon. Before long St Mary's could boast of thirty transplants with only one death, very good figures indeed. Thomas himself served as a theatre assistant for the operations. However, his application for recognition remained in abeyance, largely because if a new transplant centre were approved, funding across Britain would have to be reorganized. But he hasn't given up yet. Collaborating with geneticists at Oxford, and using MRC funding, he began investigating genetic determinants of liver disease, including the possibility of a genetic predisposition to alcoholism.

Thomas gathered around him a team of liver specialists, including John Summerfield, who now holds a personal chair in experimental medicine. Summerfield specialized in the innate immune system, which operates through the complement system and identifies bacteria by the sugars that coat them. In 1988, the year he came to St Mary's, Summerfield cloned a gene that has subsequently been found to cause chronic illness in children. The disease was discovered in the mid-1960s, but the cause could only be identified once Summerfield had cloned the gene. His current line of research, which also has therapeutic implications, aims at knocking out and replacing the gene responsible for the disease, using specially bred transgenic mice, by means of homologous recombination.

AIDS research was another molecular line. The disease was found to be caused by a retrovirus – a newly discovered form of virus that reproduced itself by reverse transcriptase. At St Mary's, Tony Pinching was developing new lines of research into cell immunity. Normally the host responds to a viral invasion by sending macrophages that ingest the bug. T-cells in the bloodstream then "switch on" the macrophage (by means of gamma interferon) so that it can recognize and destroy the virus. Most previous work blamed the immuno-suppression on a reduction in the number of T-cells. Using MRC funds, Pinching began to investigate whether the macrophages were themselves abnormal.

By the mid-1980s St Mary's could claim to be at the forefront of molecular biological research. In October 1985 school officials asserted, "Our record here belies the widely accepted view that effective research can only be pursued in large institutions."[16] Whereas the school's UGC income rose very slowly, from £4 million to £4.7 million between 1982 and 1987, research income doubled from £2 million to £4.4 million. St Mary's looked impressive. But it was uphill work convincing university officials of this fact. Government planning was intended to anticipate future changes. No matter how loudly and proudly school officials trumpeted its successes, they couldn't counter arguments that the school *might* become uncompetitive in the future. In Parliament in 1987 Lord Quinton denounced units of research "in small puddles here and there." Predictions by economists and sociologists of the future need for economies of scale carried more weight than the descriptions by scientists of their work.

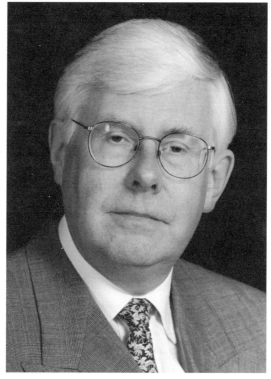

Howard Thomas. Collection of Howard Thomas

St Mary's could compete ably against other medical schools, but the real competitors were the university science departments. Here the medical schools were handicapped by their clinical responsibilities. Nor could they compete with postgraduate specialist institutions like the RPMS which did not have to teach hundreds of undergraduates. Yet in the brave new world of university financing, the medical schools would have to measure up against university science and postgraduate departments. Beginning in the spring of 1985 the UGC warned that selectivity of research funding was coming.[17] The announcement coincided with the retirement of Stanley Peart, which left St Mary's without a single FRS on staff, at a time when research credentials were needed.

Imperial College

All the small schools in London felt the threat, and they cast about for powerful allies. For St Mary's there were only two doors in West London worth knocking on: the RPMS and Imperial College of Science and Technology. Lord Flowers had suggested a closer affiliation with both institutions. All through the early 1980s representatives from the three schools met for discussions, but the RPMS dragged its heels, fearing (as it had replied to the Flowers report) a "dilution" of its research credentials. That left Imperial College. It had been founded in the early twentieth century on the model of German technical universities by a group of scientists and politicians concerned that Britain's laissez-faire attitude to science and technology was losing it the race for political and technological suprema- cy. These men included Lord Haldane as well as such supporters of Alm- roth Wright as Max Bonn and A.J. Balfour. Imperial College was created by a merger of three institutions of some standing and maturity: the Royal School of Mines, the Royal College of Science, and the City and Guilds College. By the late twentieth century Imperial College was one of the most powerful and wealthy schools in the land. Whereas Mary's had 250 full- time-equivalent staff in 1986, Imperial College had more than 2,000. If, as Richards remarked to Keith Lockyer, safety for St Mary's lay in getting under the guns of a battleship, here was a battleship indeed. But what would Imperial College gain by merging with a small and endangered med- ical school? When Richards approached Lord Flowers, the rector of Impe- rial College, early in the 1980s and again in 1985, Flowers replied that the time was not ripe.

In the mid-1980s, the mood at Imperial College changed, largely as a consequence of the molecular revolution. Unless it could incorporate bio- medicine and biotechnology, it would no longer find itself at the cutting edge of British science.[18] The same factors that made medical research unsustainable in small schools led university departments to covet it. Its methods had become as quantitative and rigorous as anything in the "hard" sciences, while the practical applications seemed endless, ranging from monoclonal antibodies to artificial joints (developed at Imperial with clini- cal collaboration). As well, Imperial College was under pressure to attract more women students and more private funding for research. A medical school would instantly ease both these problems. Medical schools were near parity in admission by sex (St Mary's would be the first to exceed parity in 1989), and they also attracted considerable private funds from pharmaceu- tical companies and research trusts such as the Wellcome, the Nuffield, the Imperial Cancer Research Campaign, and the Heart Foundation.

There was a change in leadership at Imperial College when Lord Flow- ers left to become vice chancellor of the University of London in September 1985. He was replaced by Professor (later Sir) Eric Ash. Coming from Uni- versity College, where biological and medical sciences were integrated with science and technology departments, Ash found Imperial strangely lacking, like a three-legged dog. He was convinced that "the important science of our time, and for the next century, would be the life sciences." People were spending more on health and demanding that their governments do the

same, so that "the only way a government can get itself elected is by reacting to that sentiment." Political and economic support for health research
would grow, and Imperial College would grow with it.

In January 1986 Richards went back to Imperial College. Alan Swanson,
a professor of biomechanics and pro-rector at the college, recalled that
Richards "pushed it quite hard at me." Swanson was lukewarm about the
idea, but Ash, whom Richards invited to St Mary's for lunch one day, was
more keen on it, Richards recalls: "And I said, 'Eric,' as we got to our last
sandwich, 'Would you be interested in a medical school?' And he said,
'Yes,' he said, 'I think that would be rather a good idea.'"[19] In May,
Richards advocated a merger to the Academic Board at St Mary's on political and economic grounds: "A merged institution of Science, Technology
and Medicine would be a force within the University of London considerably stronger than the sum of the parts and such a merger would be in tune
with the rationalisation and regrouping currently underway within the University."[20] St Mary's and Imperial College set up a joint working party,
chaired by Swanson, to investigate the proposal.

At St Mary's, reception of the idea was mixed. But, as Ash admitted, "St
Mary's wasn't really the problem. The real problem was Imperial College."
Though he had some powerful allies, notably Roy Anderson, a biologist
specializing in the behaviour of populations and epidemics, others were opposed. Some "hard" scientists and engineers complained that medical science wasn't rigorous enough – a concern that had scuttled plans to merge
with another school. Others worried that the medical school would absorb
a growing share of the college's finances.

To meet these criticisms, Richards attended the meeting of the Governing Body at Imperial College on 19 June 1987. He pointed out that St
Mary's had high ratings for its research and that, head for head, the school
had had more Nobel laureates and FRS than Imperial College. It was also
financially solvent (more so than Imperial, some said). Swanson's working
party confirmed the claims. Both institutions earned 29 per cent of their income from research grants. St Mary's drew 27.5 applications for every
place, while Imperial College had only 4.5. To please the critics, finances
would be kept apart for five years. Imperial's Board of Studies and Governing Body finally voted overwhelmingly in favour of the merger. So did
St Mary's.

Things now began to move quite quickly. In order to take effect in 1988,
the bill to amend the charter of Imperial College had to be lodged before
Parliament by November 1987. Most of the work fell on the secretaries of
the two institutions, John Smith and Keith Lockyer, two very competent

and good-natured men. John Smith had a distinguished career in the colonial service, eventually becoming a colonial governor before he took up post at Imperial College, so the diplomacy required of him came easily. Brian Lloyd Davies, who later became secretary to the St Mary's delegacy, also played a key role in smoothing negotiations and drawing up the parliamentary bill. Matters were in capable hands.

Where Mary's students worried about losing their identity – a concern that was met by restricting Wilson House to them for ten years – many at Imperial College were ignorant or indifferent. Bibulous students interviewed in January 1989 exclaimed, "We're doing you a great favour – especially the nurses." When asked, "What is the typical Mary's person?" replies came back ranging from "Mary who?" to "Everyone plays Rugby," to the following disquisition: "All I know is what was on that telly programme. It seems that all the Med. students are pissed for two-and-a-half terms and then stay up all night in the last three weeks before the exams."[21]

According to the terms of the merger, St Mary's became the fourth constituent college of Imperial, which was now renamed "Imperial College of Science, Technology, and Medicine." It had its own "Delegacy," chaired by Evelyn de Rothschild, which, while represented on the Governing Body of Imperial College, was largely self-governing. Undergraduate medical education remained firmly situated on Praed Street, though opportunities for combined BSc teaching did increase. Indeed, because the changes were largely formal, they were effected smoothly. Those in favour of the merger believed that it would evolve over time; those who opposed it presumed that it wouldn't amount to much. The bill was drawn up to make the least possible change to the college's charter, and a year later in October 1988 the merger was ceremoniously effected. Student musicians sweetened the air with music, the chancellor of the university, Princess Anne, was in attendance, and a ball followed. The occasion was marked by some jocularity. When St Mary's won the rugby cup earlier that year, John Smith had sent Richards a congratulatory note, observing that the ease and virility with which the victory had been achieved belied the school's role as a demure bride, and anticipating a honeymoon battle over the trousers. Richards now replied with a list of accomplishments, academic and sporting, that promised to challenge Imperial everywhere, even in its greatest strength: the boat club.

At St Mary's Hospital the flag flew at half-mast. Some consultants, shielded from university financial cuts by their NHS salaries and their private practices, objected to the merger. They feared that the traditional balance between academics and consultants would be overturned. Many had trained at St Mary's or worked there for decades. They cherished the fa-

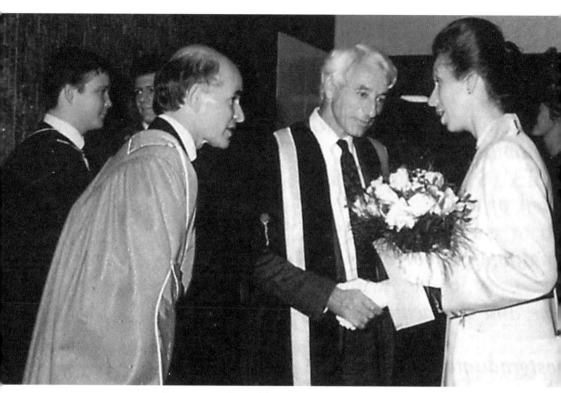

Peter Richards, Sir Eric Ash, and Princess Anne celebrate the merger of St Mary's and Imperial College. St Mary's Hospital NHS Trust Archives

mously friendly atmosphere and feared to lose it. It would be wrong to exaggerate the differences of opinion between NHS consultants and academic staff. Some of the consultants were enthusiastic supporters of the merger, and one didn't need to be an academic to be engaged in front-line research which might benefit from the association with Imperial. But there was, nonetheless, a thought-out and coherent argument against the merger and against any further concessions to Imperial once the merger had been agreed to. A close look at the experiences and the arguments of this group provides a clear view of just what was lost in the merger, and in the reconfiguration of London medicine more generally. "Upon such sacrifices," one might say with Shakespeare, "the gods themselves throw incense."

The spokesman for the traditionalist viewpoint was Alasdair Fraser, consultant gynaecologist and one-time president of the rugby football club. An athlete and the son of a practitioner in Wales, Fraser was admitted in 1947. "Never ever in a month of Sundays would I have got in nowadays," he

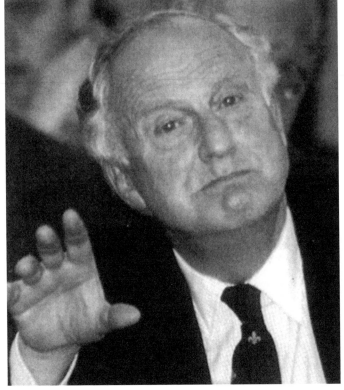

Alasdair Fraser. St Mary's Hospital NHS Trust Archives

reflects. His student days were happy ones, filled with swimming, rugby, and other extracurricular activities. When asked who influenced him as a student, he painted a portrait of a school still largely dominated by the traditional hospital honoraries rather than the salaried academics:

If you went to a musical society or a dramatic society production, or any student activity, you would find a dozen or so different consultants supporting them. They didn't just turn up at rugby matches. Every student club had an enthusiastic president from the staff, and a group of other supporters. So it wasn't just rugby, it was all the other ... the music and dramatics. Long before Peter [Richards] came, the music society was tremendously popular. The debating society, the medical society, all these clubs and societies had consultant participation. And that was the great thing about Mary's then, and right up until now, really, that the school and the hospital were so close together that it was the hospital staff who backed up the students and all their activities. And, of course, you were much more aware of consultant medical staff than you were of academic staff.

I mean, even now, the bulk of the clinical teaching is not done by academic university staff, but by hospital consultant staff. And in those days, apart from the professors of medicine and surgery, all the teaching, clinical teaching, was done by NHS consultants. Now, in your first two and half years you're in the Medical School, and this was done by preclinical teachers, but after that, it was hospital staff. So, if you like, unless I was going to become an academic in a preclinical subject, it was the hospital staff who influenced me and it was those who you got to know and see around, helping students, as much as anything else, and helping undergraduate bodies.[22]

Fraser enjoyed himself so much that he failed his examination and had to resit it. He obtained a house job with Carmichael Young, who had been president of the swim club in the year Fraser captained that club. Eventually he became a consultant gynaecologist at St Mary's. Like other Mary's-trained consultants, he became an important intermediary between the school and the students, presiding over various clubs and serving as director of clinical studies. It was this hospital-centred, friendly atmosphere that Alasdair Fraser sought to protect.

Oscar Craig, consultant radiologist and soda-siphon wielder, seconded this view of the proper relations at a teaching hospital. Each year he welcomed the fresher students with a lecture on the history of St Mary's, which was also a reflection on the activity of being a doctor. Long after his retirement he continues to be asked back each year to give the lecture to the Imperial College School of Medicine. When his name comes up in the bar, affectionate exclamations fill the air. Like Fraser, Craig sees serious purpose in the friendly relations and even the tomfoolery of the soirée. He describes the annual skit as an important model for staff-student relations:

You can be fierce, you can examine them, you can be strict with them, you can teach them, but at the same time, you're able to let your hair down with them, in going on the stage acting the fool. And that's important. It is also important that there is a proper relationship between the two. You can't bring the soda siphon act onto the ward, and I can't explain it any better than that. But the soda siphon has a place, and by God, it has a place! But its place is where it is, and it's great fun. I think that that staff/student relationship was absolutely marvellous at St Mary's. And I think this is one of the things which marks St Mary's out as being different. I don't think that it went on in any other teaching hospital in London. People were surprised when they heard that we did this. So, you know, the consultants that went on stage and acted the fool were great, and the soda-siphon act was great, in terms of what it meant to be a corporate body of people.[23]

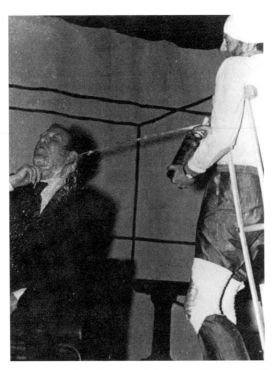

"The Soda-Siphon Sketch," by Oscar Craig: "When Dr Harold Edwards was dean and Dr Oscar Craig was director of clinical studies, they appeared in a sketch at the students' Christmas soirée. This sketch was repeated with variations each year, and always ended by one or other being squirted with the contents of a soda siphon. The students requested this soda-siphon act year after year. Perhaps the best of the sketches was when Harold Edwards appeared on stage alone and said, 'I regret to tell you that Oscar Craig has had an accident on his way to the soirée tonight. Thankfully he is not seriously injured but cannot be with us.'

"There was a hush in the audience. Harold continued, 'This leaves a gap in the program which I've been asked to fill. I've always been interested in bird life, and tonight I'm going to give you some interesting bird calls' … It had been arranged to have recordings of bird songs to which Harold would mime. He raised his head, opened his mouth and tapped with his hand on his throat to the accompaniment of the recorded bird songs. The effect was dramatic, and the audience astounded, amused and perplexed by what they saw and heard from their dean.

"Oscar Craig, back stage, was bandaged around the head and limbs and leaning on a crutch. As the bird songs were in progress he slowly and painfully came from behind the curtains and staggered towards Harold's back with the soda siphon in view. Harold continued apparently unaware of the approaching soda siphon, while the audience erupted into laughter and encouragement, which the dean acted as though in appreciation of his performance. At the appropriate moment, prolonged to get maximum effect, the soda siphon was used to drench him from head to toe, while he continued his warbling. The curtain descended to wild enthusiasm and the familiar – 'More … More … More!'"

In a series of letters published in the *Gazette*, Fraser warned of the threats to St Mary's as he saw it. Student facilities like the Beaverbrook sports ground at Teddington, the climbing hut in Wales, the swimming pool – none of these was definitely secured, nor was the school's very name, he pointed out in 1988. In April 1989 another letter observed that the latest University of London calendar reduced Mary's to a single letter, listing it as "IC (M)." In October 1989 a further letter complained when the words "St Mary's" weren't printed on student diplomas. In January 1991, describing himself as "the last of the Mohicans," Fraser remarked that the exam results recently published in *The Times* neglected to mention St Mary's. Imperial College officials responded to the complaints and repaired omissions.

Generally, good humour was maintained in these disputes about identity. In 1992 staff and students engaged in a friendly debate for and against the motion "that the concept of the Mary's Man is dead and should be buried." The outcome, the *Gazette* observed, was never in any doubt: defeat was unanimous.[24] Similar debates are still held from time to time with mixed results. In 1995 Alasdair Fraser and Oscar Craig lost a debate on the motion "that the future of St Mary's is as bleak as its history is great." An amusing speech by a Cambridge clinical student who insisted that the Mary's man should go the way of the dodo was the clear favourite at another such confrontation in 1997.

The general tone was good humoured because, on the whole, St Mary's had not lost very much. Peter Richards seemed to have achieved minimal change with maximum protection. His solution to the threat posed by the growing academicization was, like Moran's academic units, nominal: it left most activities at St Mary's intact. However, Fraser and others, including Frank Loeffler, Robin Touquet, and some student leaders, correctly diagnosed the situation. The actual, immediate change was minimal, but St Mary's had relinquished real power to Imperial College. If it were to change its mind about leaving St Mary's be, the school would find it difficult to resist. This was precisely what happened during the 1990s. With another change of rector, with new political pressures given focus by Sir Bernard Tomlinson's shake-up of the hospitals, and not least, with a change of opinion at St Mary's itself, the school did lose its name, its dean, and more besides.

The new regime was ushered in by the Tomlinson report of 1992. Insofar as the merger had been undertaken to protect a vulnerable, freestanding St Mary's Hospital Medical School from closure, it was successful. Tomlinson approved of the merger. But he liked the arrangement so much that he recommended extending it to include Charing Cross and Westminster, which would, with St Mary's, form one large undergraduate medical

school with an annual intake of three hundred. Three postgraduate institutes – the RPMS, the Institute for Cancer Research, and the National Heart
and Lung Institute – should also join. The story of this second merger is not
yet history. Relationships have not yet fallen into patterns, and there is still
much jockeying for position among the schools, colleges, and institutes.
What follows is a memo; serious analysis must await a future historian.

Another Merger: Administrative Pressures

Imperial College did not rebuff the recommendations, but it set a price on
its cooperation. Officials had little desire for a far-flung empire of struggling medical schools and institutes. This would be a genuine merger of the
three undergraduate schools and a genuine integration with the college.
The state would erect a new building at South Kensington to house the
merged preclinical departments. Clinical studies would continue to be
taught on the wards, in the teaching hospitals, but the scientific work
would be consolidated at South Kensington. In 1998 the building, named
for Sir Alexander Fleming, was inaugurated by the queen, and the new intake of three hundred students attended their class together in its spacious
lecture theatre.

Until the second merger St Mary's *was* Imperial College School of Medicine. Afterwards it was just one constituent of it, and not the most influential one. That position belonged to the RPMS with its unparalleled
research facilities. Several things had occurred to weaken the position of St
Mary's in the interim. Above all, the RAE of 1992 did not confirm the earlier UGC approval of the high standing of St Mary's. All the London teaching hospitals, saving University College, received low scores, reflecting their
heavy clinical and pedagogical responsibilities. Even where they could
boast of higher grants, as, for example, St Bartholomew's could over the
London School of Hygiene, they still obtained lower scores. Graduate institutions received a higher level of base support for research.

The RAE served well the politicians, bureaucrats, and scientists seeking to
discipline the London medical schools. Had Haldane only been able to
stage a comparable exercise in 1910, the process of concentration would
have been over that much sooner. He hadn't because the scientific and clinical elite refused to relinquish their monopoly on judgment of standing.
They insisted that it required fine discrimination of character, skill, and
grasp, which only insiders could make. But a century of increasing bureaucratization of research funding had generated new standards – bibliometric
ones such as the number of publications or citations, which claimed to
measure scientific reputation objectively. Even politicians could now judge

research programs. Researchers and clinicians still make fine discrimina-
tions of character, skill, and grasp among themselves, and they can be heard
to denounce the RAE as a "blunt instrument." The RAE left some untoward
casualties, such as Bob Williamson, a man who helped to put British medical molecular biology on the map. His work was later recognized by his
scientific colleagues with an FRS, but to accept it, Williamson had to fly in
from Australia, where he now directed a research institute with five hundred staff and a budget of $30 million.

Richards had led the move towards large, multi-faculty schools, but
other schools had caught up and, indeed, overtaken St Mary's. This became
apparent during the many reviews of medical service and medical education
of the early 1990s. For example, John H. James coordinated a review of
cardiac services, and he recalls that when the review panel asked Richards
what difference the merger had made to the experience of a St Mary's student, the dean replied that it made little or none. For other schools the picture was quite different and Richards's admission was a damaging one. It
suggested the presence of obstacles to integration, obstacles that must be
ferreted out and removed. To the political and academic masters of Imperial College, medicine seemed to be a "problem" that had to be fixed. The
second merger provided an opportunity to fix it.

Flowers had left the question of merging to his successor, so that Ash
might have a free hand. Now Ash himself stepped down, and Sir Ronald
Oxburgh was named rector. The obvious task for the new rector was to
"sort out medicine." This included integrating the new schools and convincing St Mary's to relinquish its special status. There still existed a vocal
party at St Mary's jealous of the school's special status and very much opposed to any further integration. Which way would Richards fall: with the
NHS consultants who wanted to keep their distance, or with the scientists
on staff who wanted, if anything, even closer ties with Imperial?

In fact, Richards enthusiastically urged the merger from the beginning.
He realized that it was inevitable, and, he told the *Gazette*, better to lead
than to drag along behind.[25] He had advocated wider merger to the other
medical schools years earlier, and he helped bring round Imperial College
even before the Tomlinson report. In December 1994 Imperial College announced that a merger had been agreed in principle between itself and
Charing Cross-Westminster, the RPMS, and the National Lung and Heart
Institute. Preclinical facilities would be built at South Kensington. As for
the clinical, "It is agreed that an academically led and staffed hospital will
form the principal clinical research base; initially and for the foreseeable future this principal clinical research base will be the RPMS at the Hammersmith Hospital." The same press release did say that undergraduate

teaching would not be concentrated at the principal clinical research base, but still, the news seemed bad for St Mary's. With preclinical sciences moved to South Kensington and the academic clinical base at the Hammersmith, Mary's would become a place where science was applied rather than made, a district general hospital.

The *Gazette* that carried the story also announced that Richards was leaving the school.[26] By the time the second merger took effect in 1998, he had left Imperial College, in the first instance to become medical director at Northwick Park Hospital, subsequently to become president of Hughes Hall Cambridge. Richards had been dean for more than fifteen years, and even at St Mary's, some people wanted a change. He himself felt that a new head was needed for the new school and that he was too thoroughly identified with St Mary's to be acceptable to the other schools. By the mid-1990s he had occupied a shrinking middle ground between two polarized camps. Many resented the merger, and they filled the *Gazette* with manifestos demanding that the fine Mary's traditions be preserved. Yet among some of the academic and scientific workers at St Mary's, Richards seemed to control too tightly the channels of communication with Imperial College and to slow down the pace of integration. These men and women welcomed greater collaboration. They regularly visited colleagues south of Hyde Park or at the Hammersmith to ask scientific advice, to use the equipment, or to work together in administrative committees. As Richards and Oxburgh grew at odds over details of the merger, Oxburgh found others at St Mary's willing to cooperate more fully. Thus it was that in 1994–95, Richards left to be replaced by a Mary's man of a different stripe, John Caldwell, who served as dean until the position was abolished in 1998.

Caldwell is a scientist, not a clinician. He studied pharmacy at Chelsea College and fell under the influence of people who had worked with Tecwyn Williams at St Mary's. When, in 1969, Caldwell applied to St Mary's to do a doctorate in drug metabolism, Williams put him to work on comparative amphetamine metabolism. Caldwell describes his overarching research agenda as providing quantitative measures of qualitative differences between species. Drug researchers must be able to give a drug to one species, perhaps a mouse, and then be able to predict its impact upon other species, such as a dog or a monkey or a human. Maguire's crude experiments in 1905 on rabbits and humans were a shot in the dark; Caldwell observes that a science achieves maturity when it can predict how phenomena will behave. He succeeded R.L. Smith as professor of pharmacology and toxicology, and his skills are much in demand by the pharmaceutical industry. He has built up a flourishing research program and trained dozens of doctoral students. As a laboratory scientist, he had more in common with colleagues at Imperial College than on Praed Street. This was also true of other scientists at St Mary's, including the professor of physiology, Charles Michel, who works on the biophysics of white blood cell circulation and their entrapment in the capillaries of the feet in varicose veins.

By the time Caldwell relinquished the deanship and moved across to the new building at South Kensington, becoming head of the basic medical science division, a new chain of command had been installed. In 1995 Christopher Edwards was named principal of Imperial College School of Medicine. He had strong research credentials, coming from Edinburgh where he was a professor of clinical medicine, dean of the faculty of medicine, and provost of the faculty group of medicine and veterinary medicine. He also had positions at the MRC and the Wellcome Trust, where he was a governor. Each campus was assigned a vice-principal to make the merger work on the ground – the St Mary's man was Malcolm Green, vice-principal for graduate affairs. Green had followed a career in NHS medicine with a stint overseeing the London Post-Graduate Medical Federation.

Sir Ronald Oxburgh, Christopher Edwards, and Malcolm Green, along with counterparts at other campuses, set about making the merger a physical and organizational reality corresponding to Imperial College's sense of identity. This meant constructing a research-led school. Principal Christopher Edwards explained the object: "What we wanted to do was to make sure that the formation of this medical school had real added value, that we had integration and cohesion, and very particularly, that we then built bridges between this new school and the real science and technology strengths within Imperial College." In order to get research funds from bodies like the MRC and the Wellcome Trust, he went on to argue, research groups have to achieve a "critical mass" and to prove that they have both clinical skills and basic sciences. "It is the ability to bridge between the molecule and man, between the bench and the bedside, which is key. And if you have people who are simply on one or the other side, then you don't get the link, you don't get the synergy, you don't get the vision which is required to prosecute really major quality research." The new School of Medicine (now renamed the Faculty of Medicine) has all that and more.

Edwards gently pokes fun at the traditional London teaching hospitals, which, "to be slightly pejorative, were rather like Noah's Ark. The consultants went in two by two: there were two gastroenterologists, two haematologists, two cardiologists. And, of course, that was very appropriate. It allowed the delivery of service, it allowed the teaching of those subjects. But the research profile was really very limited."[27]

Imperial College had to reform the medical schools. On its own it would have ranked third in the RAE of 1992, but the low marks received by St Mary's dropped it back to sixth, and Charing Cross/Westminster scored even worse in clinical sciences. They had to be brought up to standard. The undergraduate medical schools received low grades because they spread themselves too thinly. They might sustain one or two strong departments, supported with major research grants, but alongside these were many small departments, with just a handful of staff to do the teaching and the hospital work. Now that the RAE had been established to identify and weaken still further these small departments, Imperial College could not afford to maintain them. By introducing a division of labour and concentrating departments on sites where they were strongest, the school could demand that every department be big and strong in research. The Hammersmith would be the focus for the clinical sciences, and the other hospitals and school establishments would become more specialized institutes, with an international reputation in two or three fields, like the graduate institutions that Malcolm Green had previously overseen.

The RAE was only one concern. The MRC and the Wellcome Trust were dispensing fewer but larger grants, again to the detriment of small departments. Lurking in the background was the threat of reorganization on the NHS side. NHS research funds remain heavily concentrated in North and West London. If political pressure for redistribution emerges, the hospitals under the aegis of Imperial College will be vulnerable. The only possible defence will be greatness. Politicians may not venture to dismantle or relocate departments that are internationally famous for their clinical research, especially when they have themselves defined the standards of greatness through the RAE. Imperial College is playing for high stakes. St Mary's could not have survived in this world. At the same time the foundation for new growth was well laid by Peter Richards. In the late 1980s and early 1990s, the school had begun to rebuild areas of traditional strength, including Almroth Wright's old field of infection and immunity.

Infection Science at Imperial College Faculty of Medicine,
St Mary's Branch: Three Case Studies

MENINGITIS

Under Tom Oppé the paediatrics department, as a community service, was strong, but from the perspective of an RAE, it wasn't strong enough. It produced research publications, but it wasn't integrated into a large-scale, interdisciplinary, laboratory-centred research program. Richards decided that when Oppé retired, he needed a paediatrician who could transform the department along those lines. He settled upon Michael Levin, a South African who had trained at Northwick Park, Oxford, and Great Ormond Street, where he became the sole consultant responsible for infectious diseases, with a growing caseload of AIDS patients. When Richards approached him,

Levin turned him down flat, noting that, for lack of a paediatric intensive care unit, St Mary's had to transfer its seriously ill patients to Great Ormond Street. Richards's response was to ask, "So what would we have to do?" Levin replied that he would need two senior lecturers, an intensive care unit, and funds to sustain them.

Once he started to think about it, Levin could see good reasons for considering St Mary's. Great Ormond Street had no casualty department of its own, its cases were exclusively referrals, and its intensive care unit was so full that it turned away a third of all referrals. St Mary's would offer a more heterogeneous case load, a relationship with the local community, and superb support in infectious diseases like AIDS. A week later Richards telephoned Levin to say that he had found the money, £100,000, to fund the project. The Regional Health Authority had recognized the need for the service. Then, the local NHS authority balked at the appointment. Rather than an expensive referral service catering to patients from outside the district, it wanted a community paediatrician to meet local needs. Richards argued that the University of London, not the NHS, must determine appointments, and he finally won his case. In 1990 Levin came to St Mary's, along with senior lecturers Parviz Habibi (ICU) and Sam Walters (infection).

It soon turned out that £100,000 didn't go very far. Levin had to find other sponsors. One line of work was developed with funding from a drug company, Centocor, for a new treatment for meningococcal infections. The paediatricians did a clinical trial of the drug and began to receive meningococcal referrals. The early treatment of meningitis is crucial. Thus, rather than using ordinary ambulances, Levin developed an American system of sending out a team to stabilize patients and bring them back. The disease causes haemorrhages under the skin and in organs across the body, and if the delicate blood vessels around the brain and spinal cord are damaged, then death, brain damage, or paralysis can result. In the extremities, circulation can be so impaired as to cause gangrene, requiring amputation. Treatment is a delicate balance, because meningitis causes swelling, so fluids must be restricted, but if septicaemia occurs, then fluids must be given. Because the disease is so rare, amounting to three thousand cases annually, few hospitals see enough cases to develop expertise in recognizing and treating it, let alone doing research. Only a specialist referral centre could do that, and indeed the development of such centres, like that built up at St Mary's, have had great results. Quick and expert response to the disease has reduced mortality from 30 per cent to 6 per cent on the St Mary's Unit.

The making of the department was a television show by Channel Four. The mother of a child who died from meningitis had contacts with the media, and thanks to her efforts a *Cutting Edge* program described the new rapid response unit and exposed the lack of paediatric intensive care beds.

Weeks later, a child died after being turned away from the three paediatric intensive care units in London, all of them full. Journalists descended on the hospital, and Levin told them that he had warned politicians of the situation. One week later the Department of Health increased the funding. Levin's department was further strengthened by the appointment of Simon Kroll as a second professor of paediatrics.

As Levin remarks, the story shows the close relationship that must exist between the NHS and the University of London. The University of London established the department, and the NHS responded with funds to develop the clinical work, once the need had been demonstrated. The department treats more meningococcal infection than any other in the country, and the disease accounts for one-quarter of the intensive care caseload. AIDS and tuberculosis are other clinical and research strengths. The clinic now serves as a sturdy basis for a very large academic superstructure. Levin told Christopher Edwards that children were spending too much time in taxis and ambulances being transferred from one specialist service to another. A review of West London paediatrics was organized, and as a result West London paediatric services will be concentrated at St Mary's, by reason of its intensive care unit.

Thanks to a bold appointment by Peter Richards in the late 1980s, St Mary's quickly became a leading centre for paediatrics. Moreover, strength in that department provided good grounds for centralizing research into infection and immunity more generally on Praed Street.

GENITO-URINARY MEDICINE

Jonathan Weber provided another reason for moving infection and immunity to St Mary's. Weber came into a strong department, but he has made it still stronger. A prize-winning Cambridge student, he first came to St Mary's as a registrar to do the clinical investigations for the AIDS cohort study. On advice from the Wellcome Trust, he then spent three years studying cancer virology under Robin Weiss, a specialist in retroviruses, at the Institute for Cancer Research, and three more years at the Hammersmith studying the immunology of the AIDS virus, as a prelude to the development of a vaccine. In 1991 Weber took up a chair in genito-urinary medicine at St Mary's funded by a private research foundation that Jefferiss and Harris had developed. As with paediatrics, high-flying science merged with a strong clinical service to create a department that couldn't easily be moved, either by the NHS or the University of London, or even by Imperial College.

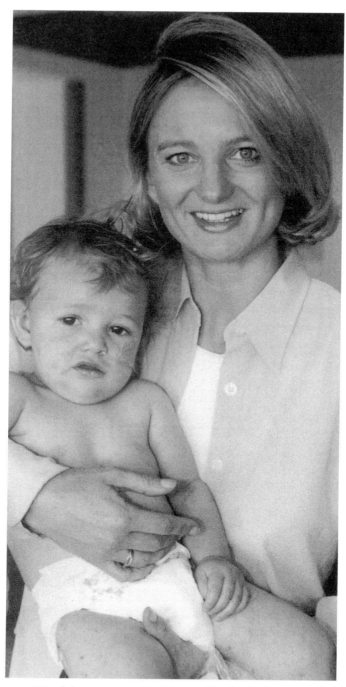

BBC *Watchdog* presenter Alice Beer with Elizabeth MacGinnis, recovering from meningitis at St Mary's. BBC Picture Library.

CREUTZFELD-JACOB DISEASE

By the early 1990s Bob Williamson's biochemistry team had moved on to Alzheimer's. In 1991 John Hardy and Alison Goate announced that they had identified the genetic cause, locating a genetic mutation seen in families with a history of the disease and in susceptible individuals within those families. Almost immediately the two were invited to the United States to join large, well-funded research teams, at salaries far better than the puny £21,000 St Mary's could offer. They didn't hesitate to accept. There was a wave of outcry at the loss to British science, and a private sponsor, the David and Frederick Barclay Foundation, approached Richards with £800,000 to keep the research team in Britain. Richards couldn't keep Hardy and Goate, but he could offer the Barclay Foundation something just as good: John Collinge's work on bovine spongiform enecephalopathy (BSE) and its human form, Creutzfeld-Jacob Disease (CJD).

CJD and BSE are both prion diseases. The prion was a new hypothesis and a radical one. It had been thought that a living pathogen – such as a virus or a bacteria – needed nucleic acid, genetic material, in order to reproduce itself. Bacteria reproduced themselves, whereas viruses could only reproduce by combining their RNA with the DNA of the host cell. Prions contain no nucleic acid: they are composed of protein (the name stands for proteinaceous infectious agent).

The hypothesis of infection by prion was first suggested in 1967, but not given much credence until the early 1980s, when new technologies of investigation identified a protein that was resistant to proteolytic degradation and could cause scrapie (ovine spongiform encepalopathy). In humans the prion protein was found to be the product of a cellular gene on chromosome 20. If injected into normal protein, the protease-resistant protein sets off a chain reaction and converts the normal protein into the pathological form. CJD is a sporadic prion disease that occurs in people who are homozygous with respect to a common polymorphism in the prion protein. Another prion disease, kuru, is seen in Papua New Guinea among people thought to have acquired the disease through cannibalism.[28]

During the 1990s prion diseases became big news in Britain. The entire British cattle herd was found to be riddled with BSE after diseased animals were made into feed. Moreover, scientists discovered a new variant of CJD with unusual characteristics. It struck teenagers, and these showed anxiety and depression and experienced limb and facial pain unlike that of ordinary CJD. Like kuru but unlike CJD, there were abundant prion amyloid plaques in their brains. Early in 1996 it was suggested that this variant of Creutzfeld Jacob Disease (VCJD) was transmitted from cattle afflicted with

BSE. Countries outside Britain suspended their beef purchases, and the British government embarked on a systematic slaughter of cattle. Roy Anderson, a population biologist, estimates that approximately one million cattle were infected, and 700,000 of those were eaten by humans.

John Collinge has done much of the work to show the relationship between VCJD and BSE. Manifestly, they are two diseases. Because one cannot infect humans experimentally, and the incubation period of kuru has been more than fifty years, proving transmission across the species barrier is not easy. The Mary's team studied phenotypes of CJD and found that the amino acids fall into four distinct alignments, representing four phenotypes. New variant CJD showed an alignment distinct from ordinary CJD and kuru. Another line of research was pursued using transgenic mice, that is, mice bred to be vulnerable to the human rather than the murine form of prion disease. As Collinge told the Association of Physicians of Great Britain in April 2000, "We believe these mice are as sensitive to human CJD as are we." The team exposed the mice to CJD, VCJD, and BSE, and found that in the clumping pattern in mice, VCJD looked more like BSE than it did CJD, showing distinctive nuclear magnetic resonance spectrums.

Collinge was initially funded by the Wellcome Trust, but confronted with the spectre of a major epidemic in Britain, the MRC awarded his group the status of a research unit, while the NHS funded a CJD service clinic. Almost by accident, thus, St Mary's became identified with the research and treatment of an important disease. During the late 1990s, at a time when the Hammersmith Hospital seemed to be casting St Mary's in the shadows, Collinge's prion unit helped to sustain academic morale and clinical research on Praed Street. And, while the sudden political importance of BSE and VCJD was, to some extent, unpredictable, the development of a first-rate research unit investigating some of the most complicated and uncharted biological phenomena at St Mary's was no accident. The work developed from a department of biochemistry that had enjoyed high standing for decades. The school that Richards had inherited and passed on has provided a sturdy foundation for the more grandiose structure that Imperial College now seeks to erect.

Epidemiology at Imperial College Faculty of Medicine, St Mary's Branch

Infection and immunity is one line of work that the college aims to develop at St Mary's. Another is medical statistics and epidemiology: the "Geoffrey Rose Initiative." Rose relinquished his academic position at St Mary's in 1977, but he maintained a cardio-vascular clinic there (which continues as the Peart-Rose clinic), and he still taught advanced students in the medical unit. Two of Rose's students carry on the work at St Mary's.

Neil Poulter was an archetypal St Mary's student of the 1960s. He limped into the interview, having dislocated his patella playing rugby, and was offered an open scholarship. His first year was spent learning biology and doing research for Donald Barltrop, a paediatrician studying lead poisoning. He went round houses in Paddington, "some of the most unpleasant, grotty housing you'd seen,"[29] collecting samples of the peeling paint and sending it back for analysis. But much of his time was devoted to sports: he played rugby, cricket, tennis, and water polo, and he went on five sporting tours.

Just before his qualifying exams, thanks to a Mary's connection, he went to work in the Wellcome Trust tropical metabolism research unit in Jamaica for a year, studying malnutrition and enjoying the local Rasta culture. Back at St Mary's he passed the conjoint exam but failed obstetrics and gynaecology, in part because he was unfamiliar with the inter-uterine monitoring equipment which the new professor, Richard Beard, had introduced. He did an orthopaedics house job under George Bonney, resat the ob-gyn exam with Alasdair Fraser as his examiner ("Presumably he had to chat the external examiner up furiously to get me through," Poulter says), and then learned practical medicine in busy general hospitals in Somerset and at Harrow Road. Peter Sever sent him to do field work measuring hypertension, first in Jamaica, then in Kenya, where he spent five years.

On his return, Geoffrey Rose, an advisor for the Kenya project, suggested that Poulter do an MSc in epidemiology with him at the London School of Hygiene. Simultaneously, Michael Marmot, an epidemiologist at UCL, invited Poulter (who now had a reputation for fieldwork) to help set up an international study of the contraceptive pill. Once he had completed the MSc, Poulter moved into Marmot's department, though, like Rose, he still saw patients in the cardiovascular clinic at St Mary's. In 1997, with the pill study completed, he took up a chair at St Mary's and at the time of writing is developing an international study of 19,000 hypertensive patients. It is an enormous project, involving twenty-one staff at St Mary's, nineteen of them full-time researchers on the project. He also participates in the annual Health Survey for England and has recently published the "rule of two thirds," showing that two thirds of people are under-treated for blood pressure.

Another recent hiring is Paul Elliott, who has held the chair of epidemiology at St Mary's since 1995. As he trained in mathematics (at Cambridge) and medicine (at UCL), epidemiology seemed an obvious route. Rose and Peart sponsored his work. During the late 1980s, with Rose and a group of American collaborators, Elliott managed an international study of salt consumption and excretion that definitively linked salt to heart disease. Current projects that Elliott is supervising at St Mary's include a study of 47,000 people in four countries, examining what they eat and excrete for two periods of twenty-four hours. The logistics of the study are enormous, and Elliott oversees a department of 150 staff, fourteen of them academics. Another line of investigation is the Small Area Health Statistics Unit, which collects vital statistics by area code and then investigates possible causes of morbidity, such as the vicinity of a waste dump.

The Geoffrey Rose and the Wright Fleming initiatives are still being developed, with new appointments being made almost daily. In May 2000 it was announced that Roy Anderson, who left Imperial College for the Linacre chair at Oxford, would come to St Mary's as professor of infectious disease epidemiology. Anderson integrates statistical and laboratory investigation into infectious disease. He brings a research team including Professor Brian Spratt; the two are the first FRS on staff at St Mary's since Peart's retirement.

On the day his appointment was announced, Anderson was at St Mary's to give a lecture in the Almroth Wright lecture series, in which he described some of the work on BSE and hazarded some estimates as to the size of the anticipated epidemic of vCJD. The St Mary's molecularists, including Howard Thomas, Leslie Brent, Jonathan Weber, John Collinge, and tropical specialist Geoffrey Pasvol, turned out in force to engage in some friendly jousting over his figures. Afterwards they shared a bottle of wine in the Wright-Fleming library. The old Inoculation Department and offices vacated by the basic scientists in their move to South Kensington ring once again with arguments over the nature of infection and the possibilities of prevention.

In December 2001 the results of a new Research Assessment Exercise were announced. Imperial College had moved up to second place in the United Kingdom for quality of research. The Faculty of Medicine distinguished itself by obtaining the highest grade (a 5*) in both clinical-laboratory and hospital-clinical subjects. The two subfields based at St Mary's, Cardiovascular Medicine and Infection and Immunology, both obtained the 5* rating. The new rector of Imperial College, Sir Richard Sykes, expressed himself as "absolutely delighted" with the results.[30]

The structure of medical research in London is still undergoing enormous change, and much remains unsettled. The ramifications of all this long-term structuring are difficult to predict in their entirety. British academe has always sustained an eclectic mix of talents. Not everyone is an Almroth Wright or a John Collinge. Most people do sound, even imaginative work, without ever being likely to become an FRS or a Nobel laureate. Some fields of science attract larger sums of money than others. The MRC prefers to fund high-tech laboratory work, leaving other medical sciences to forage in the private sector or look abroad. Fields can go in and out of fashion.

Haematology has done just that. On the eve of World War II when haematology was a glamorous new field, the MRC set up research units. After half a century of intense academic activity, haematology is no longer at the top of the MRC list of research priorities, outside of a few areas such as the thalassaemias (the subject of an MRC unit in Oxford). Sunitha Wickramasinghe became professor of haematology at St Mary's in 1979, when he succeeded Mollison. He obtained an MBBS from the University of Ceylon in 1964 and a PhD from Cambridge, where he co-authored an article published in *Nature* on the proliferation of erythropoietic cells in pernicious anaemia. After a stint as a researcher in Leeds, Wickramasinghe applied to a position at Guy's, but was advised to go to St Mary's instead, because Mollison's MRC unit had a better research program and Wickramasinghe was obviously a researcher. In 1970 he came to St Mary's as a lecturer and senior registrar and worked his way to the top. The atmosphere was very good, he recalled: there was enough money for curiosity-driven research, and Pat Mollison was a "real academic and a gentleman, and it was easy to work with him."[31] Wickramasinghe's research interests have been in the pathophysiology and ultrastructure of the bone marrow in anaemic diseases. Among the contributions to research made by his team are the description of new forms of dyserythropoietic anaemia and an account of how folic acid deficiency affects the DNA of bone marrow cells. Coming to Paddington, he had many patients referred to him for abnormally large red cells, which can be due to vitamin B12 or folic deficiency or alcohol abuse, and he began to work on the mechanisms of alcohol toxicity. While it was known that liver cells metabolized alcohol, the damage to the red blood cells only made sense if the bone marrow was also metabolizing alcohol. Wickramasinghe and his team found that macrophages were responsible for the metabolism. Other research was undertaken to help other departments: for example, the haematologists investigated the way in which the immuno-suppressive drugs used for transplantation damaged the bone marrow. Wickramasinghe was regularly supported by project grants from the MRC, and he produced more than two hundred papers and several monographs.

Wickramasinghe also oversaw the hospital haematology service, and he chaired the pathology sciences division in the medical school until that position was abolished in a merger of all the pathology divisions in 1997. From 1995 to 1997 he was deputy dean of St Mary's. Wickramasinghe has been a workhorse for St Mary's and his official positions within the school, with his other professional appointments, suggest that he has won the esteem of his colleagues. All in all, his seems a career to reflect back upon with satisfaction. But Professor Wickramasinghe feels no such satisfaction. Though one of the first to welcome closer ties with Imperial College, he has found in the new school a chilly climate and subtle pressures. His brand of science is thought "gentlemanly," rather than glamorous or lucrative. He is now leaving St Mary's to take up a position at the unit in Oxford as a visiting professor.

Wickramasinghe is not the only scientist to feel uncomfortable with the new regime. Victoria Cattell, reader in experimental nephrology, is a Mary's woman through and through – she trained there in the 1960s and married there – twice. She took up histopathology after being encouraged by transplantation pathologist Ken Porter, a friendly sponsor and a stimulating teacher of critical thinking. Like so many of the best teachers at St Mary's, Porter taught students to approach medicine as an intellectual puzzle rather than as a set of facts. Cattell became an academic histopathologist, with teaching and clinical duties, and all the while studied renal phagocytosis, inducing immune responses in animals and studying their effects on the kidney. By the late 1990s, however, she was feeling fed up. Under the NHS Trust the clinical work had increased until it seriously encroached on her research time, and her main clinical interest, nephrology, was due for transfer to the RPMS. On the academic front, she says with a wry smile, "There's really not room in the system for people like me, who work with small groups and are very independent ... What we're being told is the model of research is, now, large groups. Really, I think they're talking about forty people. Now, I've never had more than five, six people maximum here, working on this topic." Rather than join a large, number-crunching group, she took early retirement.[32]

The atmosphere at St Mary's has changed in recent years. Even those professors who are most pleased with the new arrangements feel it. One blamed an American model of academic structure that aims at making research staff feel insecure so that they work harder. Others regret that the informal and interdisciplinary discussions that used to occur in the corridors and the senior dining room have been sacrificed. Now, the senior dining room is deserted. One floor below, the students too have abandoned the student bar to study for their exams, though these exams never seriously lowered bar takings before. The bartender shakes his head in puzzlement.

Some suggest that the students are the real losers in the merger. With an intake of three hundred each year, there is little chance for teachers and students to get to know one another and every chance that the students may get lost in the shuffle. Because the students are based at South Kensington for their initial, premedical courses, the hospital consultants who traditionally took an interest in their activities no longer do so. Most agree that the new school will attract a different kind of student, one driven by intellectual ambition. This may mean that Imperial College won't train GPs, or that GPs will be more intellectually ambitious than they have been, rather than the well-rounded and sociable individuals that St Mary's has produced throughout its history. Some worry that the quality of medical care in the community may suffer. Still, the school attracts twenty applicants for every place.

Most people agree that if the changes really work, if they prove to be the saving of British medical research, then they are worthwhile. Christopher Edwards speaks of the need to bolster "UK Plc." and to reverse the decline of British research, seen in the diminishing frequency with which British research is cited. The old ways could not be sustained forever. And the truth is that St Mary's is undergoing a change rather than a crisis. In the hospital, morale is good, better than it has been in some time. The school has a new-found purpose and the resources to pursue that purpose. In terms of equipment, colleagues, and staff, many of the academic staff have never had it so good. The new building in South Kensington provides state-of-the-art research laboratories, though there are still many bugs in the system (such as faulty fume cupboards likely to set off fire alarms). More importantly, the development of infection and immunity and epidemiology bodes well for a continued academic presence on the St Mary's site. Where once Imperial College spoke of developing its clinical resources most fully at the Hammersmith, in the year 2000 Christopher Edwards planned to develop "our major laboratory research sites [at] the Hammersmith Hospital and Paddington Basin."[33]

The Paddington Basin development to which Edwards referred is far greater in scope than the Rose and Wright-Fleming initiatives. The shake-up at Imperial College provoked a rethinking of the local hospitals. If academic departments were to be concentrated in specialized sites, what would be the implications for clinical services? Could similar rationalization and concentration be effected there also?

Edwards raised the question with officials at the North-West Thames Regional Office, and the result was the West London Partnership Forum, which provides an arena for the academics and the NHS officials in West London to discuss matters of common interest. The forum established three specialist committees to advise on the organization of tertiary care in nephrology, paediatrics, and cardiovascular medicine. Nephrology, it was decided, would be relocated to the Hammersmith. As a result St Mary's stands to lose its kidney transplantation unit, though it will remain a centre for dialysis. As for paediatrics and cardiovascular medicine, the forum had to choose between Fulham Road (based upon Chelsea/Westminster

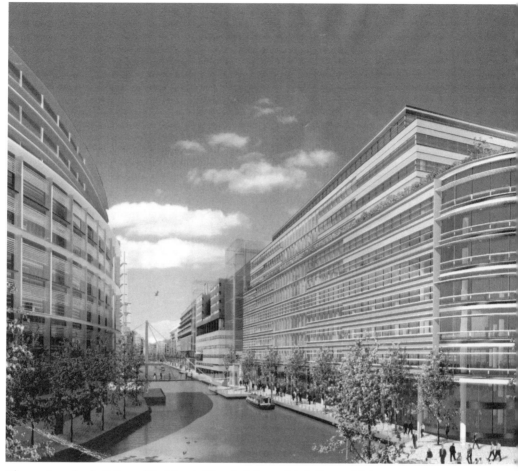

The projected rebuilding of St Mary's Hospital. Imperial College of Science, Technology, and Medicine

and the Brompton Hospitals) and St Mary's as centres for concentration. The project is a mammoth one that will involve relocating the Harefield Hospital, a centre for heart and lung transplantation, and the Royal Brompton Hospital with its associated National Heart and Lung Institute. In February 2000 the forum chose St Mary's.

When the Brompton and Harefield hospitals are moved to the St Mary's site, they will be part of a multi-billion project to regenerate the Paddington Basin. The area remains remarkably unchanged since the Victorian era. The canal is a muddy backwater where rusting shopping carts collect. On the other side, along North Wharf Road, the dustyards remain, though the stables have been replaced by fleets of rubbish trucks. The shops on Praed street are pokey and drab. Beyond the railway station lies the goods yard, and acres of vacant land.

When the bishop offered the hospital founders a plot on which to build, his was only the first of a series of failed attempts at regenerating this neighbourhood. But, finally, the new millennium has brought new hope. At the end of the 1990s a fast rail link to Heathrow airport was developed, creating new possibilities for tourism and business. Hotels developed massive programs of expansion, and glamorous chains began to bid to put their shops in Paddington, while developers have submitted plans for "high specification housing." An area the size of Soho will be redeveloped at a cost of billions.

The expansion of Paddington will pay for the expansion of St Mary's. To raise the £300 million pounds needed to bring in the Brompton and Harefield, most of the existing hospital fabric will be sold for redevelopment. The original hospital and all the subsequent developments (except for the Clarence facade, which has listed building status, and the Queen Elizabeth the Queen Mother (QEQM) wing) will be torn down. Paddington Station will extend towards the canal, atop the old Mint wing. Office blocks will cover the existing Cambridge wing and nurses' home, though Moran's school will remain. And on South Wharf Road along the canal basin, new hospital buildings will go up.

There is still a long way to go. There has been public protest against the move, by patients loyal to Harefield, for example. Nonetheless, the economic and the scientific arguments for concentration were incontrovertible. St Mary's will be rebuilt. A teaching hospital will continue to flourish next to the canal basin for a long time to come.

∞ 15

The Changed Hospital 2
Hospital Culture

THROUGHOUT THE TWENTIETH century, doctors and politicians wrestled for control of the clinical encounter. Once medicine had begun to advance a creditable claim to explanatory power and therapeutical efficacy, ratcheting up successes, and once the middle classes began to demand admission to hospitals, the state began to take an interest in the equitable distribution of this resource. The result was an enormous improvement in the quality and quantity of medical care provided to the English population. But some of the qualities that the best, most privileged doctors could offer their patients – personal interest, constant care, state-of-the-art remedies – could not be sustained in this levelling upward. The state's interest in medicine was impersonal and bureaucratic, and it forced medical institutions into strange, new, impersonal, and bureaucratic configurations. To the London teaching hospitals, which occupied the pinnacle of the pre-war medical hierarchy in Britain, the National Health Service came as a life preserver, but it sometimes seemed a yoke that weighed more and more heavily.

Successive ministers of Health imposed an ever more stringent financial discipline upon hospitals to curb what Enoch Powell, Health minister from 1960 to 1963, described as an "infinity of demand." It was Powell who observed, "The unnerving discovery that every Minister of Health makes at or near the outset of his term of office is that the only subject he is ever destined to discuss with the medical profession is money."[1] During the 1960s the state had no other form of disciplining medicine than the financial. Only in the 1970s and '80s did civil servants and politicians develop a comprehensive discourse of their own that permitted them to undercut that of the medical profession. Battle was engaged. Hospital officials fought to defend their institutions against state officials trying to starve them into closure. St Mary's, like the other teaching hospitals, won some battles and lost others.

Patients seemed sometimes to be caught in the crossfire, as the accusations and the jargon flew. Hospitals had always appeared as vast and intimidating institutions to many of their impoverished and sick patients; now they became all the more so. The twin forces of scientization and bureaucratization made medicine more alien and impersonal in its language and rituals. In London the Blitz and then the NHS had made people feel that hospitals belonged to them as familiar, even well-loved institutions. Half a century later with control of the hospitals devolved upwards, away from the local inhabitants, and with enormously increased turnover of patients and staff, this sense of familiarity can be endangered. The crisis is not simply a crisis in funding or in the clinical encounter: it strikes at the heart of sociability itself. Though relations between citizens have changed enormously since the founding of St Mary's Hospital in 1851, a concern for the well-being of others remains central to them. A bureaucratically entrenched callousness in regards to the provision of medical care may undermine notions of duties or rights of citizens in society as a whole.

Happily, we are not there yet. In the absence of a painless means of rationing health care, the state and the medical profession do collaborate to ensure that medicine is as equitable and caring as they can make it, with each side policing the other to ensure it doesn't abnegate its part. Equally important are the limits of their powers. Neither political nor professional bodies can entirely determine the clinical encounter. Agency flows upwards as well as downwards. Life on the ward is constructed by patients, nurses, and doctors who learn to accommodate one another through shared experiences. Often, this shared culture reflects years of tradition, which can never be entirely eradicated by the rationalizers. A wise governor won't govern against the grain of tradition and human nature. This final chapter explores life on the ground, in the wards at St Mary's. While it casts sober glances towards current conditions in the hospital, it focuses on past rather than present relations. The gist of the argument is that a survey of the traditions at St Mary's over the last century, of the rules and of the people who broke the rules, provides considerable reassurance that the human element remains in the present day a robust foundation for the daily renewal of the social contract.

Until the Thatcherite reforms there was always a clear and personal centre of gravity to whom lay, medical, and nursing staff all ultimately looked: the house governor. The first task of a house governor was to be impressive. Thomas Ryan, who had the post from 1887 to 1920 (having come

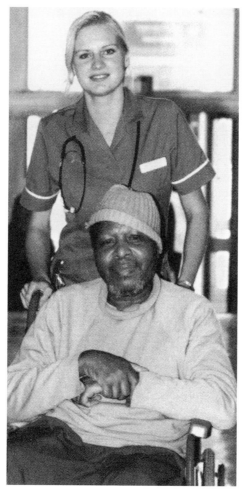

Life on the wards.
St Mary's Hospital NHS Trust Archives

from Queen Charlotte's Hospital) was a "stockily built gentleman in a frock-coat with a definite air of self-importance who walked slowly down the centre of the corridor with legs slightly apart."[2] His successor from 1920 to 1949 was Colonel Walter Parkes, a military man with a fine bearing who lost a lung in the First World War. His porters were old soldiers, and a memorial to the Fifth Army adorns the hospital gate. Its general, Sir Hugh Gough, was a governor and deputy chairman at St Mary's. A favourite of Sir Douglas Haig's, he was given the command of the army, composed largely of depleted battalions. In 1918 at Passchendaele the British Expeditionary Force suffered its first true defeat of the war, and the French, blaming the Fifth Army, insisted it be broken up. In peacetime Gough laboured to restore its honour: St Mary's was the field of operations, and Parkes his faithful helper.[3]

With the aid of only a secretary, a steward, two clerks, and four porters, Colonel Parkes ran St Mary's for three decades. According to Arthur Dickson Wright,

Presiding over a community something like two thousand strong, five hundred of whom were sick, there must have been no end to the permutations and combinations of trouble that came his way. A patient would have a harsh time in casualty from a new houseman overcome by qualification and would communicate his troubles to a hospital benefactor, who would threaten a redistribution of his largesse. In this situation Parkes was at his best and with consummate guile and tact would persuade the patient that firm handling was indicated for her especial complaint, would convince the houseman that his Napoleonic tendencies would be excellent if reserved for the certain later day when he would be on the hospital staff. The only rueful person would be the benefactor who after it was all over, found himself filling in a cheque for twice his usual amount.[4]

Parkes's successor was Alan Powditch, who came to St Mary's in 1938 and worked his way up to the governorship in 1950.[5] He adapted to the NHS in the 1940s but was less able to adapt to the strikes and bureaucracies of the 1970s.

Medical governance was in the hands of the consultants, who virtually dictated terms to the lay governors. The whole of the senior staff met at the Medical Committee, while a smaller chairman's committee did the serious work. This happy arrangement ended with the reorganization of the NHS. The chairman's committee was abolished and the Medical Committee found its proceedings trumped by district-wide committees, often on financial grounds. The clinicians could only plead, as Richard Beard did in 1976, that "the decision as to where reductions would be implemented was a medical one and not for the administration."[6] The vogue for expert management receded at the end of the 1980s, and in the 1990s local governance revived. Clinicians are equal partners on the board of trustees that runs the St Mary's NHS Trust. The system is intended to be less confrontational, on the principle that doctors will be more cooperative if they can help to make decisions. Doctors are the essential intermediaries between administrative necessity and public demand.[7] The concept of clinical governance lies at the heart of this new attitude. Clinical governance addresses the clinical encounter as a whole, to ensure that patients receive the best medical care according to their own wishes, with established mechanisms of accountability. What is new is the government's determination to police it, rather than letting the medical profession police itself. The state now sets formal mechanisms of accountability, such as evidence-based medicine (which requires clinicians to produce evidence in favour of the treatments that they

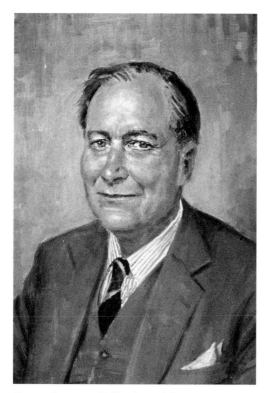

George Bonney. Collection of George Bonney

adopt), clinical audit (which requires them to study their own results), and a forum to hear patients' concerns and complaints. Much of the best self-policing by doctors still occurs informally, by means of a "three wise men" system introduced by orthopaedic surgeon George Bonney. A commandingly tall and urbane man with a dry sense of humour, Bonney trained and worked at St Mary's, serving as chair of the Group Medical Committee from 1971 to 1974 and chair of the District Hospital Medical Committee from 1974 to 1977. Some thought him a busybody, always reforming aseptic or admitting procedures, but it is busybodies like Bonney who ensure that St Mary's continually mends its ways.

Among the old centripetal forces to disappear was the medical superintendent. For the better part of a century two long-standing medical superintendents, Matthew Mitchell Bird and Henry ("Cocky") Cockburn, served as a mortar binding together the bricks of a common hospital culture. A shy, furtive figure with a drooping moustache and a sonorous voice, Mitchell Bird qualified at St Mary's in 1887 and the following year was named medical superintendent, a post he held for thirty-two years. He coped with epidemics, decrepit staff, raw students, and troublesome patients. St Mary's was his whole life, and when he died, he left his estate to the hospital. At his funeral it was said that if Mary's men were known throughout the world as men of character, this was largely due to Mitchell Bird.

After his departure in 1920 the post reverted to a short-term office for junior men in need of a salary. Then Henry Cockburn again turned this marginal position into one of considerable influence wholly through the strength of his personality. Cockburn came to St Mary's in the 1930s as one of Moran's rugby players, and while he lacked scientific ambition, his quiet competence made him indispensable. He was medical superintendent from 1955 until his retirement when the post was abolished. Like Mitchell Bird, Cockburn became a surrogate father of the students and nurses, disciplining them, caring for them, finding practices for them, and inculcating Moran's philosophy of character. He dominated the rugby team in the 1930s, and in later years his influence over the students only grew. Tony Roberts, who came to St Mary's during the 1960s on a scholarship, was a first-rate hockey player, but as St Mary's had no reputation for hockey he decided to play for more promising teams. One by one, friends came up to him and said quietly that Cocky thought he should play for Mary's. Roberts led St Mary's to a cup win in hockey. When he qualified, Cockburn found him a general practice near Beaconsfield with Jeremy Carless.

On Cockburn's departure nurses mourned him deeply. As one ward sister, Christine Rose, said, "Mary's needed him like hell. He was the spirit of Mary's. He was a calm centre." On days when she was "rushing around like a scared hen," Cockburn would walk in with his unfailing deadpan expression and a glimmer in his eyes, call a coffee break, and sort out the problems. "He wasn't encroaching on the others. He knew where the stress points were, he appeared, and he made you laugh." For many nurses, Cockburn was the alpha and the omega of St Mary's, the first face they saw at the interview panel and the last one they still recognized when they returned, later in life, for a visit to their old hospital. Evangeline Karn recalled, "if you didn't pass the Dr Cockburn test, basically, you didn't come to St. Mary's. And he would say something like, 'Not St Mary's,' you know. There was a sort of ... I don't know whether it's a myth or not, but there was a sort of idea that there was a sort of girl that was suitable for St Mary's. Not, perhaps, highly ambitious, not, perhaps, highly intellectual – perhaps they would go to St Thomas's. But really caring, good fun, good practical nurses."[8] Cockburn arbitrated and taught character as Moran would have recognized it.

A measure of the change that Cockburn's departure marked was the appointment of a specialist consultant to the Accident and Emergency department. Until the 1980s the department was supervised by the orthopaedic surgeons but largely run by nurses and students, with Cockburn as a mediator. Until Cockburn retired and until the inadequate facilities could be expanded, there seemed no real necessity for a specialist in A & E medicine, and St Mary's was the last London teaching hospital to appoint one.

When Robin Touquet was named to the post in 1986 he found that people expected him to fill Cockburn's boots. Touquet trained at the Westminster and then worked as a GP in Kent for a year, but abuse of the system – he was called out to a trivial case in the middle of the night by a man scheming to have his damp walls repaired – drove him back to the hospital. With his GP and surgical experience and training, Touquet could well have become a de facto medical superintendent as some expected of him, but instead he determined to build up the A & E department as a place of "real-time" specialty teaching. When he arrived, the department consisted of himself and five senior house officers. For five years he was constantly either present or on call until a second consultant, Jane Fothergill, was named in 1991. Touquet, Fothergill, and their junior colleagues have made the place a leading exponent and centre for the development of A & E medicine, a fitting "shop window" to the hospital. It is home to new initiatives such as the "Paddington Alcohol Test," which provides counselling for alcohol abusers who are seen repeatedly, and a resuscitation training service developed by Fothergill. A series of papers published on the Notting Hill Festival enabled Touquet to produce statistics showing that the festival was becoming less, not more violent. The A & E has become a service closely tuned to the needs of the local population. As well as emergency care, it provides a safe haven for homeless families, elderly, immigrants, refugees, and young runaways.[9]

On 5 October 1999 the A & E department had its greatest test. Early that morning two trains collided head-on at Ladbroke Grove outside Paddington Station. Compounding the crush injuries – the fractures and lacerations – were serious burns caused by a fireball that swept through the front carriage. Thirty people died at the scene, and dozens more were critically injured. Even before it had been officially notified, the St Mary's A & E department initiated its "Major Incident" procedures devised by Fothergill, having been warned of the crash by a nurse on another carriage who called them on her mobile phone. Staff leaving at the end of the night shift were kept on, the fresh staff were assigned to emergency stations, and burn experts were called in from Chelsea-Westminster. By the time the first patients arrived, all was ready and waiting for them, and every patient was seen by a consultant-led team. It was a harrowing day for the staff, coping with fifty-one patients, some horribly hurt, but by the end of it they could congratulate themselves on a job well done.

Specialization in the A & E department reflects specialization across the

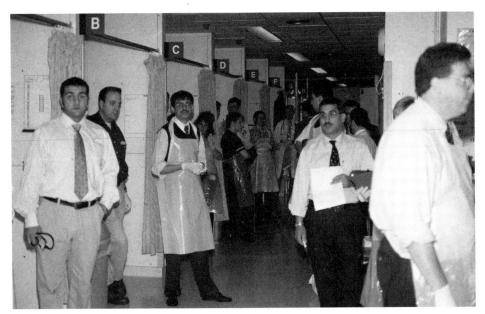

Paddington Rail Disaster: At the ready stations. Collection of Robin Touquet

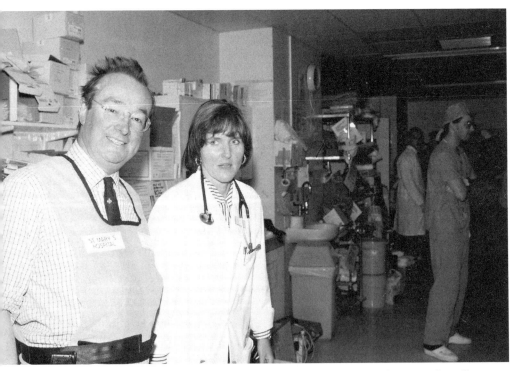

Paddington Rail Disaster: Consultants Robin Touquet and Jane Fothergill
at the end of the day. Collection of Robin Touquet

hospital. Standards of care have never been higher, but the division of labour among large teams of doctors, students, and nurses requires enormous planning and organization. In practice the oldest solution to the problem of continuity of care remains the best: namely, rounds.

Rounds

For much of the history of St Mary's, doctors and surgeons were not much in attendance, spending several hours doing rounds twice a week. Moran only came in on Saturday mornings, and would teach "brilliantly" on patients he had never seen before. One exception was Arthur Dickson Wright, who frequented the hospital at all hours, often operating through the night. (Ultimately his difficult manner and long hours were unconducive to a happy home life, and his marriage failed;[10] after a crippling stroke, he spent his last years in the Lindo Wing and died in the hospital where he had spent his life.) Dickson Wright loved to infuriate the nurses by ducking around the back staircases so he could burst in and surprise them. But for most consultants, ward rounds were highly ritualized. Patients were trussed by tight sheets so they could hardly move, and they dared not call for a bedpan.[11] A specimen of the traditional round is described by Jack Litchfield, a dresser to Sir William Willcox in the 1930s: "The round was conducted with some formality. Sir William, Justin Bartlett [the house physician] and Sister headed the procession, followed by three nurses and the clerks. The first nurse carried a tray with tendon hammer, ophthalmoscope etc.; the second a chair which was presented to Sir William at suitable moments and the third acted as a runner and would hand to sister the enamelled pots containing stools, which Sir William liked to inspect."[12] The pomp and ritual of the ward round bolstered the mystique of medical authority. In 1920 Luff advised the students that the doctor should seem an "oracle" to his patients.[13]

Consultants now spend more time in the hospital, and their manner is more casual. But even without the pomp, a consultant can still strike terror into the souls of junior staff and patients on a ward round. Neil Poulter was George Bonney's house surgeon for a stretch in the 1960s, and the experience remains with him. "For example, you had to have the x-rays on the ward round. And there was no question about, 'I'm terribly sorry, I couldn't get them.' You had to get them. And so you spent half your life on your knees, pleading with radiographers to take x-rays which were not acute." One memorable day Bonney "stood there at the end of the bed whilst we explained to him that this wasn't ready, and that hadn't been done, and these were things that were out of your control, you know. And he nodded, and he just turned to Mrs. Whatever, and said, 'Mrs. ___' he said, 'I'm terribly sorry, it appears we're not doing anything at all for you,' and just walked out. So there's the patient looking at you, and you say, 'It's okay, it's okay! I'll be back. I'll explain.' And then you'd run off to the next disaster."[14] Jenny Large, Sister Manvers during the 1970s, described the routine in the 1970s of Hugh Dudley, who took a minor teaching round on Thursday and a major one on Tuesday. "That round would take you all morning, basically, because the whole entourage, all his team – the junior doctors, the SHOs, the junior and senior registrars, usually the physio and the nurses – would go round bed by bed. And if he wanted to know something, like a blood result, he wanted it then. He didn't want to know that it hadn't come back from the lab, he wanted it then, and that was it. And if the junior didn't know about it, it was, 'Just get off my ward round, and don't you come back until you know what you're doing.' And you would often start a ward round with ten or twelve people, and end up with you and Prof. Dudley, because all the rest would have been thrown off it!"[15]

If ward rounds permitted consultants to terrorize junior staff, grand rounds were a more even form of combat, pitting consultant against consultant. Early in the century they were called the "clinico-pathological conference" and chaired by the pathologist, but he humiliated the clinicians so ruthlessly that they refused to participate. At mid-century, meetings were revived by W.D. Newcomb, E.H. Kettle's successor as professor of pathology until 1954. An outstanding clinical pathologist, he introduced the idea of the "total post-mortem." (He was also an avid gardener, the excellence of his tomatoes "reputedly due to the liberal application of blood clot."[16]) Students listened as surgeons and physicians battled over disciplinary boundaries, and they wrote the cases up in the *St Mary's Hospital Gazette*.

Surgeons often attacked the physicians for not referring patients to them. In 1948 even the mild-mannered Pannett openly criticized the medical unit when it persisted in treating by transfusions a man with a duodenal ulcer, who was vomiting blood. "The patient had been treated according to the best medical opinion, but he did not think this was right." All those transfusions, Pannett commented, "might throw the metabolism out of order."[17] Physicians in their turn criticized the surgeons for operating precipitously. In 1951 a man operated on for abdominal cancer seemed to be doing well, but as Charles Rob said, "Good morning, Mr X, how are you?" and took the man's wrist to feel for his pulse, the patient suddenly died under the horrified gaze of the ward. "It was assumed that a medical catastrophe had occurred at that instant." Was the operation to blame or had the man a preexisting coronary condition? The pathologists found a coronary embolus, but they weakened their case by losing the corroborating slide.[18]

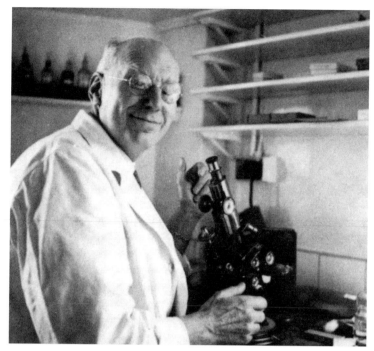

W.D. Newcomb. St Mary's Hospital NHS Trust Archives and the
Royal College of Surgeons of England

Newcomb made merry at the clinicians' expense. In 1949 when they misdiagnosed a miner with carcinoma as syphilitic, "Prof Newcomb gets up
and says that it is all very difficult. He is very anxious to support the clinicians, but the histology is completely against them."[19] Another time, when
clinicians failed to diagnose periarteritis nodosa, a member of the medical
unit asked "where the fat comes from in lipoid pneumonia." A "shocked"
Newcomb explained:

"It is endogenous." He found that some people still did not know this and
quoted an examiner who was recently instructed in the subject by a Mary's student! We were gradually educating people, he said, but he couldn't think how
Dr. Ackroyd could have needed enlightenment.

Dr. Ackroyd, who professed himself corrected and deeply humiliated, asked
if babies were endogenous.

Prof. Newcomb: "No they are medicinal and are inhaled."

At this point most of us felt grateful to Dr. Brooks for his unambiguous
explanation that he had always presumed the fat in lipoid pneumonia came from
degenerate polymorphs.[20]

At the end of the twentieth century, grand rounds were held each Friday lunchtime, chaired by professors of the medical unit Howard Thomas or John Summerfield. They modelled their meetings after the celebrated rounds at the Hammersmith, which both attended. The atmosphere was friendly, even playful, as the senior staff jibed with one another. But though the tone can sometimes be light, grand rounds are a serious business, where difficult cases are brought forward for diagnosis, or an unexpectedly fatal outcome is reviewed with the idea that another treatment might be provided next time. Grand rounds are designed to teach junior staff to be open to critical scrutiny and to talk about their difficult cases. They also provide a forum for addressing the hospital staff generally, to discuss matters of policy. Pinching and Weber used grand rounds to present an early AIDS patient and show the staff that "this wasn't just a strange disease that we read about in the journals with a strange sort of people who do bizarre things." Pinching clearly recalls the "drawing-in of breath, the hush that descended."[21] At grand rounds, the staff collectively reflect upon what they are up to and how well they achieve it.

Most clinical departments have their own rounds. Often they have more clinical staff than did all of St Mary's when it opened, so they must cultivate teamwork to ensure continuity of care. The early vascular meetings exemplify their efforts. These meetings are descended from the audit introduced by Hugh Dudley, who insisted on a regular review of all untoward outcomes and campaigned for a national database of statistics showing surgical outcomes. The tradition of audit was maintained after his departure, and at the end of the century Averil Mansfield presided over the vascular meetings, held early on Tuesday mornings.

Vascular surgeons at St Mary's take in referrals from across the country, and they perform some drastic operations. Together they and the surgeons-in-training decide who can be operated on successfully and how to go about it. Occlusion of the blood vessel is a matter of degree, and the surgeons must decide if the occlusion is too far advanced or not yet advanced enough for surgery. Another day, presented with a man showing occluded carotid arteries whose condition is complicated by a neurological disease damaging the brain and thickening the artery wall, the surgeons wonder whether he is a good risk or whether he should be treated conservatively. They turn for advice to Felix Eastcott who, although retired, still attends the Tuesday morning meetings.

Fifty years earlier, discussion concerned the scope of operations that surgeons could perform – how deeply they could penetrate the human body, how much they could safely excise. Nowadays, discussions search for better routes to similar outcomes, with an eye to making surgery less rather than more heroic. Vascular surgeon Nick Cheshire comments:

I think there's absolute recognition that what you can do with a knife and fork, we're at the limits of it. There is no more advance to be made in that. And some of the operations we do here, like thoracico-abdominal aneurysm repair, we're more or less unique in this country. This is where the aneurysm affects the chest and the abdomen. And it is the limits of what most patients can withstand, you know, the complications and mortality are high, but then you're playing for high stakes, you know, they die if you don't fix it. So I think everybody knows there's not an awful lot more can be done. Most people would agree. If you're looking for advance in surgical technique terms, it's now all about the applications of technology, whether that's keyhole, laparoscopic, x-ray guided, it's some way of doing the operation in a less insulting way. And that's usually technology-based.[22]

Cheshire spoke as the vascular surgeons had just finished comparing the outcome of operations performed with and without a pump to bypass the heart and lungs. As initial experiences working without the pump succeeded, more and more operations have been done without the by-pass equipment. Cheshire explained that the new technologies have considerably improved the capacity for pre-operative discussion of patients: "Every patient needs something slightly different doing, even with the same pathology. And imaging is so good now that even without seeing the patient, your colleagues in the same subject can get a very good idea of what you're talking about, when you put your x-rays up at the x-ray meeting." Before the new imaging equipment was introduced at St Mary's, visual inspection of lesions was often only possible on the operating table itself or in the mortuary.

Also addressed at clinical meetings is the relationship between research and clinical care. Surgeons wishing to try out a new therapy or technique will usually set up a clinical trial. Once upon a time patients might be blindly allocated one treatment or another and then the protocol would remain rigidly in place until the trial ended. Nowadays clinicians monitor patients closely and remove them from the trial if they notice an adverse effect. At clinical meetings the staff review the progress of patients, as of the trial itself, and perhaps discuss alternative trials.

Nursing

Another traditional force for continuity of care in the hospital is the nursing staff. Nurses have acquired new responsibilities and powers. To take one example, Touquet and Fothergill established a wholly nurse-run clinic for minor injury at St Charles Hospital in North Kensington. Nurses are no longer the untutored helpmates of doctors, and nursing has become the specialized profession Florence Nightingale dreamed of. St Mary's Hospital was at the forefront of the change.

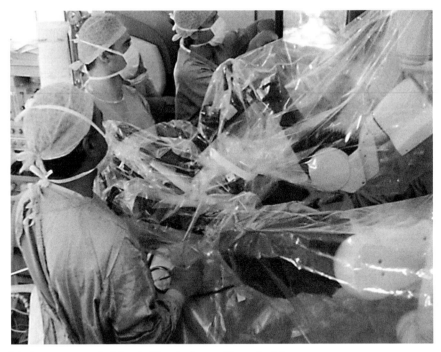

Modern surgery. St Mary's Hospital NHS Trust Archives

From the establishment of the nursing school in the 1870s until the First
World War, training consisted wholly of ward work, supplemented with occasional lectures by consultants. The probationer nurse reported to the
wards from her first day. Her early months were spent scrubbing floors and
sluices, then providing bedpans and bed-baths (known as "backs and bot-
toms"). Rose Anderson, née Smith, spent four years from 1919 to 1923
learning nursing at St Mary's. She most disliked polishing the brass plates
honouring patrons who had endowed beds: "Oh, those brass plates – acrid
fumes from the Great Western Railroad turned them black, the elbow
grease needed was colossal – if only the donors had realised the work they
involved." Many students dropped out, but others queued up to replace
them. After a year Rose Smith shucked off her humble muslin cap and
donned a linen one. She was now allowed to assist in dressing patients, to
attend the ward rounds, and even to dispense medicines to the patients.
"Many poultices were used for pneumonia and it was a thrill to be allowed
to watch the temperature and wait for the crisis." At the end of the training course, she was subjected to a written and a practical exam performed
on volunteer boy scouts. Smith made a "lovely chest poultice" and came

away happy; her friend, though she tried to stop a cut throat with a tourniquet, passed as well.[23] The nursing students' salaries were pitifully small: only £56 for their four years of work. Men's salaries per capita were much higher. The costs of salaries at St Mary's, below £10,000 before the war, rose to £25,000 in 1926. Nurses' salary costs rose only from £4,606 to £6,079 during the same six-year period.

But women still found nursing an attractive career, imbued with a spirit of service. The young women were sternly told that "everything we touched was a sacred Trust."[24] The school drew middle- and working-class women and even the occasional aristocrat. Princess Alexandra of Connaught came to St Mary's during the First World War, when genteel women flooded into hospitals as nursing assistants. Though she found the work hard, the living rough, and the patients filthy and smelly, the atmosphere was happy: "I grew very fond of the old Hospital. It was a home from home to me, and I used often to wonder how I was going to settle down to a different kind of life when the war was over."[25] She liked the casualty department best, where "life is presented in the raw," and she learned to cope with the drunks and the police cases. The memory was still powerful more than three decades later: "The dimly-lit room, with the trolley drawn up in a corner near the sink under the one light. The mackintosh pillow, which kept slipping and sliding about; the rough brown blanket continually being kicked off. The pungent smell of stale beer and sweat." Widowed, she later took charge of casualty at University College Hospital and then founded her own nursing home.

Most nurses worked only a few years before marriage, but for some, nursing was an alternative to a wedded life. The ambitious could aspire to become a matron, a figure of tremendous dignity and importance. With an enormous cap and ruffs, she could resemble a fully rigged sailing ship as she marched through the hospital, scolding probationers for the indecorous display of an ankle during the making of a bed.[26] St Mary's had a run of distinguished matrons during the twentieth century. Two have been commemorated by archivist Kevin Brown in the *Dictionary of National Biography*: Dorothy Bannon and Mary Milne.[27] Both trained at St Thomas's during the 1910s. Bannon came to St Mary's in 1922 to replace an unpopular matron and had to improve the training course to meet the standards of the newly created General Nursing Council. She retired from St Mary's in 1928, planning to join a convent, but in 1929 she was named matron in chief of the LCC hospitals, just as the LCC took over seventy-five old infirmaries and fever hospitals, as well as schools, asylums, and sanatoria, with a nursing staff of 11,000. Bannon made the system work well.

Bannon's successor at St Mary's was Mary Milne, her junior at St Thomas's; Bannon sternly advised her to hide her short hair under an artificial bun. Milne was matron at St Mary's from 1928 to 1933 and devoted herself to getting Salton House built next to the medical school. In 1933, she joined Bannon in the LCC service, but she soon missed the practical work and took up a position in Leeds. When Matron Salton died suddenly in December 1940, Milne returned to St Mary's, to replace her and also became the matron for the Wartime Sector. Milne oversaw the nursing establishment for the whole St Mary's group and served on an NHS committee to manage the non-teaching hospitals in Paddington.

By constant self-assertion the matrons of St Mary's improved their official standing. In 1950 the matron was finally given voting rights at the Hospital Nursing Committee. She also supervised the nursing arrangements in all the constituent hospitals. In 1962 the matron of the Samaritan Hospital was suspended for failing to recognize the authority of the St Mary's matron. In practice the amount of authority that the nurses exercised depended largely on strength of character. Asserting authority required steely nerves. Ward Sister Jenny Large describes how her relationship with Professor Dudley evolved. In the evenings, if he'd been operating that day, she says, Dudley would "pop in and say, 'Do you want me to see anybody?' When he first started, he would never say that. He would just come in and in a very bombastic way would go and see everybody, and cause mayhem!" But, Large explains,

We built up a trust between each other, particularly after I hit him one day! He had a terrible habit of wandering through the ward, ripping dressings off wounds to have a look at it, poking his fingers around the wound, and just walking off to the next bed and ripping the next dressing off. I used to say to him, "There's a wash-basin over there, use it, please, because all you're doing, if there's any infections, you're moving it up my ward, and I won't have it in my ward ... And he kept doing it, and so one day, I went round with an 18-inch perspex ruler, which I kept down by my side, and I said, "Wash-hand basin," and he didn't go to it, so I hit him over the back of the knuckles with it! And he looked at me in this horrified way, and the rest of the team sort of melted away, knowing that Mount Vesuvius was about to erupt. He just grinned at me, and he said, "In future, I'll just look at the wounds that you wish me to see, Sister." I said, "That's fine by me." And he never did it again.[28]

Doctors, nurses, and students fraternized together despite prohibitions that were in place until the Second World War. In 1941 the medical students lived in the hospital, taking turns fire-watching. Because of the blackout, there wasn't much to do when they weren't fire-watching, and two brothers, John and Rollo Ballantyne, went to the house governor and proposed a musical society of nurses and medical students. Parkes conferred to the matron, who asked him, "The nurses work with the men, so why shouldn't they play with the men?" Parkes capitulated with the stern remark, "Be it on your own head if anything untoward happens." Nine months later, a dramatic society was also formed.[29]

But students and nurses had always met illicitly. "We weren't allowed to speak to med students, but of course we did," said Sister Brown, who was at St Mary's from 1929 to 1965.[30] One shocking match was that of Dora Fletcher, Sister Thistlethwayte, a lively woman who trotted around the hospital in high heels. In 1927, already dying of breast cancer, she married a newly qualified doctor many years younger. Sister Dora is said to haunt the wards of St Mary's, and on busy nights, patients have reported being given bedpans by "the Sister with the crooked strings and long dress"– a reference to the old habit of tying the cap strings to the right rather than under the chin.[31] Another interwar marriage was that of Sister Allcroft and a ward houseman. Their daughter, Christine Harrington, herself became a ward sister at St Mary's. Her father spoke admiringly of his wife's efficient governance of the nurses, telling Christine, "When those nurses did something wrong, she just humiliated them ... She flicked off her cuffs, she'd roll up her sleeves, and she showed them how it should be done, and they never did it wrong again."[32] Theirs was a well-ordered household.

Conditions for nursing students began to improve at the end of World War I. Other jobs with shorter hours and higher wages opened up, and women began to leave nursing. Into the 1930s shop clerks could only work eight hours per day while nurses worked eleven.[33] The nurses began to professionalize. The campaign to reform nursing by creating independent professional bodies had begun in the late nineteenth century. From the 1880s a group of reform-minded women, led by Ethel Bedford Fenwick, formed a British Nursing Association and agitated for a system of state registration of nurses that would, Fenwick argued, protect the public against inadequately trained nurses.[34] Worried at the prospect of losing their supply of cheap labour, the voluntary hospitals resisted the reforms. In 1907, for example, the board of St Mary's told the Royal British Nurses' Association that it saw no advantage to either the public or to nurses in its proposed examinations and diplomas.[35] The hospital's own qualification was quite sufficient.

But the nurses persisted, seeing how professionalization had benefited the doctors. At the end of the First World War, nurses began to join in the industrial unrest that swept the country. To the government and the middle-class reformers like Fenwick, registration and a central nursing body would stave off a less genteel and more militant unionization. A registration bill was enacted in 1919, and a General Nursing Council was finally established. The GNC set a standard of three years training in a general hospital (though it was still possible to practise with lesser qualifications), but the voluntary hospitals kept their own superior standard of four years. Those who completed the full four at St Mary's received a special badge, the "Mary's Penny."

The early 1920s saw the introduction of a preliminary training school at St Mary's, which was initially held in Norfolk Square, subsequently moving to Joyce Grove. For three months probationers were taught such basics as how to make beds and starch their caps. Professional relations were further cemented within the Past and Present Nurses' League, formed by Miss Bannon in 1922 "to allow Past and Present members of the Training School to meet; & to allow past members to keep in touch with their Hospital." Members subscribed two shillings and sixpence. The subscriptions went towards social and sporting events and a charity fund for nurses fallen on hard times. Later, the league also paid dues to professional organizations, established scholarships, and, from 1967, published a journal. Meetings were held twice a year, and at the first meeting seventy-seven applications were approved for membership. Gatherings might be enlivened by a bazaar, a lecture, a swim in Moran's pool, or a tour of Salton House (the nurses home for which the nurses raised money), and by plates of sticky buns.

Though conditions undoubtedly improved, St Mary's remained hardpressed to attract nurses. In 1948 Matron Milne advised the governors that something had better be done at St Mary's to attract and keep happy and productive junior nurses.[36] Despite improvements, ranging from better salaries (above £100 per annum by this time), shorter hours, better housing, and larger helpings of salad and Spam,[37] the number of students declined. About 1,200 nurses applied each year, 300 were interviewed and 120 admitted, forming a school of forty every four months. But many wouldn't show up, and the matron had difficulty filling the spots.[38] Into the 1960s it became harder to fill staff positions as well. At mid-decade, when the senior nurse tutor resigned, the post sat vacant for eighteen months until the matron, Miss Gardiner, finally hired Stanley Holder. That she appointed a man revealed the shortage of qualified women. Although men were beginning to make some headway in the nursing hierarchy in provincial hospitals, they had not yet done so in the London teaching hospitals.

Stanley Holder, having spent five years as principal nurse tutor in the now-defunct Hackney Hospital and then working in journalism, decided to return to practical work at St Mary's.[39] He found a conservative atmosphere and poor morale. Facilities were minimal: the library was in a corridor, the staff room had four chairs, and there was one practical room, one seminar room, and one classroom. But before he could reform the teaching, he had to improve working conditions. With help from the ward sisters, he developed standard ward procedure and policy books. He also made the nursing school functionally independent of the hospital when he persuaded the governors to let him decide where the probationers should be placed. Then Holder reformed the nursing school. He introduced a diploma course leading to a degree program. He began to recruit male nurses. He reduced lectures by consultants to focus teaching on nursing practice. He created a clinical skills course which the medical students clamoured to enter: they too wanted to learn how to do a lumbar puncture or pass a tube. He persuaded the hospital to erect a new school in the Mint Wing. In 1969 Queen Elizabeth the Queen Mother officially opened the new wing, culminating a hectic but very fruitful couple of years.

Meanwhile Holder became involved in nursing policy. The Department of Health was wrestling with the crisis in nursing. In the mid-1970s, nursing management was reconstructed in the image of factory line management, with numbers rather than titles to distinguish rank. Matrons became "Chief Nursing Officers." Responsibilities were formally defined, with a definite pay scale attached to them for the first time. The old culture of nursing, rooted in shared, tacit knowledge, camaraderie, and rigid hierarchies, was swept away. But the new culture never took hold of the nurses' hearts as the old had done, and it made the hiring crisis all the worse. At St Mary's, assigning everybody numbers "was death to the thing, really, because everybody hated to be a number." Nor did the nurses like the way that clinical responsibilities and pay scales were linked. Previously, according to Holder, "a sister was the sister was the sister. She might have had six patients, or she might have had sixteen patients. She still got paid the same." The new scheme was "foreign to nurses. Quite foreign. It undermined all their professional understanding of themselves, you know, as a person who had to be controlled through a financial subvention. Oh, terrible! And they found it very foreign, and they couldn't come to terms with that. And they couldn't come to terms with seeing each other having different levels of pay, because of different grades. And they suddenly felt that their service had been downgraded."

During the 1980s the DHSS tried another tack: instead of being like an industry, nursing would be like a learned profession. In 1983 the General Nursing Council was replaced by a "United Kingdom Central Council for Nursing, Midwifery, and Health Visiting," which included Holder. Demographers predicted a critical shortage of nurses by the year 2000, and the committee was told to make nursing more attractive by infusing it with academic interest and encouraging nurses to develop intellectual curiosity and independent judgment. The scheme, called Project 2000, was intended to overcome what historian Anne Marie Rafferty describes as the "deep anti-intellectual prejudice"[40] attached to nursing. Schools of nursing were to be affiliated with universities, and the students were to be completely liberated from their traditional service responsibilities, which would be done by low-paid nursing assistants. In 1989 a pilot project was begun at St Mary's Hospital, and then Project 2000 was introduced throughout the NHS

Nurses who worked in hospital wards during Project 2000's introduction describe its impact as "dreadful." They lost keen young workers who had acquired considerable preliminary knowledge. The replacement workers were so untrained as to be almost useless, and their numbers were far fewer than what was needed. The chronic shortage of nursing was immediately exacerbated and, as a result, more agency nurses were hired than ever, so that nursing bills rose. Morale and intellectual scope diminished rather than increased, because the nurses working the wards could hardly wait to finish their shifts and get away to their second, agency-paid shift elsewhere. Defenders of Project 2000 reply that stinginess on the government's part caused these problems but that the principle itself was sound. The retort might be that the government's stinginess was so thoroughly to be expected that the reformers should have planned for it. As one of the consequences of the reform of both nursing and the NHS, the St Mary's nursing school was relocated to Thames Valley University and renamed the North West of London College of Nursing and Midwifery. The college still trains students at St Mary's but has no specific connection with the hospital.

Some indication of the human side of the reforms can be seen in the early career of a student who entered St Mary's in 1989, the first class in the country to experience Project 2000. Justin Gaffney chose nursing over medicine because he wanted to work with patients.[41] Reading journals like the *Nursing Times*, Gaffney had realized that nursing was changing and that St Mary's was at the vanguard of the change. The hospital was small but big enough to have a variety of services, and it was known to have a friendly atmosphere. And so he came to St Mary's and enjoyed himself there and did well. Like medical students a generation earlier, the student nurses were told to "think critically": teachers "kept using this term, 'critical thinkers,' that these would be people who questioned everything that was going on, and didn't just accept a face value." The course was modular, including heavily theorized units on the art and science of nursing and on social policy, as well as the biological sciences and the practical training. Gaffney also joined nursing politics, attending the annual congress of the Royal College of Nursing. His first placement was in a vascular ward that saw some of the sickest patients in the hospital, with enormous open chest wounds or unstable aneurysms. Just as in Hugh Dudley's day, the surgeons and the nurses often had different ideas about how to dress wounds and keep them sterile.

Gaffney then became interested in sexual health, and after specialized training, took up a position at King's College Hospital on a ward with AIDS beds. There his progress through the ranks was quick. Before long, however, a new position came up at St Mary's, running the Working Men Project, a sexual health clinic. The post was a senior one, G grade (a "ward sister in the old style"), but though Gaffney lacked experience, he had been thoroughly trained in sexual health and in research techniques. He got the job, having moved from qualification to a senior grade in eighteen months. In 2000 he was working towards a PhD, though he had no plans to leave clinical work. He was full of enthusiasm and plans for improving the clinic. His is a success story.

And yet a fast track to responsibility is not the exclusive property of nurses trained under Project 2000. The old system had its successes too. One exemplar of this success is Tess Cann, who decided to become a nurse after finding she enjoyed a temporary job in a nursing home. She trained in Nottingham just before the introduction of Project 2000. She has no regrets: "I absolutely loved my training ... the emphasis was very much on the practical, and the clinical. And I think, you know, with hindsight, it may have been nicer to have more time put aside for formalized study, but the actual content of the course, from the clinical point of view, when we came out after three and a bit years, we were ready to go on the wards."[42] Senior students taught junior ones, so learning was infused with a sense of camaraderie. She came to London to specialize in colo-rectal nursing, working at King's College Hospital and then St Mark's, where she was a ward sister, weighed down with administration. When an opening came up at St Mary's, she applied.

The colo-rectal clinic at St Mary's is unusual. At its head is Ara Darzi, the professor of surgery. Darzi has introduced technologies that enable him to delegate much of the colo-rectal work to nurse practitioners in the surgical unit – that is, to nurses specially trained and encouraged to enter into territory traditionally occupied by the medical profession. A nurse practitioner can perform a rigid video endoscopy in a clinic at St Charles Hospital, sending the visual information back to Darzi's office at St Mary's for confirmation of her diagnosis. As a result, more patients are seen much more quickly and economically. The unit has two nurse practitioners, Tess Cann and Paula Taylor. Taylor, who was hired first, in 1996, pioneered the video clinic and other advanced practices in colo-rectal nursing. In 1998 she was named British nurse of the year, and in June 2000 she became the first nurse consultant at St Mary's. She too was conventionally trained. She and Cann manage two nurse-led colo-rectal clinics. One clinic provides a one-stop service for people with rectal bleeding who are at a low risk for cancer; once cancer has been ruled out, they are treated for minor complaints (major ones are referred to Darzi) and advised how to improve their diet and lifestyle to ward off piles. The other clinic is aimed at people with a high risk of cancer. They are given a thorough examination and, if the results show cancer, they can be in Darzi's clinic within two days.

It is not yet clear what lies ahead for the ambitious nurse or nurse practitioner. The nurses studied here all seem good candidates for new heights of academic or consultant standing. All show tremendous enthusiasm for their work. Cann exclaims, "I'm motivated to learn, and I make sure I do, all day, every day. And I always have."[43] Keenness is crucial to maintaining a buoyant nursing profession. As for education, this too must have an important place, though one difficult to assess during a period of change. Even self-styled "critical thinking" can become a new orthodoxy that can imprison thought as securely as hoary routine. The Stanley Holder Nursing Library (which recently merged with the medical school library) is full of books with such titles as *Paradigms of Nursing Theories*, wherein students have dutifully underlined passages and circled diagrams that provide snappy answers to potential exam questions about the definition of thought itself, definitions which philosophers would find absurd. The markings stop well before the end of the book. To some extent, good nursing, like good medicine, can only be taught where there is a good teacher, a keen student, and a conducive atmosphere. And, of course, a willing patient.

The Patient

Patients do as much as nurses or doctors to set the atmosphere on the ward. The London voluntary hospitals admitted the London working classes, and the wards echoed with the lively sounds of a shared culture. In 1900 H. Stansfield Coller told the students that in the London poor they would find "perhaps the most intelligent and interesting poor people in the world": filthy, yes, but also patient, self-denying, loving, and even heroic. He instanced the dying woman who fumbled for a handkerchief to protect his fingers from her sweat, the "common little slum child" on the operating table who said, "Kiss me first, doctor," and the cabman who, when rebuked for cruelty to a horse, joked that there could be no worse cruelty than being a patient "at St. Mary's 'Orspital, and under the care of Mr Collier." Rose Anderson recalled that the patients of the 1920s were always

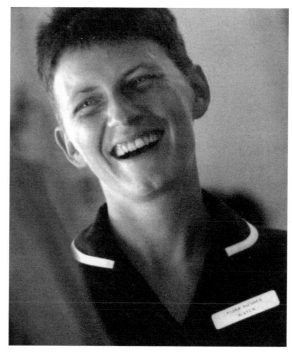

Nurse Fiona Hughes.
St Mary's Hospital NHS Trust Archives

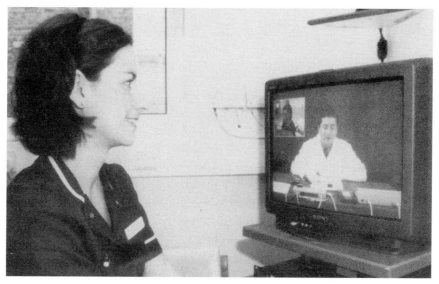

Nurse practitioner Paula Taylor. St Mary's Hospital NHS Trust Archives

making jokes. If they liked a nurse, they would greet her with a chorus of "Bottle please, nurse," instead of "Good morning," so long as Sister wasn't around to scold.[44] As a class, these patients were vulnerable and disempowered. Nonetheless, on the wards they couldn't be treated impersonally but remained as idiosyncratic as all the other denizens of St Mary's. They demanded treatment on their own terms and often received it. Relationships in the hospital were thus never wholly medicalized; they remained irreducibly social.

One former student at St Mary's who was hospitalized in the early 1950s was amused by the spectacle of competitive "patientmanship." During the exam season when students prowled the wards in packs, one such group made for the bed opposite the observer's.

A sharp faced, lean customer occupied it. They grouped themselves round him and one of them said something I could not catch. The effect was electric. In a trice he had tossed off the blankets, exposed himself, bared a leg which was decorated with a bandage, and was proceeding to demonstrate himself with an energy, enjoyment and lack of reserve which drew my interest. I think his audience asked a "question" or so; at any rate, whether they did so or no, they were entertained to a lecture lasting some fifteen minutes on his symptoms and history, from youth onwards. I can't tell you much about his condition, except that I heard him say he had, among other troubles, a swollen testicle. His audience politely examined him, listened, felt and observed. Finally, they thanked him and left. After they had gone, he lay back for a moment resting, as well he might. He then slowly pulled his clothing together and gathered the blankets round him. And then, turning to the ward at large, he said: –"Ah well! Yer just 'ave to 'umour them – just like children they are!"[45]

Patients could bring a cheerful stoicism to the hospital. Geoffrey Rose was fascinated by one of his early cases, seen when he was a registrar in Pickering's medical unit. In 1956 Rose admitted a sixty-three-year-old man who had spent a varied life, working as a collier, kitchen porter, usher, cleaner, barman, porter, and a knacker's yard attendant. "His summers were commonly spent 'on the road'; his preference was to winter in hospital." For nearly fifty years the man had rarely drunk less than ten pints of beer each day. Early in May 1956 he came to St Mary's by bus after he began vomiting vast quantities of blood, which the unit replaced by transfusion. In two weeks he received fifty-three pints of blood. Throughout the ordeal his general condition remained "remarkably good," and when asked how he felt, he always replied, "Champion." The surgeons tried to locate the bleeding, investigating first the oesophagus and then the stomach. "Of the pleasures which life affords, few can better the removal of an oesophagoscope; and of its disappointments, can any exceed the replacement of an oesophagoscope by a gastroscope? Mr. H., however, bore it all with much fortitude, and continued to feel 'champion.'" The physicians decided not to send the man for surgery – operative mortality was high for those with massive bleeding – so they continued with the transfusions, adding streptomycin, and they stopped feeding him by mouth. Under this regime the perforated ulcer finally healed itself and soon the man was on the road again, with an invitation to return that winter for a partial gastrectomy.[46]

There were many other patients to whom St Mary's became a temporary home at certain seasons. Jenny Large, Sister Manvers, recalls the

old favourites who would turn up at Christmas time and come in for a bed. And I used to have two or three old boys on Manvers that would turn up, and one of them used to have a varicose ulcer on his leg, and he would turn up into Casualty, on Christmas Eve, like a prayer every year, having scratched this until it bled. And then he'd say, "Ring Manvers, and speak to Sister Large, she knows about my poorly leg. It always gets bad in the winter, and I usually come in for two or three days." And they'd ring me up and say, "It's old so and so." And I'd say, "Oh yeah, send him up," because you could do those sorts of things in those days. And he would get admitted for two or three days while we dressed this ulcer, that didn't really need it anyway. And he would unpack his little suitcase, and he'd still have his pyjamas there from the previous year, with the tinsel all round the neck, you see, ready for Christmas. And he'd say, "Do they still come carol singing in the evening? And do we still get sherry and brandy, and Guinness?" "Yes!" And he'd stay, he'd have his Christmas meal on Christmas Day, and then he'd finish all the bits of niceties up on Boxing Day, and then he'd go home, "Thank you very much," and you'd never see him again until the next Christmas!

Large concludes with an exclamation, "But that doesn't happen any more, I'm sure!"[47]

Patients negotiated their status and their use of the hospital with its staff in a dialogue rather than a monologue. They could draw upon a common culture, and they could band together in self protection in their dealings with the officialdom that St Mary's represented. As a houseman at Paddington General in the 1960s, Jeremy Carless had a lesson in this culture of solidarity when he listened to a group of Irishmen, treated for stab wounds, confound a police officer with an elaborate explanation as to how they had all tripped onto their "kirks."

The introduction of middle-class patients ruptured this easy ward culture. Rose Anderson, an orphan who began nursing at St Mary's in 1919 shortly before a means test was introduced, said, "I was astounded at the catty behaviour of some of the better-offs. They constantly demanded everything immediately, and were always complaining about something." Two paying patients demanded to share the chicken diet given to a seriously ill woman on the ward and so distressed the non-paying patient that she died, according to Anderson, whom the two reported for rudeness.[48] The creation of the Lindo Wing separated the wealthy from the rest, while the introduction of the NHS restored equality of condition to patients on the public wards. The Lindo Wing continues to attract some of the wealthiest people in the world. George Pinker, obstetrician at St Mary's, was also consultant obstetrician to the royal family, and at his insistence the royal princes William and Harry were born in the Lindo Wing, the first royal births in a public hospital.

Relations between patients and doctors or nurses at St Mary's continue to be mediated by lay volunteers, and there remains considerable scope for philanthropic work. Until 1974 the governing body combined medical staff and "public" men and women: people with public offices or prominent in business. The most eminent governors were city bankers. Some of the illustrious banking families who have supported St Mary's include Ernst Cassell and Baron Revelstoke of Barings (both donors), Viscount Bearsted of M. Samuel & Co. (a board member, 1956–74), Henry Sporborg of Hambros (chairman of the board from 1964 and a generous benefactor to the hospital), and the Rothschild family.

The relationship between St Mary's and the Rothschilds began in 1891, when Alfred de Rothschild, a member of the banking firm N.M. de Rothschild and the first Jewish director of the Bank of England,[49] was named a life governor. In 1893 he became treasurer to St Mary's and donated or secured tens of thousands of pounds for the hospital. He told his fellow governors that it was the egalitarianism of the hospital that most appealed to him: "Ever since my earliest days I have felt that no form of charity appeals so entirely to one's sympathies as the London Hospitals, for they distribute amongst the poor and the needy, spontaneously & without remuneration, the same treatment, the same luxuries, and if necessary the same dainties, as are within the reach of the wealthy, when it is they who are stricken down by disease or accident."[50] Though expressed in Victorian language, this is Lear's cry, "O! reason not the need. Our basest beggars are in the poorest thing superfluous. Allow not nature more than nature needs, Man's life is cheap as beast's." When Alfred de Rothschild died in 1917, his nephew Anthony replaced him as treasurer (but only after being reassured that the office was not a taxing one). Anthony, who inherited the family firm, served as chairman of the governing board from 1944 to 1957, and four years later he died in the Lindo Wing.

Not all of the supporters of St Mary's are rich or famous: people of all rank have involved themselves from one end of the hospital's history to the other. A series of associations have existed to help the hospital by making clothing for patients or raising money for other extras such as flowers. At first there was a St Mary's Aid Society, which in 1906 became the St Mary's Hospital Ladies Association. This was primarily run by the wives of the hospital consultants. To join, one had to pay a small subscription and make two items of clothing. During the 1920s flower stalls and children's tea parties were held. In 1927 the Ladies Association organized a ball that brought in £1,219, and they also donated three hundred linen sheets, three hundred twill sheets, three hundred pillow cases, and other items that they had made. In 1945 the association raised £695 from subscriptions and donations and made up over 13,400 garments and 24,000 surgical dressings. In 1953 it held a tombola to raise £1,500 and equipped every bed with a radio receiver.

Fifteen years into the NHS, the Ladies Association, presided over by Lady Moran, was still flourishing, with 230 members and more than £10,000 raised during those fifteen years. They ran a trolley service to sell sweets, stationery, and cosmetics, and by means of jumble sales, wine and cheese parties, and a dress show had provided curtains for cubicles, electric fans, and other amenities.[51] In 1974 they became the Friends of St Mary's, and in 1985, four hundred strong, the Friends spent £26,000 on gifts and equipment, raised at the flower and sweet shops and an annual bazaar.

Intermediaries like the Friends try to make life better for the patients. The government has also tried to empower patients by insisting on their rights. A patient's charter sets limits to, for example, waiting times. If patients don't like the service, they can complain to the hospital or demand an independent review by the NHS. The complaints system has become a bureaucracy all its own: in 1997–98, the hospital heard 989 complaints and ten requests for an independent review. Medical errors occur, as they always have done and always will do. In July 1999 a settlement of £2.5 million was reached in a case where a delivery went wrong, resulting in cerebral palsy. Sometimes St Mary's is censured, as in the case of a man brought in dead who was cremated before his family learned of the death. Sometimes the investigation identifies larger problems. In 1997 one young man tragically slipped between the cracks of the welfare system: he suffered from mental disorder and refused his medication, but he could appear entirely rational on examination. After one violent episode landed him at Harrow Road police station, St Mary's psychiatrists recommended the man be compulsorily committed for in-patient care, but the court psychiatrists disagreed and the man was released. The psychiatric team at St Mary's wasn't told of his release and, troubled by "staffing difficulties and high workload pressures," it did not follow up his case. The man's condition deteriorated, and he fatally stabbed a policewoman. An inquiry exonerated St Mary's but had stern recommendations for the Health Authority welfare officers.[52]

Of all the forces that shape the patient's experience of St Mary's, that of "high workload pressures" is foremost. The hospital now sees ten times as many in-patients each year as it did a century ago, and five times as many out-patients, while tens of thousands more patients come in for day surgery, where once they might have stayed a week. It took nearly fifty years to see the first million patients at St Mary's; now it takes only three to four years. Under these circumstances the sense of "community" experienced by patients and carers must be thin indeed. This atomization is increased by the large-team approach to clinical care: as one consultant observed, in a hospital the consultant may be the 375th person to see the patient.

It was very different a few decades ago. Patients might stay for months and even years, even when there was no clear medical need, but rather a human need for familiar and friendly faces. When June Opie was admitted with polio in the late 1940s, her situation rapidly became so serious that she could move nothing but her eyelid, and only the newly introduced iron lung saved her life. The doctors and nurses had never seen anyone so badly stricken, and it seemed something of a miracle when she began to recover. Opie had only just arrived in London from New Zealand, so she had nowhere else to go and few friends. She stayed at St Mary's for nearly three years, slowly learning to use her body again. Though an orthopaedic case, she lived in a medical ward at her own insistence, so that she could be near the ward sister she first saw on admission and whom she felt she needed.

Opie wrote a book about her time at St Mary's, which she described as a happy and entertaining place. Entertainment might take the form of watching the senior physician slip on the polished floor and "make a three point landing under a patient's bed" or the annual Christmas pageant when the students performed an uproarious "*danse des arbres*," which was a "whirl of tipsy branches." But above all it was the banter on the wards that she recollected most vividly, a banter that helped to make light of her dreadful illness. When a plaster cast was made of the front of her body, the students and nurses were so amused by its curves that they all tried it on, sauntering around the ward, and a house surgeon painted a bikini on it. One medical student, visiting her late at night, dived under the bed to escape the night sister on her round, and then couldn't prise himself out of the cast stored there. Another encounter between Opie and one of her doctors also conveys the irreverent atmosphere:

"June, can you lift your head yet?"

I shut my eyes, clenched my teeth, and endeavoured to set some machinery going inside my brain that would make my neck take the weight of my head. But there was nothing except a grunt of unrewarded effort. I opened my eyes. "I tried."

"You don't need to tell me."

"Why? Did you see something move?"

"No. But you look just like a choking chicken."[53]

It takes time for relationships to develop that permit this sort of teasing. And yet, somehow, these human relations must be maintained. They are the guarantee that healing will remain subsidiary to humanity, that the tail will not wag the dog.[54] If the medical encounter becomes so streamlined that patients become mere objects for medical knowledge and practice and doctors and nurses are merely purveyors of that knowledge and practice, then the hospital will not serve social cohesion but will teach people, doctors, nurses, patients, and lay workers to meet as Eliot's "committee members," and as self-absorbed members at that. That would end a very long tradition of medicine and of sociability which has been seen in Paddington almost since people first began to live there.

Abbreviations

A & E	Accident and Emergency Department (formerly Casualty Ward)
AHA	Area Health Authority
BJVD	*British Journal of Venereal Disease*
BMA	British Medical Association
BMJ	*British Medical Journal*
BSE	Bovine Spongiform Encephaly
CJD	Creutzfeld-Jacob Disease
CMAC	Contemporary Medical Archives Collection at the Wellcome Library for the History and Understanding of Medicine
CMO	Chief Medical Officer
COS	Charity Organisation Society
DHSS	Department of Health and Social Services
DSO	Distinguished Service Order
ECG	Electrocardiograph
FRCP	Fellow of the Royal College of Physicians of London
FRCS	Fellow of the Royal College of Surgeons of England
FRS	Fellow of the Royal Society
GMC	General Medical Council
GNC	General Nursing Council
JHM	*Journal of the History of Medicine and Allied Sciences*
JMAC	Joint Medical Advisory Committee (of the University of London)
LCC	London County Council
LMA	London Metropolitan Archives
MOH	Medical Officer of Health
MRC	Medical Research Council

MRCP   Member of the Royal College of Physicians of London
MSC   Medical School Committee of St Mary's Hospital Medical School
NHS   National Health Service
OPD   Out-Patient Department
PRO   Public Record Office
RAE   Research Assessment Exercise
RAMC   Royal Army Medical Corps
RAWP   Resource Allocation Working Party
RCP   Royal College of Physicians of London
RCS   Royal College of Surgeons of England
RHB   Regional Hospital Board
RMO   Resident Medical Officer
RPMS   Royal Post-Graduate Medical School
SMHA   St Mary's Hospital NHS Trust Archives
SMHG   *St Mary's Hospital Gazette*
UCCA   University Central Council on Admissions
       (now the UCAS: University and Colleges Admissions Scheme)
UCH   University College Hospital
UCL   University College London
       (including University College Hospital Medical School)
UGC   University Grants Committee
VCJD   New Variant Creutzfeld-Jacob Disease
WA   Westminster Archives
WFI   Wright-Fleming Institute

Notes

Introduction

1 On the Crystal Palace, Jeffrey Auerbach, *The Great Exhibition of 1851: A Nation on Display* (New Haven: Yale University Press, 1999); also the discussion in E.A. Heaman, *The Inglorious Arts of Peace: Exhibitions in Canadian Society during the Nineteenth Century* (Toronto: University of Toronto Press, 1999).

2 Susan C. Lawrence, *Charitable Knowledge: Hospitals, Pupils, and Practitioners in 18th-Century London* (Cambridge: Cambridge University Press, 1996).

3 Quoted in W.F. Bynum, *Science and the Practice of Medicine in the Nineteenth Century* (Cambridge: Cambridge University Press, 1994), 105.

4 Leading social historians of mid-Victorian medicine have pointed out that the history of "medico-scientific activities" has yet to be written: see Jean M. Peterson, *The Medical Profession in Mid-Victorian London* (Berkeley: University of California Press, 1978), 172; Irvine Loudon, *Medical Care and the General Practitioner, 1750–1850* (Oxford: Clarendon, 1986), 281.

5 Some more probing histories of medical schools outside London have recently been written: Mark Weatherall, *Gentlemen, Scientists and Doctors: Medicine at Cambridge, 1800–1940* (Cambridge: Cambridge University Press, 2000); Jack Morell, *Science at Oxford: Transforming an Arts University* (Oxford: Clarendon Press, 1997); see also Lindsay Granshaw, *St Mark's Hospital: A Social History of a Specialist Hospital* (London: King Edward's Fund, 1985). As well, Steven Sturdy, Michael Barfoot, Christopher Lawrence, and Andrew Hull are producing studies of Scottish medical institutions.

6 Zachary Cope, *The History of St. Mary's Hospital Medical School, or A Century of Medical Education* (London: Heinemann, 1954).

7 For example, R.J. Minney, *The Two Pillars of Charing Cross: The Story of a Famous Hospital* (London: Cassell, 1967); W.R. Merrington, *University College Hospital and Its Medical School: A History* (London: Heinemann, 1976); Douglas Ranger, *The Middlesex Hospital Medical School: Centenary to Sesquicentenary, 1935–1985* (London: Hutchinson Benham, 1985) (the sequel to H. Campbell Thomson, *The Story of the Middlesex Hospital Medical School* (London: John Murray, 1935); A.E. Clark-Kennedy, *The London: A Study in the Voluntary Hospital System* (London: Pitman, 1962); Charles Cameron, *Mr Guy's Hospital* (London: Longman's, 1954); Lindsay Granshaw, "St Thomas's Hospital, 1850–1900," (PhD thesis, Bryn Mawr, 1981).

Chapter One

1 Roy Porter, *The Greatest Benefit to Humanity: A Medical History of Humanity from Antiquity to the Present* (London: HarperCollins, 1997), 198; David Owen, *English Philanthropy, 1660–1960* (Cambridge, Mass.: Belknap Press, 1965). Other studies include Günter B. Risse, *Hospital Life in Enlightenment Scotland: Care and Teaching at the Royal Infirmary of Edinburgh* (Cambridge: Cambridge University Press, 1986); John V. Pickstone, who observes that "Voluntary hospitals were, pre-eminently, community institutions," in *Medicine and Industrial Society: A History of Hospital Development in Manchester and Its Region, 1752–1946* (Manchester: Manchester University Press, 1985); Mary E. Fissell, *Patients, Power and the Poor in Eighteenth-Century Bristol* (Cambridge: Cambridge University Press, 1991); Hilary Marland, *Medicine and Society in Wakefield and Huddersfield, 1780–1870* (Cambridge: Cambridge University Press, 1987).

2 F.H. Davies, *Paddington in 1665, the Year of the Great Plague* (London: J. Morton, 1874).

3 William Robins, *Paddington Past and Present* (London: Caxton, [1853]), 132.

4 *Bayswater Chronicle*, 29 November 1900.

5 V.A.C. Gattrell, *The Hanging Tree: Execution and the English People, 1770–1868* (Oxford: Oxford University Press, 1994).

6 Augustus Cove, *The Tocsin Sounded* (London: M. Jones, 1813; 2nd ed.); see Stanley A. Holland, "Augustus Cove and the Grand Junction Canal Company," *The Journal of the Friends Historical Society* 58 (1997): 37–43.

7 Alan H. Faulkner, *The Grand Junction Canal* (Newton Abbot: David & Charles, 1972), 80; John Hassell (ed. John Cranfield), *A Tour of the Grand Junction Canal in 1819* (London: Cranfield & Bonfiel, 1968).

8 Jack Simmons, *The Victorian Railway* (London: Thomas & Hudson, 1991), 39.

9 Robins, *Paddington: Past and Present*, 195.

10 Peter Thorold, *The London Rich: The Creation of a Great City from 1666 to the Present* (London: Viking, 1999), 202.

11 Graily Hewitt, *The Sanitary Condition of Paddington* (London: John Churchill, 1856).

12 The sale list is held at the British Library.

13 Loftus Slade, *Paddington As It Was and As It Is* (London: West End Printing Works, 1877).

14 Westminster Archives (WA), PV239, meeting, 1 May 1820.

15 WA, PV239, meetings, 20 and 27 July 1820.

16 This board of guardians preceded the more formal body created by the Poor Law of 1834. It was named specifically to assist the overseers in providing (and denying) relief. The Select Vestry Minutes and the papers of this board of guardians are held at the Westminster Archives. The papers of the board of guardians formed under the Poor Law are held at the London Metropolitan Archives (hereafter LMA).

17 Parish of Paddington, *Cash Account for the Year Ending April 1833* (London: William Davy, 1833), 17.

18 P.F. Aschrott, *The English Poor Law System, Past and Present* (London: Knight & Co., 1902); William C. Lubenow, *The Politics of Government Growth: Early Victorian Attitudes towards State Intervention, 1833–1848* (Newton Abbot: Archon Books, 1971), 48.

19 The figures are not quite accurate because food and clothing given to outdoor paupers were billed to the workhouse account; this would have helped to account for the savings in the workhouse expenditure. Parish of Paddington, *Cash Account for the Year Ending April 1833* (London: William Davy, 1833), and subsequent volumes.

20 LMA, K BG, Kensington Board of Guardians, 1, 98.

21 WA, PV, 238, 77–8.

22 Norah H. Schuster, *The Western General Dispensary, St Marylebone* (London: St Marylebone Society, 1961).

23 The records of the workhouse are at LMA, PA BG, Paddington Board of Guardians.

24 Robins, *Paddington Past and Present*, 156.

25 LMA, PA BG 002, 258–9.

26 Hewitt, *The Sanitary Condition of Paddington*.

27 *Drainage and Sewerage* (London: John Churchill, 1847). The association's treasurer was Joseph Toynbee, future aural surgeon to St Mary's and aspiring medical officer of health.

28 Third Earl Fortesque, *To the Representative Vestries of Marylebone, St Pancras, and Paddington* (n.p., 1858).

29 J. Burdon Sanderson, *Paddington, Sanitary Report for the Year 1856* (n.p., n.d.), 11.

30 Charles Murchison, "Contributions to the Etiology of Continued Fever," *Medico-Chirurgical Transactions*, n.s. 23 (1858): 273–4.

31 *An Address on the Necessity for a New Hospital in the North-Western Quarter of the Metropolis* (London: n.p., 1842).

32 Hewitt, *The Sanitary Condition of Paddington*, 35.

33 Martin J. Wiener, *Reconstructing the Criminal: Culture, Law, and Policy in England, 1830–1914* (Cambridge: University Press, 1990), 19. See also Mitchell Dean, *The Constitution of Poverty: Toward a Genealogy of Liberal Governance* (London: Routledge, 1991).

34 Joachim Schlor, *Nights in the Big City*, trans. P.G. Imhof and D.R. Roberts (London: Reaktion, 1998), 47.

35 *The Paddington Tragedy: A Circumstantial Narrative of the Lives and Trial of James Greenacre, & The Woman Gale, for the Murder of Mrs. Hannah Brown, His Intended Wife* (London: Orlando Hodgson, [1836]).

36 Robins, *Paddington Past and Present*, 170.

37 Ibid., 68.

38 Charman Edwards, *Tall Pines in Paddington* (London: Ward, Lock & Co., 1949), 7. He continues: "Paddington an idea! And when a man girds up his loins and is amove with the restlessness in him, by what physical bounds shall his idea be limited?"

39 T.T. Carter, *Richard Temple West, A Record of His Life and Work* (London: John Masters, 1895), 112. He was describing the 1860s.

40 In Wiener, *Reconstructing the Criminal*, 31.

41 Marshall Tweddell, *Fourteen Years in a London Parish: A Memoir of St. Saviour's Paddington* (London: Burt & Sons, 1897), 28–9.

42 Parent Duchâtelet's treatise appears in the inventory of books of James Beatty, the railway engineer.

43 William Acton, *Prostitution Considered in Its Moral, Social & Sanitary Aspects, in London and Other Large Cities* (London: John Churchill, 1857), 16.

44 William J.E. Bennett, *A Sermon, Preached at the Opening of the Temporary Chapel, Preparatory to the Building of the Church of S. Mary Magdalene, Paddington on February 14th 1865* (London: J.T. Hayes, 1865), 5.

45 *An Address on the Necessity for a New Hospital.*

46 *Bayswater Chronicle*, 2 January 1864.

47 Society for the Promotion of Christian Knowledge, *Original Family Sermons* (London: John W. Parker, 1833) 5, 115–6. See Richard Allen Soloway, *Prelates and People: Ecclesiastical Social Thought in England, 1783–1852*

(London: Routledge & Kegan Paul, 1969).

48 Gertrude Toynbee, ed., *Reminiscences and Letters of Joseph and Arnold Toynbee* (London: Henry J. Glaisher, n.d.), 38–9.

49 J. Hassell, *Memoirs of the Life of the Late George Morland* (London: James Cundell, 1806).

50 [Augustus Cove], *Thomas Payne Defended & Completely Justified; or, A Reprimand for the Grand Junction Canal Company* (London: Barton & Harvey, 1809). A copy held by the British Library has Cove's handwritten notes in the margin, claiming authorship and recording Payne's death.

51 Association for the Improvement of London Workhouses, *The Management of the Infirmaries of the Strand Union, the Rotherhithe and the Paddington Workhouses* (London: For the Association, 1867), 47.

52 Ruth G. Hodgkinson, *The Origins of the National Health Service: The Medical Services of the New Poor Law, 1834–1871* (London: Wellcome Historical Medical Library, 1967).

53 Ibid., 275.

54 Weiner, *Reconstructing the Criminal*, 49.

55 Edward Sieveking, "On Dispensaries and Allied Institutions," in F.D. Maurice, ed., *Lectures to Ladies on Practical Subjects* (Cambridge: Macmillan, 1857; 3rd ed.), 97–8.

56 *An Address on the Necessity for a New Hospital*, 8.

57 Gareth Stedman Jones, *Outcast London: A Study in the Relationship between the Classes in Victorian Society* (Harmondsworth: Penguin, 1984), 249–50.

58 Virginia Berridge, "Health and Medicine," in F.M.L. Thompson, ed., *Cambridge Social History of Britain* (Cambridge: Cambridge University Press, 1990), 204; and see the article by Frank Prochaska, "Philanthropy," in the same collection. 356–93.

59 *Lancet* (1858) 2: 13–14.

60 Ibid., (1856) 2: 203–4.

61 J.H. Gurney, *An Address to the Inhabitants of St Mary's District, Marylebone* (n.p., 1852), 22–3.

62 G. Elliott, *Sermons on the Charitable Institutions of the District of Trinity, Marylebone* (London: James Darling, 1847), 21–2.

63 *Report from the Select Committee of the House of Lords on Metropolitan Hospitals, &c.* (London: Hansard, 1890), 140. See also Zachary Cope, *The History of St Mary's Hospital Medical School, or, A Century of Medical Education* (Toronto: Heinemann, 1954), and R.R. James, *The School of Anatomy and Medicine adjoining St George's Hospital, 1830–1863* (London: George Pulman & Son, 1928).

64 Roy Porter, *London: A Social History* (Harmondsworth: Penguin, 1994), 212.

65 *Times*, 27 March 1843; *An Address on the Necessity for a New Hospital*; St Mary's Hospital NHS Trust Archives (SMHA), SM AD 1/1, 21–31.

66 Roger Fulford, *Royal Dukes: Queen Victoria's Father and "Wicked Uncles"* (1933; reprint, London: Pan Books, 1948), 317; Frank Prochaska, *Royal Bounty: The Making of a Welfare Monarchy* (New Haven: Yale University Press, 1995), 25.

67 Charles E. Rosenberg, "'Inward Vision and Outward Glance': The Shaping of the American Hospital, 1880–1914," *Bulletin of the History of Medicine* 53 (1979): 485–506.

68 St Mary's Hospital, *Annual Report* 1 (1852), 42–3.

69 SMHA, SM AD 1/6, 396–7.

70 Karel Williams, *From Pauperism to Poverty* (London: Routledge, 1981), 132–5.

71 Harold Perkin, *The Rise of Professional Society: England since 1880* (London: Routledge, 1989). Morris Vogel has remarked of American hospitals in this period that they were "undifferentiated welfare institutions" with little medical about them. See "The Transformation of the American Hospital, 1850–1920," in Susan Reverby and David Rosner, eds., *Health Care in America: Essays in Social History* (Philadelphia: Temple University Press, 1979), 105.

72 Stefan Collini, *Public Moralists: Political Thought and Intellectual Life in Britain* (Oxford: Clarendon Press, 1991).

73 SMHA, SM AD 1/1, 150, 170.

74 Cited in Brian Abel-Smith, *The Hospitals, 1800–1948: A Study in Social Administration in England and Wales* (London: Heinemann, 1964).

75 The term comes from Charles E. Rosenberg, "Florence Nightingale on Contagion: The Hospital As Moral Universe," in Charles Rosenberg, *Explaining Epidemics and Other Studies in the History of Medicine* (Cambridge: Cambridge University Press, 1992).

76 SMHA, SM AD 1/1, 166–7.

77 *Bayswater Chronicle*, 12 June 1875.

78 SMHA, SM AD 1/2, 78–9.

79 SMHA, SM AD 1/2, 349–53.

80 *Lancet* (1851) 2: 60–1.

81 The soup kitchen was connected with the church rather than the hospital, although the governors supported it with a subscription.

82 *BMJ* (1859), 1047.

83 *Lancet* (1958) 1: 166.

84 *SMHG* 8 (1902): 153–6 and 9 (1903), 2–6.

85 *BMJ* (1873) 2: 157.

86 Ibid., (1869) 2: 389–90.

87 Surgeon Walter Pye, addressing the incoming students, *BMJ* (1880) 2: 584–5.

88 *St. Mary's Hospital, Extracts from Speeches Made at a Public Meeting Held in the Vestry Hall, Paddington, on Wednesday, December 11, 1861* (London: John Elliot, n.d.).

89 T.K. Chambers, *The Renewal of Life* (London: John Churchill, 1862), 21.

90 SMHA, SM AD 1/7, 545.

91 Ibid., SM AD 1/3, 148.

92 Ibid., SM AD 1/7, 117–18.

93 *SMHG* 6 (1900): 11–12 and 8 (1902): 153–6.

94 Ibid.

95 *SMHG* 3 (1897): 82.

96 SMHA, SM AD 1/3, 522–3.

97 Ibid., 1/4, 153–5.

98 *SMHG* 3 (1897): 81–3.

99 Jean M. Peterson, *The Medical Profession in Mid-Victorian London* (Berkeley: University of California Press, 1978).

100 SMHA, SM AD 1/8, 547–8.

101 Donald Winch, *Adam Smith's Politics: An Essay in Historiographic Revision* (Cambridge: Cambridge University Press, 1978); J.W. Burrow, *Whigs and Liberals: Continuity and Change in English Political Thought* (Oxford: Clarendon Press, 1988), 38.

Chapter Two

1 *A Manifesto by the Medical and Surgical Association of the Borough of Marylebone* (London, n.p., 1844).

2 S.E.D. Shortt, "Physicians, Science, and Status: Issues in the Professionalization of Anglo-American Medicine in the Nineteenth Century," *Medical History* 27 (1983): 63.

3 Ivan Waddington, *The Medical Profession in the Industrial Revolution* (Dublin: Gill & Macmillan, 1984), 19.

4 Geoffrey Rivett, *The Development of the London Hospital System, 1823–1982* (London: King's Fund, 1986), 35.

5 Adrian Desmond, *The Politics of Evolution: Morphology, Medicine, and Reform in Radical London* (Chicago: Chicago University Press, 1989), 112; Jean M. Peterson, *The Medical Profession in Mid-Victorian London* (Berkeley: University of California Press, 1978), 141–2.

6 Richard Drayton, *Nature's Government: Science, Imperial Britain, and the Improvement of the World* (New Haven: Yale University Press, 2000), 132, 197.

7 Edwin Lee, *Hospital Elections and Medical Reform* (London; John Churchill, 1848), 2–3.

8   On the Royal Society, see Dwight Atkinson, *Scientific Discourse in Sociohistorical Context: The Philosophical Transactions of the Royal Society of London, 1675–1975* (New Jersey: Lawrence Goldbaum, 1999).

9   *Testimonials Submitted to a Committee of the Governors of St. Mary's Hospital by John Rose Cormack*, MD FRSE, FRCP *Edinburgh* (n.p., December 1850); bound in the *Aberdeen Tracts*, vol. 10, no. 14, at the Wellcome Library for the History of Medicine. Also *Lancet* (1845) 2: 489–91, 515–7. Cormack was prohibited from taking students on the wards, and he criticized the governors' lack of support for scholarly activity.

10 Lorraine Daston, "Baconian Facts, Academic Civility, and the Prehistory of Objectivity," in Allan Megill, ed., *Rethinking Objectivity* (Durham: Duke University Press, 1994), 37–64; Steven Shapin, *A Social History of Truth: Civility and Science in Seventeenth-Century England* (Chicago: University of Chicago Press, 1995).

11 See the discussion in W.J. Reader, *Professional Men: The Rise of the Professional Classes in Nineteenth-Century England* (London: Weidenfeld & Nicolson, 1966).

12 *Lancet* (1857) 2: 10.

13 *Lancet* (1845) 2: 76.

14 *Lancet* (1853) 1: 1–3.

15 Recent history of societies is scanty but see Jacqueline Jenkinson, *Scottish Medical Societies 1731–1837: Their History and Record* (Edinburgh: Edinburgh University Press, 1993).

16 W.F. Bynum and Janice C. Wilson, "Periodical Knowledge: Medical Journals and Their Editors in Nineteenth-Century Britain," in W.F. Bynum, Stephen Lock, and Roy Porter, eds., *Medical Journals and Medical Knowledge: Historical Essays* (London: Routledge, 1992), 30. See also the other articles in the collection, especially Jean Loudon and Irvine Loudon, "Medicine, Politics, and the Medical Periodical, 1800–1850," 49–69, and Peter Bartrip, "The British Medical Journal: A Retrospect," 126–45.

17 Peter Bartrip, *Themselves Writ Large: The British Medical Association, 1832–1966* (London: BMJ, 1996), 12. See also his *Mirror of Medicine: A History of the British Medical Journal* (Oxford: Clarendon and BMJ, 1990).

18 Norman Moore and Stephen Paget, *The Royal Medical and Chirurgical Society of London Centenary, 1805–1905* (1905), 97.

19 *Lancet* (1860) 2: 334–5.

20 The phrase in quotation marks is from Benedict Anderson, *Imagined Communities: Reflections on the Origins and Spread of Nationalism* (London: Verso, 1991).

21 Sir Morrell Mackenzie told the Select Committee of the House of Lords that St Mary's was founded by doctors, with the help of benevolent lay persons.

See *Report from the Select Committee of the House of Lords on Metropolitan Hospitals, &c.* (London: Hansard, 1890), 140. See also Cope, *The History of St Mary's Hospital Medical School* (London: Heinemann, 1954), and R.R. James, *The School of Anatomy and Medicine adjoining St George's Hospital, 1830–1863* (London: George Pulman & Sons, 1978).

22 *SMHG* 10 (1904): 78.

23 *Lancet* (1861) 2: 265.

24 Lindsay Granshaw, "'Fame and Fortune by Means of Bricks and Mortar': Specialist Hospitals in Britain, 1800–1948," in Lindsay Granshaw and Roy Porter, eds., *The Hospital in History* (London: Routledge, 1989): 199–220.

25 SMHA, SM AD 1/8, 375–6.

26 Royal College of Physicians of London, Thomas Buzzard papers, letter to Gowers, 6 December 1905.

27 *Lancet* (1847) 1: 385.

28 *Dictionary of National Biography* (London: Oxford University Press, various dates), passim.

29 *SMHG* 10 (1904), 79.

30 *Lancet* (1882) 2: 510.

31 *SMHG* 9 (1903), 2–6.

32 W.M. Ord, ed., *Collected Works of Francis Sibson* (London; Macmillan, 1881).

33 Bodleian Library, University of Oxford MS Acland d63; John Burdon Sanderson papers MS AD 179 at University College London Archives. See A.H.T. Robb-Smith, "Medical Education," in M.G. Brock and M.C. Curthays, eds., *History of the University of Oxford in the Nineteenth Century* (Oxford: Clarendon Press, 1997), vol 1, 563–82.

34 R. Scott Stevenson and Douglas Guthrie, *A History of Oto-Laryngology* (Edinburgh: E & S Livingstone, 1949), 65–7.

35 *Lancet* (1857) 2: 614. "His colleagues told him 'he must be clearly understood to be solely responsible for the results. They – i.e., the surgical staff – washed their hands of ovariotomy.'"

36 Ornella Moscucci, *The Science of Woman: Gynaecology and Gender in England, 1800–1929* (Cambridge: Cambridge University Press, 1990), 171–2.

37 *BMJ* (1859): 15–17. On Marshall Hall, see Diana E. Manuel, *Marshall Hall (1790–1837): Science and Medicine in Early Victorian Society* (Amsterdam: Rodopi, 1996).

38 *Lancet* (1859) 1: 581–8.

39 *Lancet* (1857) 2: 624–6.

40 Baker Brown, *On the Curability of Certain Forms of Insanity, Epilepsy, Catalepsy, and Hysteria in Females* (London: Robert Hardwicke, 1866).

41 *Lancet* (1867) 1: 434 and passim.

42 *A Manifesto by the Medical and Surgical Association of the Borough of Marylebone*, 5–6.

43 See, for example, the somewhat antediluvian defence of this position in Allan Bloom, *Love and Friendship* (New York: Simon & Schuster, 1993).

44 *Lancet* (1850) 1: 659. On the debate and on Tyler Smith and modesty, see Ornella Moscucci, *The Science of Woman*, and Mary Poovey, "'Scenes of an Indelicate Character': The Medical Treatment of Victorian Women," in Catherine Gallagher and Thomas Lacqueur, *The Making of the Modern Body: Sexuality and Society in the Nineteenth Century* (Berkeley: University of California Press, 1987), 137–68. On Baker Brown, see also Ann Dally, *Women under the Knife: A History of Surgery* (London: Hutchinson, 1991).

45 *Lancet* (1850) 1: 595–7.

46 *Lancet* (1856) 1: 426–7.

47 *Lancet* (1856) 1: 30.

48 *Lancet* (1847) 1: 321–3.

49 The doctors could discuss genitalia without prurience, but they could offend sexual morality either by teaching the women themselves to speak about their genitalia or by permitting men like Baker Brown to trade on the fact that women could not speak about their genitalia.

50 George Weisz, *The Medical Mandarins: The French Academy of Medicine in the Nineteenth and Early Twentieth Centuries* (Oxford: Oxford University Press, 1995); John Harley Warner, *The Therapeutic Perspective: Medical Practice, Knowledge, and Identity in America, 1820–1885* (1986; reprint, Princeton: Princeton University Press, 1997).

51 John Harley Warner, *Against the Spirit of System: The French Impulse in Nineteenth-Century American Medicine* (Princeton: Princeton University Press, 1998), 251.

52 John V. Pickstone, *Ways of Knowing: A New History of Science, Technology and Medicine* (Manchester: Manchester University Press, 2000), 112.

53 On the distinction, see David Edgerton, ed., *Industrial Research and Innovation in Business* (Cheltenham: E. Elgar, 1996) and "From Innovation to Use: Ten Eclectic Theses on the Historiography of Technology," *History and Technology* 16 (1999): 111–36.

54 Thomas Kuhn, *The Structure of Scientific Revolutions* (Chicago: Chicago University Press, 1970; 2nd ed). Robert Anderson has argued that research only came to the Scottish universities in the late nineteenth century: see Anderson, "Ideas of the University in Nineteenth-Century Scotland, Theory versus Reality," in Martin Hewitt, ed., *Leeds Working Papers in Victorian Studies* 1 (1998): 1–13.

55 Quoted in A. McGehee Harvey, *Science at the Bedside: Clinical Research in American Medicine, 1905–1945* (Baltimore: Johns Hopkins University Press, 1981), xi.

56 This question is posed by Shapin, *The Scientific Revolution*, 4.

57 Robert Anderson, "Ideas of the University"; Joseph Ben-David, "Scientific Productivity and Academic Organization in Nineteenth-Century Medicine," *American Sociological Review* 25 (1960): 828–43; Arlene Marcia Tuchman, *Science, Medicine, and the State in Germany: The Case of Baden, 1815–1871*. (Oxford: Oxford University Press, 1993); see also the essays in Andrew Cunningham and Perry Williams, eds., *The Laboratory Revolution in Medicine* (Cambridge: Cambridge University Press, 1992).

58 *Lancet* (1860) 2: 185–6.

59 Miles Weatherall, "Drug Therapies," in W.F. Bynum and Roy Porter, eds., *Companion Encyclopedia of the History of Medicine* (London: Routledge, 1993), vol. 2, 921.

60 *Lancet* (1858) 2: 533–4, 562.

61 *BMJ* (1859) 1: 102–4, for example. On inhibition, see Roger Smith, *Inhibition: History and Meaning in the Sciences of Mind and Brain* (London: Free Association Books, 1992).

62 A. Forbes Sieveking, *In Memoriam: Sir Edward Henry Sieveking*, MD, LLD, FRCP, FSA (London: n.p., 1904).

63 Charles Handfield-Jones and Edward H. Sieveking, *A Manual of Pathological Anatomy* (London: John Churchill, 1854).

64 Royal College of Physicians of London, Papers of Sir Edward Sieveking.

65 Neville M. Goodman, "Medical Attendance on Royalty: The Diaries of Dr. Edward Sieveking," in F.N.L. Poynter, ed., *Medicine and Science in the 1860s* (London: WIHM, 1968): 127–36.

66 Reviewing the second edition of Markham's manual, *Lancet* (1860) 2: 139.

67 See Terrie Romano, "Making Medicine Scientific: John Burdon Sanderson and the Culture of Victorian Science" (PhD dissertation, Yale University, 1993).

68 Held at the National Library of Scotland.

69 A list of his papers, more than two hundred, is provided in Walter Broadbent, ed., *Selections from the Writings Medical and Neurological of Sir William Broadbent* (London: Henry Froude, 1908).

70 *SMHG* 5 (1899): 80–6.

71 Bodleian Library, University of Oxford, MS Acland d63, 6–10.

72 On different kinds of physiology and physiologists, see Stephen Jacyna, "Theory of Medicine, Science of Life: The Place of Physiology in the Edinburgh Medical Curriculum, 1790–1870," in Vivian Nutton and Roy Porter, eds., *The History of Medical Education in Britain* (Amsterdam: Rodopi, 1995), 141–52.

73 *Collected Works of Francis Sibson*, vol. 3, 255.

74 W.B. Cheadle, *On the Principles and Exact Conditions to Be Observed in the Artificial Feeding of Infants* (London: Smith, Elder & Co., 1889); see the

Cheadle papers at the Royal College of Physicians of London.

75 The examples are taken from Broadbent, *Selections from the Writings*.

76 M.E. Broadbent, *The Life of Sir William Broadbent* (London: John Murray, 1909).

77 *Selections from the Writings*, 219.

78 Christopher Lawrence, "Incommunicable Knowledge: Science, Technology and the Clinical Art in Britain, 1850–1914," *Journal of Contemporary History* 20 (1985): 503–20.

79 *SMHG* 13 (1907): 79–80.

80 *SMHG* 14 (1908): 13–14.

81 SMHA, SM AD 35/9, 51.

82 On Smith, see Carleton B. Chapman, "Edward Smith (?1818–1874), Physiologist, Human Ecologist, Reformer," *Journal of the History of Medicine and Allied Sciences* 22 (1967): 1–26.

83 *BMJ* (1857): 349–50; (1859): 600.

84 Jürgen Habermas, *The Structural Transformation of the Public Sphere: An Inquiry into a Category of Bourgeois Society* (Cambridge: MIT Press, 1989).

85 *BMJ* (1859): 600.

86 *Lancet* (1911) 1: 212.

87 *Final Report of the Royal Commission on University Education in London* (Parliamentary Papers, vol. 11, 1913). On neurology, see Edwin Clarke and L.S. Jacyna, *Nineteenth-Century Origins of Neuroscientific Concepts* (Berkeley: University of California Press, 1987).

Chapter Three

1 *Lancet* (1845) 2: 380.

2 LMA, PA BG 74/1, 430.

3 Thomas Neville Bonner, *Becoming a Physician: Medical Education in Britain, France, Germany and the United States, 1750–1945* (New York: Oxford University Press, 1995), 194. Other sources on English medical education include Charles Newman, *The Evolution of Medical Education in the Nineteenth Century* (London: Oxford University Press, 1957); Vivian Nutton and Roy Porter, eds., *The History of Medical Education in Britain* (Amsterdam: Rodopi, 1995); F.N.L. Poynter, *The Evolution of Medical Education in Britain* (London: Pitman, 1966). See also Zachary Cope, *The Royal College of Surgeons of England: A History* (London: Anthony Bled, 1959) and George Clarke, *A History of the Royal College of Physicians of London* (Oxford: Clarendon Press, 1964).

4 Edward S. Crisp, *The Examination of a Rejected Candidate at the Royal College of Physicians of London, December 21st 1848* (London: John Churchill, 1849).

5 *SMHG* 14 (1908): 68–73.

6 *SMHG* 46 (1935): 31–3.

7 SMHA, SM AD 1/5: 81–2.

8 J.B. Morrell, "The Chemist Breeders: The Research Schools of Liebig and Thomas Thomson," *Ambix* 21 (1972): 1–46 and, more generally, J.B. Morrell, *Science, Culture and Politics in Britain, 1780–1820* (Aldershot: Ashgate, 1997). See also David Knight and Helge Kragh, eds., *The Making of the Chemist: The Social History of Chemistry in Europe 1789–1914* (Cambridge: Cambridge University Press, 1998).

9 Russell Maulitz, *Morbid Appearances: The Anatomy of Pathology in the Early Nineteenth Century* (Cambridge: Cambridge University Press, 1987).

10 SMHA, SM AD 1/4, 461.

11 See Jacob W. Gruber, *A Conscience in Conflict: The Life of St George Jackson Mivart* (New York: Columbia University Press, 1960).

12 SMHA, SM AD 1/9, 253.

13 James Edgar Strick, "The British Spontaneous Generation Debates of 1860–1880: Medicine, Evolution, and Laboratory Science in the Victorian Context" (PhD dissertation, Princeton University, 1997), 95. Cope seems to have his dates wrong.

14 SMHA, MS AD 1/1, 92–5.

15 *SMHG* 3 (1897): 116–9. Shepherd is quoted in Paul K. Underhill, "Science, Professionalism, and the Development of Medical Education in England: An Historical Sociology" (PhD dissertation, University of Edinburgh, 1987), 494.

16 *SMHG* 5 (1899): 133–4.

17 SMHA, MS AD 1/1, 92–5.

18 *Lancet* (1851) 2: 319.

19 *SMHG* 17 (1911): 19–25.

20 SMHA, SM AD 1/13, 16–17.

21 *Past and Present League of Nurses Journal* 8 (1971): 22–7.

22 Ruth Richardson, *Death, Dissection, and the Destitute* (Harmondsworth: Penguin, 1988).

23 SMHA, SM AD 1/9, 434–5; MS AD 1/1, 405–6 and 544–6.

24 Robert Tyre, *Saddlebag Surgeon: The Story of Murrough O'Brien, M.D.* (Toronto: J.M. Dent, 1954).

25 SMHA, SM AD 1/14, 575–7 and 583–4. Lawson is invited to "see the necessity of relieving the School from a serious responsibility."

26 *SMGH* 16 (1910): 62.

27 SMHA, MS AD 1/3, 223.

28 SMHA, SM AD 2/1.

29 *SMHG* 15 (1909): 64–6.

30 *SMHG* 7 (1901): 83–5.

31 Tyre, *Saddlebag Surgeon*.

32 *SMHG* 14 (1908): 121.

33 *BMJ* (1878) 2: 522–3.

34 *SMHG* 9 (1903): 105.

35 *BMJ* (1871) 2: 409.

36 Zachary Cope, *History of St Mary's Hospital Medical School* (London: Heinemann, 1954).

37 *BMJ* (1873) 2: 484, for Owen's report. Page welcomed Lister to London and praised his work when he gave the inaugural lecture in 1877, but the *Lancet* edited out that portion of the speech. *Lancet* (1877) 2: 489–90; *BMJ* (1877) 2: 484. See Thomas Keller, "Railway Spine Revisited: Traumatic Neurosis or Neurotrauma?" *Journal of the History of Medicine* 50 (1995): 507–25, and Erich Michael Caplan, "Trains, Brains, and Sprains: Railway Spine and the Origins of Psychoneurosis," *Bulletin of the History of Medicine* 69 (1995): 387–419.

38 *SMHG* 7 (1901): 65–6.

39 *SMHG* 9 (1903): 154–5.

40 Maguire's failing is recorded in the margins of a copy of Cope, *The History of St Mary's Hospital Medical School* held by the Wellcome Library. It belonged to Sir Arthur MacNalty, who was Maguire's houseman at the Brompton and initialled the note.

41 According to Arthur Dickson Wright, *Past and Present Nurses' League Journal* 8 (1971), 26.

42 Andrew Cunningham and Perry Williams, eds., *The Laboratory Revolution in Medicine* (Cambridge: Cambridge University Press, 1992).

43 Patricia Helen Bracegirdle, "The Establishment of Histology in the Curriculum of the London Medical Schools, 1826–1886" (PhD dissertation, University of London, 1996).

44 SMHA, MS AD 1/3, 228–9.

45 University College London Archives, John Burdon Sanderson Papers, MS ADD 179. See Stella V.F. Butler, "Science and the Education of Doctors in the Nineteenth Century : A Study of British Medical Schools with Particular Reference to the Development and Uses of Physiology" (PhD dissertation, Manchester University, 1981). See also Gerald L. Geison, "Social and Institutional Factors in the Stagnancy of English Physiology, 1840–1870," *Bulletin of the History of Medicine* 46 (1972): 30–58; W.F. Bynum, *Science and the Practice of Medicine* (Cambridge: Cambridge University Press, 1994), 114.

46 W.J. O'Connor, *British Physiologists, 1885–1914: A Biographical Dictionary* (Manchester: Manchester University Press, 1991), 201. Previously it had met only at Oxford, Cambridge, UCL and King's College London. See also Sharpey-Schafer, ed., *The History of the Physiological Society during Its First Fifty Years, 1876–1926* (Cambridge: Cambridge University Press, 1927).

47 SMHA, MS AD 1/3, 540.

48 J. Burnett, "The Origins of the Electrocardiograph As a Clinical Instrument," in W.F. Bynum, C.J. Lawrence, and V. Nutton, eds., *The Emergence of Modern Cardiology* (London: Wellcome Institute, 1985): 53–76; also Robert G. Frank, "The Telltale Heart: Physiological Instruments, Graphic Methods, and Clinical Hopes, 1854–1914," in William Coleman and Frederic L. Holmes, eds., *The Investigative Enterprise: Experimental Physiology in 19th-Century Medicine* (Berkeley: University of California Press, 1988), 211–90.

49 See John E. Senior, "Rationalising Electrotherapy in Neurology, 1860–1920" (PhD dissertation, Oxford University, 1994).

50 A.H. Sykes, "A.D. Waller and the University of London Physiological Laboratory," *Medical History* 33 (1989): 217–34.

51 SMHA, MS AD 1/3, 255.

52 Ibid., 330.

53 Ibid., 318.

54 Ibid., 277.

55 On the place of games in the Victorian university, see Andrew Warwick, "Exercising the Student Body: Mathematics and Athleticism in Victorian Cambridge," in Christopher Lawrence and Steven Shapin, eds., *Science Incarnate: Historical Embodiments of Natural Knowledge* (Chicago: University of Chicago Press, 1998), 288–326.

56 *SMHG* 4 (1898): 7–9. William became a noted actor, and when he was murdered in 1898, St Mary's mourned him as its own. His brother gave up medicine for a bohemian life mostly spent fishing.

56 *BMJ* (1868) 2: 374–5.

57 *Bayswater Chronicle*, 9 October 1876.

58 *SMHG* 3 (1897): 76.

59 SMHA, MS AD 1/3, 178.

60 *SMHG* 5 (1899): 143–5.

61 *SMHG* 6 (1900): 30.

62 *SMHG* 2 (1896): 39–41.

63 *SMHG* 4 (1898): 106–8.

64 W.W. Sargant, *The Unquiet Mind* (London: Heinemann, 1967), 21.

65 T.S. Eliot, *Notes towards the Definition of Culture* (London: Faber and Faber, 1948), 47.

66 *BMJ* (1872) ii, 420.

67 Philip Mason, *The English Gentleman: The Rise and Fall of an Ideal* (London: Deutsch, 1982).

68 On liminality, see Victor Turner, "Variations on a Theme of Liminality," in Sally F. Moore and Barbara G. Meyerhoff, eds., *Secular Ritual* (Amsterdam: VanGoram, 1977), 37–9.

69 *SMHG* 3 (1897): 65–6.

Chapter Four

1 Ralph Williams, *A Plea for the Church in Our New Parish* (London: R.D. Dickenson, 1893).

2 Charles Booth, ed., *Life and Labour of the People in London* (London: Macmillan, 1892–97).

3 Jerry White, *The Worst Street in North London: Campbell Bunk, Islington, between the Wars* (London: Routledge & Kegan Paul, 1986), 48–9.

4 In 1891, 918 bricklayers, 3,347 carpenters and joiners, 889 plasterers and paper-hangers, 1,230 builders, and 639 architects and engineers lived in Paddington, comprising about 3 per cent of London's total of these trades, while 4.9 per cent of London carriage-builders (1,436 in total) chose that district for their homes; 1,195 or 3.1 per cent of London blacksmiths also resided in Paddington. By comparison, Paddington accommodated only 1.1 per cent of "sundry" manufacturers, 1.2 per cent of those in the printing trades, 1.8 per cent of those in precious metals, and 1.4 per cent of those in the metal trade of London.

5 W.M. Blandford, *The Story of a Church in a Potato Shop* (London: Spottiswoode, 1889), 9.

6 Paul Lindsay, *The Synagogues of London* (London: Vallentine Mitchell, 1993).

7 *By-Laws of the Westbourne Lodge, No. 1035, of Freemasons* (London: H.M Arliss, 1858); *Astounding Disclosures in Connection with Spiritualism and the Spirit World! Supernatural Visits at the House of a Clergyman in Bayswater* (London: J Onwhyn, [1864]).

8 *Bayswater Chronicle* 1 (1860–1), 22 and passim; also 25 April 1863; Henry Taylor, *The Marylebone Readings and their Critics* (London: Marylebone Penny Readings, 1869).

9 SMHA, SM AD 1/19, 283–4.

10 SMHA, SM AD 1/9, 659–60.

11 SMHA, SM AD 1/13, 198–9.

12 Helen Bousanquet, *Social Work in London, 1869–1912* (1914; reprint, Brighton: Houghton Press, 1973), 5, 43. The papers are held by the London Metropolitan Archives, A FWA KW A5/1.

13 *Bayswater Chronicle*, 4 April 1863.

14 *Bayswater Chronicle*, 2 November 1861.

15 *Bayswater Chronicle* 1 (1860–1), 163

16 *Bayswater Chronicle*, 5 September 1861.

17 WA, *Report on the Health of Paddington during the Half-Year ending Lady-Day, 1866*.

18 WA, *Paddington, Sanitary Report for the Year 1869–70*.

19 Anne Hardy, *The Epidemic Streets: Infectious Disease and the Rise of Preventive Medicine, 1856–1900* (Oxford: Clarendon Press, 1993) and *Health and Medicine in Britain since 1860* (Basingstoke: Palgrave, 2001).

20 *Bayswater Chronicle*, 25 January and 8 March 1890.

21 *Bayswater Chronicle*, June to July 1890.

22 Sandra den Otter, *British Idealism and Social Explanation: A Study in Late Victorian Thought* (Oxford: Oxford University Press, 1996), and Michael Freeden, *The New Liberalism: An Ideology of Social Reform* (Oxford: Clarendon Press, 1986; 2nd ed.); Stephan Collini, *Liberalism and Sociology: L.T. Hobhouse and Political Argument in England, 1880–1914* (Cambridge: Cambridge University Press, 1979).

23 Jose Harris, *Private Lives, Public Spirit: Britain, 1870–1914* (London: Penguin, 1993); John Davis, "The Progressive Council, 1889–1907," in Andrew Saint, ed., *Politics and the People of London: The London County Council, 1889–1965* (London: Hambledon Press, 1989), 27–48; James Gillespie, "Municipalism, Monopoly and Management: The Decline of 'Socialism in One County,' 1918–1933," in Saint, *Politics and the People of London*, 103–26; Ross McKibbin, *The Evolution of the Labour Party, 1910–1924* (Oxford: Clarendon Press, 1974), xv.

24 *Bayswater Chronicle*, 25 January 1890.

25 Sir James Marchant, *Dr John Clifford, C.H., Life, Letters, and Reminiscences* (London: Cassell, 1924), 180–1.

26 A.M. McBriar, *An Edwardian Mixed Doubles: The Bosanquets versus the Webbs: A Study in British Social Policy, 1890–1929* (Oxford: Clarendon Press, 1987).

27 Paddington and Marylebone District-Nursing Association, for Providing Trained Nurses for the Sick Poor at Their Own Homes, *Report for the Year 1887* (London: Hutchings and Crowsley, 1888) and *Report for the Year 1888*. See Anne Summers, "The Costs and Benefits of Caring: Nursing Charities c. 1830–1860," in Jonathan Berry and Colin Jones, eds., *Medicine and Charity before the Welfare State* (London: Routledge, 1991), 133–48.

28 Keir Waddington, "Unsuitable Cases: The Debate over Out-Patient Admissions, the Medical Profession, and Late Victorian Hospitals," *Medical History* 42 (1998): 26–46.

29 SMHA, SM AD 1/14, 237–8.

30 SMHA, SM AD 1/15, 243–6, 249–55.

31 LMA, Charity Organisation Society, A FWA C A26/1 Medical Subcommittee, passim.

32 LMA, Charity Organisation Society, A FWA KW A5/1.

33 Keir Waddington, "Bastard Benevolence: Centralisation, Voluntarism and the Sunday Fund, 1873–1898," *London Journal* 19 (1994): 151–67.

34 *Lancet* (1870) 2: 457.

35 In 1893 the average consumption was 9½ ounces per patient per day. In 1902 one junior doctor commented, "One often sees in the wards patients on large doses of alcohol who are in an extremely obfuscated condition, and who, if allowed out of bed, would certainly be regarded as very drunk." SMHA, SM AD 1/17, 624–5; *SMHG* 8 (1902): 102.

36 *SMHG* 8 (1902): 100–4.

37 Frank Prochaska, *Philanthropy and the Hospitals of London: The King's Fund, 1897–1990* (Oxford: Clarendon Press, 1992).

38 LMA, A KE 258/6, King's Fund, file on St Mary's, report dated 13 July 1898.

39 SMHA, SM AD 2/2, 563–4.

40 *Bayswater Chronicle*, 26 April 1890.

41 In 1905 it was reckoned that the previous year Kensington patients had cost the hospital £4,450, while Kensington residents had subscribed only £582; for Marylebone residents the figures were £4,050 and £428 or about two shillings per patient treated. *SMHG* 11 (1905): 57–9.

42 SMHA, SM AD 2/2, 462.

43 SMHA, SM AD 35/2, 14.

44 *Practitioner* n.s. 9 (1899): 535–40.

45 *Daily Telegraph*, 21 January 1903; LMA, A KE, 258/6, loose papers.

46 SMHA, SM AD 2/3, 229–31.

47 SMHA, SM AD 2/2, 329–31 and 375–6.

48 *SMHG* 13 (1907): 14–15.

49 *Report from the Select Committee of the House of Lords on Metropolitan Hospitals* (London: Hansard, 1890), 245–7, 236–7.

50 SMHA, SM AD 2/1, 600–01.

51 SMHA, SM AD 2/3, 612–14.

52 SMHA, SM AD 2/2, 299–300.

53 SMHA, SM AD 2/3, 18.

54 SMHA, SM AD 2/2, 391–3.

55 *SMHG* 11 (1905): 80–1.

56 *SMHG* 16 (1910): 114–6.

57 Charles Rosenberg, *The Care of Strangers: The Rise of America's Hospital System* (New York: Basic Books, 1987).

58 Steve Sturdy and Roger Cooter, "Scientific Management and the Transformation of Medicine in Britain, c. 1870–1950," *History of Science* 36 (1998): 421–66; Paul Starr, *The Social Transformation of American Medicine: The Rise of a Sovereign Profession and the Making of a Vast Industry* (New York: Basic Books, 1982); Harold Perkin, *The Rise of Professional Society: England since 1880* (London: Routledge, 1989); Keir Waddington, *Charity and the*

London Hospitals 1850–1898 (Woodbridge: Boydell, 2000); Steven Cherry, *Medical Services and the Hospitals in Britain, 1860–1939* (Cambridge: Cambridge University Press, 1996).

59 Ida Mann, *Ida and the Eye: A Woman in British Opthalmology* (Tunbridge Wells: Parapress, 1996).

60 Michael Bliss, *William Osler: A Life in Medicine* (Toronto: University of Toronto Press, 1999).

61 SMHA, SM AD 2/2, 309.

62 Ibid., 661. On the new technologies like X-rays, see Joel D. Howell, *Technology in the Hospital: Transforming Patient Care in the Early Twentieth Century* (Baltimore: Johns Hopkins University Press, 1995).

63 *Bayswater Chronicle*, 22 November 1890.

64 *Lancet* (1904) 2: 1129.

65 *Lancet* (1909) 2: 767–70.

66 *SMHG* 16 (1910): 9–10.

67 CMAC, Moran papers, M B 51, 22 February 1909, to his father.

68 *Lancet* (1904) 2: 1123.

69 Christopher Lawrence, "Incommunicable Knowledge: Science, Technology and the Clinical Art in Britain, 1850–1914," *Journal of Contemporary History* 20 (1985), 503–20; see also his "Still Incommunicable," in Christopher Lawrence and George Weisz, *Greater Than the Parts: Holism in Biomedicine, 1920 to 1950* (Oxford: Oxford University Press, 1998). See also Rosemary Stevens, *Medical Practice in Modern England: The Impact of Specialization and State Medicine* (New Haven: Yale University Press, 1966) and the work of George Weisz, including "Medical Directories and Medical Specialization in France, Britain, and the United States," *Bulletin of the History of Medicine* 71 (1997): 23–68.

70 See Geoffrey Rivett, *The Development of the London Hospital System, 1823–1982* (London: King's Fund, 1986).

71 Arthur Conan Doyle, *Memories and Adventures* (London: John Murray, 1924); Sir Harold Morris, *Back View* (London: Peter Davies, 1960); Daniel Stashower, *Teller of Tales: The Life of Arthur Conan Doyle* (Harmondsworth: Penguin, 1999), 63.

72 In *SMHG* 14 (1908): 44–8.

73 SMHA, SM AD 1/17, 650–1.

74 *Report from the Select Committee*, 14703–40.

75 *SMHG* 12 (1906): 103.

76 *Report from the Select Committee*, 199.

77 *Lancet* (1894) 1: 1169–70; E.H. Sieveking, *On the Reform of the Out-Patient Department of the Hospitals* (London: T. Richards, 1868).

78 *SMHG* 3 (1897): 5.

79 In Hodgkinson, *The Origins of the National Health Service*, 482.

80 Geoffrey Rivett, *The Development of the London Hospital System 1823–1982* (London, King's Fund, 1986), 178.

81 Judith Moore, *A Zeal for Responsibility: The Struggle for Professional Nursing in Victorian England, 1868–1883* (Athens: University of Georgia Press, 1988).

82 SMHA, SM AD 1/9, 41.

83 SMHA, SM AD 1/11, 140–2.

84 Zachary Cope, *A Hundred Years of Nursing at St Mary's Hospital Paddington* (London: Heinemann, 1955); Cecil Woodham-Smith, *Florence Nightingale* (London: Constable, 1950).

85 LMA, Nightingale Papers, H1 ST NC. Courtesy of the Nightingale Museum.

86 Ibid., H1 ST NC 18 12/14–15, p. 13 (letter dated 19 June 1876).

87 Ibid., H1 ST NC3 SU/180, no. 31.

88 Susan Reverby, *Ordered to Care: The Dilemma of American Nursing, 1850–1945* (Cambridge: Cambridge University Press, 1987).

89 LMA, Nightingale Papers, H1 ST NC 18 8/5.

90 Ibid., A NFC, 88/4, has scribbled notes on the course.

91 LMA, Nightingale Papers, H1 ST NC 18 12/14, p. 22.

92 Ibid., Nightingale Papers, H1 ST NC 10 27 11.

93 Association for the Improvement of London Workhouses, *The Management of the Infirmaries ...* (London: For the Association, 1867).

94 *The Hospital* 39 (1906): 313.

95 *Bayswater Chronicle*, 21 June 1890. Mrs Charles opposed most of Savill's initiatives: the next month she tried to ban whisky from the infirmary, but the rest of the guardians, all men, refused to follow her. The cost per head of alcoholic stimulants at the infirmary was 6s. 2½d. At St Mary's it was £1.18.11.

96 Mary E. Fissell, "The Disappearance of the Patient's Narrative and the Invention of Hospital Medicine," in Roger French and Andrew Wear, eds., *British Medicine in an Age of Reform* (London: Routledge, 1991), 92–109.

97 Ida Mann, *Ida and the Eye*, 59.

98 *SMHG* 3 (1897): 143–5.

99 *SMHG* 4 (1898): 46–7.

100 *SMHG* 14 (1908): 126–34; 19 (1913): 152–5.

Chapter Five

1 Arthur M. Silverstein, *A History of Immunology* (San Diego: Academic Press, 1989). See for example, an article in the *SMHG* 3 (1897): 99–101.

2 *SMHG* 2 (1896): 4–5.

3 *SMHG* 7 (1901): 9–10.

4 *SMHG* 10 (1904): 78.

5 *SMHG* 2 (1896): 121–2.

6 SMHA, SM AD 35/2, 22.

7 *Lancet* (1903) 1: 1497–1500.

8 *SMHG* 5 (1899): 116–21.

9 *The Practitioner* 62 (1899: 430–55; and *SMHG* 6 (1900): 17.

10 *Lancet* (1902) 1: 429–31.

11 SMHA, MS AD 1/3, 376.

12 *Lancet* (1900) 2: 1136–7.

13 *Lancet* (1901) 1: 1260–5.

14 Ibid.: 532.

15 *Lancet* (1905) 1: 1352–3.

16 On Horder, see Christopher Lawrence, "A Tale of Two Sciences: Bedside and Bench in 20th-Century Britain," *Medical History* 43 (1999): 421–49.

17 SMHA, SM AD 2/4, 467–8.

18 Stephen S. Hall, *A Commotion in the Blood: Life, Death, and the Immune System* (New York: Henry Holt, 1997).

19 For biographies of Wright, see: Leonard Colebrook, *Almroth Wright, Provocative Doctor and Thinker* (London: Heinemann, 1954); Zachary Cope, *Almroth Wright, Founder of Modern Vaccine-Therapy* (London: Nelson, 1966); and the definitive new work by Michael Dunnill, *The Plato of Praed Street: The Life and Times of Almroth Wright* (London: Royal Society of Medicine, 2001), published after this chapter was written.

20 *Lancet* (1900) 2: 952.

21 *Lancet* (1900) 1: 1158.

22 Gerald L. Geison, *The Private Science of Louis Pasteur* (Princeton: Princeton University Press, 1995; Bruno Latour, *The Pasteurization of France*, trans. Alan Sheridan and John Law (Cambridge: Harvard University Press, 1988).

23 *Lancet* (1900) 1: 1360–1.

24 *Lancet* (1900) 2: 1556–61.

25 *Lancet* (1901) 1: 609–12.

26 Ibid.: 783–5, 786, and 857–8.

27 Ibid.: 1532–4.

28 Colebrook, *Almroth Wright*, 27.

29 *Journal of Vaccine Therapy* 2 (1913): 22.

30 *Lancet* (1901) 2: 1195–6. Here I am referring to the laboratory techniques and claims, rather than the typhoid vaccination which, in practice, was open to many objections, as I have shown.

31 Philip D. Curtis, *Disease and Empire: The Health of European Troops in the Conquest of Africa* (Cambridge: Cambridge University Press, 1998).

32   *SMHG* 9 (1903): 33.

33   *SMHG* 58 (1952): 94–100; SMHA MS AD 1/5, 73.

34   Anne-Marie Moulin, *Le dernier langage de la medicine: histoire de l'im-munologie de Pasteur au Sida, pratiques theoriques* (France: Presses Universi-taires de France, 1991), 86.

35   Wright, "Studies on Immunisation," 83; from *Proceedings of the Royal Soci-ety* 73 (1903).

36   "Studies on Immunisation," 102; from *Proceedings of the Royal Society* 74 (1904).

37   *SMHG* 10 (1904): 89–91.

38   *BMJ* (1904) 2: 1243–6.

39   J. Rosser Matthews, *Quantification and the Quest for Medical Certainty* (Princeton: Princeton University Press, 1995), contains a full account of the controversy.

40   *Lancet* (1904) 1: 800 and passim.

41   Cope, *Almroth Wright*; St Mary's Hospital, *Annual Report* (1907).

42   A.E. Wright, "On the Treatment of Acne, Furnculosis and Sycosis by Thera-peutic Inoculations of Staphylococcus Vaccine," *BMJ* (1904) 1: 1075–7.

43   SMHA, SM AD 2/5, 636–7.

44   SMHA, SM AD 35/1, 26.

45   St Mary's Hospital, *Annual Report* 46 (1906).

46   Michael Worboys, "Vaccine Therapy and Laboratory Medicine in Edwardian Britain," in John V. Pickstone, ed., *Medical Innovations in Historical Per-spective* (London: Macmillan, 1992), note 36.

47   W.D. Foster, *Pathology As a Profession in Great Britain and the Early Histo-ry of the Royal College of Pathologists* (London: The College, 1982).

48   Worboys, "Vaccine Therapy and Laboratory Medicine," 92–3.

49   E.M. Tansey and Rosemary C.E. Milligan, "The Early History of the Well-come Research Laboratories, 1894–1914," in Jonathan Liebenau, Gregory J. Higby, and Elaine C. Stroud, eds., *Pill Peddlers: Essays on the History of the Pharmaceutical Industry* (Madison, Wis.: American Institute of the History of Psychiatry, 1990), 91–106.

50   Steven Sturdy, "Medical Chemistry and Clinical Medicine: Academics and the Scientisation of Medical Practice in Britain, 1900–1925," in Ilana Löwy, ed., *Medicine and Change: Historical and Sociological Studies of Medical Inno-vation* (London: John Libbey, 1993), 371–93.

51   A.M. Cooke, *A History of the Royal College of Physicians* (Oxford: Claren-don Press, 1972), vol. 3, 928–9. John Ritchie, *History of the Laboratory of the Royal College of Physicians of Edinburgh* (Edinburgh: Royal College of Physicians, 1913).

52 Peter Keating, "Vaccine Therapy and the Problem of Opsonins," *JHM* 43 (1988): 281–2.

53 Keating, "Vaccine Therapy," note 81.

54 Royal Society of Medicine, *Vaccine Therapy: Its Administration, Value, and Limitations* (London: Longman's, 1910), 74.

55 Ibid., 75.

56 Ibid., 97–101.

57 *Journal of Vaccine Therapy* 2 (1913): 24.

58 Offprint of a paper "Laboratory Tests As a Guide to Inoculation Treatment," given at the BMA (printed in the *BMJ* 9 November 1912): 7.

59 *Vaccine Therapy*, 128–37.

60 "Studies on Immunisation," 109–11.

61 SMHA, SM AD 2/6, 314–5.

62 Cope, *Almroth Wright*, 104–5.

63 The minutes are held at the St Mary's Hospital Archives.

64 LMA, A/KE/532/4, printed pamphlet on "Therapeutic Inoculation," 5–6.

65 See the bundle of papers in LMA, A/KE/532/4, file "Almroth Wright."

66 A. Landsborough Thomson, *Half a Century of Medical Research* (London: HMSO 1975); Joan Austoker and Linda Bryder, eds., *Historical Perspectives on the Role of the MRC: Essays in the History of the Medical Research Council of the United Kingdom and Its Predecessor, the Medical Research Committee, 1913–1953* (Oxford: Oxford University Press, 1989).

67 Michael Worboys raises this suggestion in "Vaccine Therapy and Laboratory Medicine."

68 Notes of the discussions between Wright and MRC officials are in the CMAC, RAMC papers, Leishman collection, box 124, file 563. On research laboratories, the classic article is J.B. Morrell, "The Chemist Breeders: The Research Schools of Liebig and Thomas Thomson," *Ambix* 19 (1972): 1–46; see also Gerald L. Geison and Frederic L. Holmes, *Osiris: Research Schools: Historical Reappraisals* n.s. 8 (1993), passim.

69 SMHG 18 (1912): 96–8.

70 Claire Herrick, "Of War and Wounds: The Propaganda, Politics, and Experience of Medicine in World War I" (PhD dissertation, Manchester University, 1996).

71 *BMJ* (1915) 1: 764.

72 *BMJ* (1915) 2: 721.

73 *BMJ* (1915) 1: 825–6.

74 Herrick, "Of War and Wounds."

75 Quoted in Zachary Cope, *Almroth Wright*, 81.

76 CMAC, RAMC, 365/4.

Chapter Six

1   SMHA, MS AD 1/3, 315–6.

2   Ibid., passim.

3   In 1885 only one-quarter of students registered as university students; by 1910, two-thirds registered. Evidence given before the Royal Commission on University Education in London, *Final Report of the Commission* (Parliamentary papers vol. 40, 1913). Henceforth, Haldane Commission.

4   *Report from the Select Committee of the House of Lords on Metropolitan Hospitals* (London: Hansard, 1890), 39.

5   SMHA, MS AD 2/3, loose paper at end of volume and see the minutes for 9 November 1900, continued in 2/4, 23 November 1900.

6   SMHA, MS AD 1/5, 179–82.

7   *SMHG* 6 (1900), 108–11.

8   SMHA, MS AD 1/4, 274–5.

9   Ibid., 486–8.

10 Ibid., 351.

11 SMHA, MS AD 1/3, 303–4.

12 University of London Archives, CF 1/5/1444, letter of 7 April 1905.

13 Eric Ashby and Mary Anderson, *Portrait of Haldane at Work on Education* (London: Macmillan, 1974); Richard Burdon, Viscount Haldane, *The Nationalisation of Universities* (London: Lamley, 1921); Abraham Flexner, *Medical Education in Europe: A Report to the Carnegie Foundation for the Advancement of Teaching*, Bulletin 6 (New York, 1912).

14 Zachary Cope, *The History of St Mary's Hospital Medical School* (London: Heinemann, 1954), 163.

15 Haldane Commission, fifth report, 80–1.

16 Ibid., 156–64.

17 SMHA, MS AD 5/1, 197.

18 *SMHG* listed publications of all staff members each month.

19 *SMHG* 19 (1913): 64–7.

20 Lord Haldane would be dropped from the wartime government by reason of his pre-war German sympathies.

21 Douglas G. Browne and E.V. Tullett, *Bernard Spilsbury: His Life and Cases* (Harmondsworth: Penguin, 1951); Philip H.A. Willcox, *The Detective-Physician: The Life and Work of Sir William Willcox* (London: Heinemann, 1970).

22 SMHA, MS AD 5/2 117,

23 Flexner, *Medical Education*, 132. Contrast Steve Sturdy, "Chemical Physiology and Clinical Medicine: Academics and the Scientisation of Medical Practice in Britain, 1900–1925," in Ilana Löwy et al., eds., *Innovation in Medicine: Historical and Sociological Perspectives* (London: Jann Libbey,

1993), 352–74; Robert E. Kohler, *From Medical Chemistry to Biochemistry: The Making of a Biomedical Discipline* (Cambridge: Cambridge University Press, 1982).

24 *SMHG* 14 (1908): 92–5.

25 *SMHG* 10 (1905): 118–19, and Leonard Colebrook, *Almroth Wright: Provocative Doctor and Thinker* (London: Heinemann, 1954), 264–7.

26 *SMHG* 13 (1907): 27.

27 Colebrook, *Almroth Wright*, 268–74.

28 *SMHG* 58 (1952): 138–42.

29 *Lancet* (1900) 2: 1709–14.

30 *SMHG* 8 (1902): 67.

31 *Lancet* (1900) 2: 789–92.

32 *Lancet* (1909) 2: 1773–4.

33 D.B. Lees, *Valedictory Lecture Delivered at St Mary's Hospital, May 29 1907* (n.p., 1907), pamphlet in Royal College of Surgeons of England Library.

34 *SMHG* 13 (1907): 95–8; 17 (1911): 142–6; 14 (1912): 3–8, 70–5.

35 *SMHG* 15 (1909): 116–20.

36 *SMHG* 13 (1907): 97.

37 *SMHG* 11 (1905): 56–7.

38 *SMHG* 15 (1909): 123–4.

39 *SMHG* 11 (1905): 103–5.

40 *SMHG* 12 (1906): 110–14.

41 *SMHG* 13 (1907): 80–2.

42 *SMHG* 36 (1930): 46–50; and 38 (1932): 106–11.

43 *SMHG* 38 (1932): 133.

44 *SMHG* 14 (1908): 65–8.

45 *SMHG* 15 (1909): 96–7.

46 *SMHG* 12 (1906): 73.

47 Ibid.: 3.

48 And especially by Rous, as one piffling rhyme remarked: "Go to, go to thou bold JB nor rouse the great one's ire / Why twit ye thus a thunderbolt, why dabble ye with fire?"

49 *SMHG* 11 (1905): 117; 12 (1906): 7–8.

50 Ida Mann, *Ida and the Eye* (Tunbridge Wells: Parapress, 1996), 70.

51 SMHA, MS AD 5/1, 177.

52 *SMHG* 17 (1911): 123–4.

53 Haldane Commission, fifth report, 40.

54 *SMHG* 19 (1913), 139–42.

55 SMHA, SM AD 5/2, 117.

56 *SMHG* 26 (1920), 1.

57 Public Record Office (PRO), ED 24 1961.

58 The definitive biography is Richard Lovell, *Churchill's Doctor: A Biography of Lord Moran* (London: Royal Society of Medicine Services, 1993).

59 *SMHG* 26 (1920): 23-5.

60 CMAC, Moran papers, M5.

61 SMHA, SM AD 35/7, 56.

62 CMAC, Moran papers, L1.2, letter from Herringham to Wilson.

63 SMHA, MS AD 5/3, 41.

64 SMHA, SM AD 2/8, 330.

65 George Graham, "The Formation of the Medical and Surgical Professorial Units in the London Teaching Hospitals," *Annals of Science* 26 (1970): 1-22; Andrew Hull, "Hector's House"; see also, for example, A.E. Clark-Kennedy, *The London: A Study in the Voluntary Hospital System*, vol. 2 (London: Pitman, 1963), 207-8.

66 *Lancet* (1920) 2: 1287-90.

67 SMHA, SM AD 35/7, 56.

Chapter Seven

1   Martin Gorsky and John Mohan, "London's Voluntary Hospitals in the Interwar Period: Growth, Transformation, or Crisis?" *Nonprofit and Voluntary Sector Quarterly* 30 (2001): 247-75.

2   *Bayswater Chronicle*, 12 February 1921.

3   *SMHG* 14 (1908): 56-61.

4   Quoted in *SMHG* 12 (1906): 44.

5   *SMHG* 18 (1912): 67-9.

6   *SMHG* 14 (1908): 97.

7   The *Annual Reports* of the MOH of Paddington are published as an appendix to the Borough Council's *Annual Report*.

8   CMAC, Moran papers, A 4/2, obstetrics file, Bourne to Wilson, 24 October 1933.

9   *Lancet* (1927) 2: 1277.

10 *Bayswater Chronicle*, 13 March and 11 December 1920.

11 SMHA, SM AD 35/8, 78.

12 SMH *Annual Report*.

13 *Bayswater Chronicle*, 24 January 1920.

14 Interview with Christine Rose, July 1999.

15 *Bayswater Chronicle*, 14 May 1921.

16 *Bayswater Chronicle*, 26 March 1921.

17 *Bayswater Chronicle*, 16 April 1921.

18 *Bayswater Chronicle*, 31 January and 3 April 1920.

19 Geoffrey Rivett, *The Development of the London Hospital System, 1823-1982* (London: King's Fund, 1986) 185.

20 Lady Harris denounced "the unmerited hatred with which the lower classes looked on any class but their own." When the visiting speaker, Major Boyd Carpenter, suggested that acts of kindness could overcome this suspicion, citing his own example of giving a lift in his car to a working man who had grumbled about having to walk, "Lady Harris said she did not think such gracious acts would be much use in Paddington." *Bayswater Chronicle*, 1 May 1920.

21 Bentley B. Gilbert, *British Social Policy, 1914–1939* (London: B.T. Batsford, 1970), 205.

22 For the centre perspective, see John M. Eyler, *Sir Arthur Newsholme and State Medicine, 1885-1935* (Cambridge: Cambridge University Press, 1997).

23 See Linda Bryder, *Below the Magic Mountain: A Social History of Tuberculosis in Twentieth Century Britain* (Oxford: Clarendon Press, 1988). *Lancet* (1898) 2: 1101–03.

24 Anne Hardy, *The Epidemic Streets* (Oxford: Clarendon, 1993).

25 Paddington MOH, *Annual Report for the Year 1907*, 23.

26 F.B. Smith, *The Retreat of Tuberculosis, 1850–1950* (London: Croon Helm, 1988).

27 *Lancet* (1911) 2: 150.

28 *SMHG* 29 (1914): 3–7.

29 LMA, LCC Papers, PH Gen 4 43 contains early correspondence. Postwar correspondence is in a file labelled Paddington Chest Clinic: LCC, PH PHS 4/29.

30 LMA, LCC, PH, PHS 4/29, Memo from Dr Bentley to Dr Hewat, 9 June 1936.

31 T.K. Chambers, *The Renewal of Life* (London: Churchill, 1862), 217–21.

32 *SMHG* 10 (1904), 45.

33 David Innes Williams, *The London Lock: A Charitable Hospital for Venereal Disease, 1746–1952* (London: Royal Society of Medicine, n.d.). Background readings include Jeffrey Weeks, *Sex, Politics, and Society: The Regulation of Sexuality since 1800* (London: Longman, 1989; 2nd ed.); Frank Mort, *Dangerous Sexualities: Medico-Moral Politics in England since 1830* (London: Routledge & Kegan Paul, 1987); Roger Davidson and Lesley Hall, eds., *Sex, Sin and Suffering: Venereal Disease and European Society since 1870* (London: Routledge, 2001).

34 On the early history of the Wassermann, see Ludwik Fleck, *The Genesis and Development of a Scientific Fact*, Thaddeus J. Trenn and Robert K. Merton eds.; trans. Fred Bradley and Thaddeus J. Trenn (Chicago: University of Chicago Press, 1981).

35 SMHA, SM AD 2/10, 62.

36 This is according to his obiturist, in *SMHG* 78, no. 8 (December 1972), 27.

37 SMHA, SM AD 35/14, 162.

38 *Lancet* (1938) 2: 355–62.

39 LMA, LCC, PH HOSP/2/57.

40 G.L.M. McElligott, "The Venereal History: Truth or Fiction," *British Journal of Venereal Disease* (hereafter BJVD) 8 (1932): 292.

41 BJVD 11 (1935): 40–1.

42 Aleck Bourne, *A Doctor's Creed: The Memoirs of a Gynaecologist* (London: Victor Gollancz, 1962), 24.

43 SMHA, private information.

44 BJVD 24 (1948): 26–38.

45 A.J. Cronin, *The Citadel* (1937; reprint, Kent: New English Library, 1983), 237.

46 SMHG 45 (1939): 31.

47 SMHG 20 (1914): 32. The speaker, Clayton Green, preceded the quotation with the account of a man who came to Mary's with both his shoulders dislocated. The surgeon, surgical registrar, and sundry house surgeons failed to reduce the double dislocation and discharged the man, who came back a few weeks later having been cured by a bone-setter: "Well, he first sweated me, then he hung me up and punched me in the back until the bones went in.' And yet Science (with the University Commission's big S) would tell them that these men had no powers which the orthodox did not possess."

48 John Rhode, *The Murders in Praed* Street (London: Penguin, 1928) and *The Paddington Mystery* (London: Geoffrey Bles, 1925).

49 Almroth Wright was a favourite target of antivivisectionists, e.g., the pamphlet *The "Cooked" Statistics Concerning Anti-Typhoid Inoculation during the Recruiting for the Great War* (London: British Union for the Abolition of Vivisection, n.d.).

50 *Bayswater Chronicle*, October and November 1930.

51 See Nicolas A. Rupke, ed. *Vivisection in Historical Perspective* (London: Routledge, 1987); Richard D. French, *Antivivisection and Medical Science in Victorian Society* (Princeton: Princeton University Press, 1975).

52 Frank Honigsbaum, *The Division in British Medicine: A History of the Separation of General Practice from Hospital Care, 1911–1968* (London: Kogan Page, 1979), 130–1, 141–2, 239, 267.

53 PEP (Political and Economic Planning), *Report on the British Health Services* (London: PEP, December 1937).

54 M.A. Crowther, *The Workhouse System: The History of an English Social Institution* (Georgia: University of Georgia Press, 1981).

55 Ross McKibbin, *The Evolution of the Labour Party, 1910–1924* (Oxford: Clarendon, 1974), xv.

56 *Bayswater Chronicle*, 17 September and 1 October 1921.

57 Derek Fraser, *The Evolution of the British Welfare State* (London: Macmillan, 1984; 2nd ed.), 194.

58 Rivett, *The Development of the London Hospital System*, 199.

59 Pamela M. Graves, *Labour Women: Women in British Working-Class Politics, 1918–1939* (Cambridge: Cambridge University Press, 1994), 220.

60 Lara V. Marks, *Metropolitan Maternity: Maternal and Infant Welfare Services in Early Twentieth Century London* (Amsterdam: Rodopi, 1996), 72 and 138.

61 SMHA, SM AD 2/7, 583.

62 Irvine Loudon, *Death in Childbirth: An International Study of Maternal Care and Maternal Mortality, 1800–1950* (Oxford: Clarendon Press, 1992).

63 Graves, *Labour Women*, 194.

64 Marks, *Metropolitan Maternity*, 95; and see Loudon, *Death in Childbirth*, and Jane Lewis, *The Politics of Motherhood: Child and Maternal Welfare in England, 1900–1939* (London: Croom Helm, 1980).

65 Paddington MOH, *Annual Report for the Year 1930*.

66 *Bayswater Chronicle*, 29 March and 19 April 1930.

67 *Lancet* (1927) 2: 1276.

68 *Bayswater Chronicle*, 21 June 1930.

69 *Lives of the Fellows of the Royal College of Surgeons of England* (London: Royal College of Surgeons of England, various dates).

70 John Stewart, *The Battle for Health: A Political History of the Socialist Medical Association, 1930–51* (Aldershot: Ashgate, 1999), 38.

71 Stewart, *The Battle for Health*, passim.

72 Aleck Bourne, *A Doctor's Creed*.

73 SMHG 43 (1937): 128–9.

74 SMHG 49 (1943): 41–6.

75 Aleck Bourne, *Health of the Future* (Harmondsworth: Penguin, 1942), 137–41.

76 Harold C. Smith, ed., *War and Social Change: British Society in the Second World War* (Manchester: Manchester University Press, 1986); Paul Addison, *The Road to 1945: British Politics and the Second World War* (London: Pimlico, 1994).

77 Charles Webster, *The National Health Service: A Political History* (Oxford: Oxford University Press, 1998), 34; see also Peter Hennessey, *Never Again: Britain 1945–1951* (London: Vintage, 1993) and Nicolas Timmins, *The Five Giants: A Biography of the Welfare State* (London: HarperCollins, 1995).

78 Michael Foot, *Aneurin Bevan: A Biography* (London: MacGibbon & Kee, 1962–73).

79 Anne Chisholm and Michael Davie, *Beaverbrook: A Life* (London: Pimlico, 1993), 360.

80 John V. Pickstone, *Medicine and Industrial Society* (Manchester: Manchester University Press, 1985), 345.

81 Lovell, Richard, *Churchill's Doctor* (London: Royal Society of Medicine Services, 1993), v; CMAC, Moran Papers, L6.3, 22 March 1940.

82 CMAC, Moran papers, L 7.9.

83 Michael Foot, *Aneurin Bevan* (London: Granada, 1975), vol. 2, 131.

84 Honigsbaum, *The Division in British Medicine*.

85 Honigsbaum quotes this remark more fully as the epilogue to *The Division in British Medicine*, 319.

86 Ibid., 305.

87 *SMHG* 16 (1910): 87. See below, chapter on Moran's Mary's.

80 SMHA, MS AD 4, 54.

Chapter Eight

1 *BMJ* (1932) i, 485–7; J.J. Rousseau, *The Social Contract*, trans. G.D.H. Cole (London: Dent, 1963).

2 *SMHG* 68 (1962): 4–9.

3 AlmrothWright, *Alethetropic Logic: A Posthumous Work* (London: William Heinemann, 1953), 212.

4 Ronald Hare, *The Birth of Penicillin and the Disarming of Microbes* (London: George Allen and Unwin, 1970).

5 *SMHG* 84, 12 (1978): 12–13.

6 *Alethetropic Logic*, 98–9.

7 Ibid., 197–8.

8 There is no satisfactory account of this development. The account by Rosser Matthews leaps from Almroth Wright versus Greenwood directly to the mid-century MRC trials: *Quantification and the Quest for Medical Certainty* (Princeton: Princeton University Press, 1995); see also Alan Yorke Yoshioka, "Streptomycin, 1946 : British Central Administration of Supplies of a New Drug of American Origin with Special Reference to Clinical Trials in Tuberculosis" (PhD dissertation, Imperial College, 1998); Harry M. Marks, *The Progress of Experiment: Science and Therapeutic Reform in the United States, 1900–1990* (Cambridge: Cambridge University Press, 1997).

9 See Christopher Lawrence, "Moderns and Ancients: The 'New Cardiology' in Britain, 1880–1930," in W.F. Bynum, C. Lawrence, and V. Nutton, eds., *The Emergence of Modern Cardiology* (London: WIHM, 1985), 1–33; see also chapter 13 below.

10 The debate spans two volumes of the *Lancet*: (1917) 1: 555 (Smith), 589 (Poynton), 700–1 (Castellain), 820–1 (Mackenzie), 854 (Poynton), 891–2 (Colbeck), 927–9 (Morison), 965 (Broadbent), 1012–13 (Lewis); and (1917) 2: 24 (Broadbent), 61–3 (Mackenzie), 97 (Lewis), 172–3 (Allbutt), 255–7 (Mackenzie), 405–6 (Allbutt), and 474 (Poynton).

11 This was also the theory of Plimmer, when in 1899 he advised students at St Mary's that they would be guided by "Clinical Experience: i.e., by a collec-

tion of information about sick people and their diseases, which is derived, according to your powers, from your own observations, but principally from the recorded observations of others, which you will have to carry about with you in your memory." *SMHG* 5 (1899): 117.

12 *Lancet* (1900) 1: 731-2.

13 Wright, *Alethetropic Logic*, 208.

14 *Alethetropic Logic*.

15 Leonard Colebrook and E.J. Storer, "On Immuno-Transfusion," offprint, p 19; in *Lancet* (1923) 2: 1341.

16 These examples are taken from the Inoculation Department offprint collection, held at the Centre for History of Science, Technology, and Medicine, Imperial College.

17 Interview with Keith Rogers, 26 January 1999.

18 SMHA, MS AD 5/1, 86.

19 SMHA, MS AD 2/5, 86, 88, and 102. On virology, see Antonius Adrianus Franciscus Joseph van Helvoort, "Research Styles in Virus Studies in the 20th Century: Controversies and the Formation of Consensus" (PhD dissertation, University of Limburg, 1993).

20 André Maurois, *The Life of Sir Alexander Fleming, Discoverer of Penicillin*, trans. Gerard Hopkins (Harmondsworth: Penguin, 1963).

21 The best overview with a survey of existing literature is the biography by Gwyn Macfarlane, *Alexander Fleming: The Man and the Myth* (Oxford: Oxford University Press, 1985); see also F.W.E. Diggins, "The True History of the Discovery of Penicillin, with Refutation of the Misinformation in the Literature," *British Journal of Biomedical Science* 56 (1999): 83–93.

22 National Library of Scotland, John Burdon Sanderson Papers. The Grocers were considering diverting the funding for scholarships into a chair, as Michael Foster suggested they do, but Wright argued they could best serve science by funding young scholars.

23 Her second award was in 1922, the Henry George Plimmer Fellowship of Imperial College. Again, she was told to stay at St Mary's and "make no demands on the College." *Ida and the Eye* (Tunbridge Wells: Parapress, 1996), 164.

24 Hare, *The Birth of Penicillin*, 30.

25 SMHA, Inoculation Department minute book, 16.

26 Leonard Colebrook, *Almroth Wright* (London: Heinemann, 1954), 199.

27 Lily E. Kay, *The Molecular Vision of Life: Caltech, the Rockefeller Foundation, and the Rise of the New Biology* (Oxford: Oxford University Press, 1993).

28 SMHA, SM AD 2/9, 65-6.

29 CMAC, Moran papers, A 7/2, 22/12/50.

30 Royal Society of London, Howard Florey papers, 98 HF 36.17.1. By permission of the President and Council of the Royal Society. Gwyn Macfarlane, *Howard Florey: The Making of a Great Scientist* (Oxford: Oxford University Press, 1979) and Trevor I. Williams, *Howard Florey: Penicillin and After* (Oxford: Oxford University Press, 1984).

31 Lesley Brent, interview, 23 March 2000.

32 Frederick Ridley, "Lysozyme: An Antibacterial Body Present in Great Concentration in Tears, and Its Relation to Infection in the Human Eye," RSM 21 (1928): 55–65, Ophthalmology section.

33 Ronald Hare, *The Birth of Penicillin*; and "New Light on the History of Penicillin," *Medical History* 26 (1982): 1–24.

34 Interview with H.H. Eastcott, 25 January 1999.

35 Hare, "New Light on the History of Penicillin."

36 Wai Chen, "The Laboratory As Business: Sir Almroth Wright's Vaccine Programme and the Construction of Penicillin," in Andrew Cunningham and Perry Williams, *The Laboratory Revolution in Medicine* (Cambridge: Cambridge University Press, 1992), 245–94.

37 *Journal of Pathology and Bacteriology* 45 (1937): 472-3.

38 *Horizon* show, 8 April 1991, "The Mould, the Myth, and the Microbe."

39 Alexander Fleming and G.F. Petrie, *Recent Advances in Vaccine and Serum Therapy* (London: J. & A. Churchill, 1934), 361–2, 411–2. Petrie, a bacteriologist at the Lister, wrote the section on serum therapy and Fleming the section on vaccine therapy.

40 *A Hospital Which Has Achieved Something New* (London: Morton, Burt & Sons, 1931). A copy is in the Moran papers, CMAC.

41 The original article is in the *Lancet* of 29 May 1909; the subsequent articles are: *Lancet* (1912) 1: 1752–4; and (1912) 2: 48; 115–17 (Fleming and others); 183–5; 258–9; 336 (D'Este Emery), 408, 558 (Bassett-Smith).

42 CMAC, RAMC 365, Bowlby papers, Wright to Sir Arthur Sloggett, 12 January 1917.

43 Freeman's work is described in a series of articles collected together as the Inoculation Department reprints collection, held at Imperial College, and in John Freeman, *Hay-Fever: A Key to the Allergic Disorders* (London: William Heinemann, 1950).

44 On the GP as representing the whole-person approach, see Ann Digby, *Making a Medical Living: Doctors and Patients in the English Market for Medicine, 1720–1911* (Cambridge: Cambridge University Press, 1994), 101.

45 Hare, *The Birth of Penicillin*; *Past and Present Nurses' League Journal* 10 (1973): 376–7.

46 *Lancet* (1912) 2: 472–3.

47 *Lancet* (1912) 1: 116.

48 Wright, *Alethetropic Knowledge*, ch. 19.

Chapter Nine

1   In Dannie Abse, ed., *My Medical School* (London: Robson Books, 1978), 48.

2   Ida Mann, *Ida and the Eye* (Tunbridge Wells: Parapress, 1996), 59.

3   CMAC, Moran papers, 8/4, White to Wilson, 29 December 1932.

4   Ibid., L.2, Wright to Wilson, April 1929.

5   *SMHG* 75 (1969), 227–8.

6   For example see Steve Sturdy, "The Political Economy of Scientific Medicine: Scientific Medicine and the Transformation of Medical Practice in Sheffield, 1890–1922," *Medical History* 36 (1992): 125–59.

7   Barbara Brooks and Paul Roth, "*Rex v. Bourne*, and the Medicalisation of Abortion," in Michael Clark and Catherine Crawford, eds., *Legal Medicine in History* (Cambridge: Cambridge University Press, 1994), 314–43.

8   CMAC, Moran papers, Wilson to Beaverbrook, 18 January 1928.

9   SMHA, MS AD 1/6, 25.

10 CMAC, Moran papers, L.2., 8 May 1929.

11 Ibid., L.2.21, Wilson to Miss Kindersley, 21 May 1929.

12 Ibid., L.2.15, Wilson to Lady Kenmare, 13 May 1929. See W.R. Merrington, *University College Hospital and Its Medical School: A History* (London: Heinemann, 1976).

13 *Final Report of the [Haldane] Commission* (Parliamentary papers, vol. 40, 1913), 136.

14 Ross McKibbin, *Classes and Cultures: England, 1918–1951* (Oxford: Oxford University Press, 1998), 351.

15 Richard Holt, *Sport and the British: A Modern History* (Oxford: Clarendon Press, 1989), 228. There is a growing literature on the subject; see also John Nauright and Timothy J.L. Chandler, eds., *Making Men: Rugby and Masculine Identity* (London: Frank Cass, 1996).

16 CMAC, Moran papers, L.3.21, Wilson to Beaverbrook 20 October 1935.

17 Ibid., L.4.4 .

18 *SMHG* 1 (1895): 166–7.

19 *SMHG* 16 (1910): 87–8.

20 *BMJ* (1936) 2: 449.

21 *SMHG* 16 (1910): 5.

22 *SMHG* 14 (1908): 130–4.

23 *SMHG* 16 (1910): 94–6.

24 CMAC, Moran papers, H8/3, paper dated 1951. See Joanna Bourke, *Dismembering the Male: Men's Bodies, Britain, and the Great War* (London: Reaktion Books, 1996).

25 See Norman R. Eder, *National Health Insurance and the Medical Profession, 1913–1939* (New York: Garland, 1982), 146–7.

26 Abse, *My Medical School*, 51.

27 Interview of J. Litchfield by Alisdair Fraser, 27 November 1996, St Mary's Hospital Archives.

28 The figures are provided by Thomas King, *SMHG* 102, no. 1 (January 1996): 6. The argument is not intended to suggest that Mary's men were *more* heroic than other medical men. Comparison of this sort would be odious, impossible, and unhelpful, because Moran helped to establish a climate of ideas that pertained more widely, for example, with articles in the *BMJ*.

29 A manuscript copy is in CMAC, RAMC papers, 1042.

30 *SMHG* 51 (1945): 100-01.

31 Ann Dally, "Rejuvenation and Respectability: The 'Monkey Gland King' and the Fututre Psychiatrist," Glandular Visions conference, Wellcome Institute, 1998.

32 W.W. Sargant, *The Unquiet Mind* (London: Heinemann, 1967).

33 CMAC, Moran papers, H 11/6.

34 Ibid., A 7/2, letter to Carmalt Jones, 22 December 1950.

35 *SMHG* 68 (1962), 244–8.

36 The Lien Wu, *Plague Fighter: The Autobiography of a Modern Chinese Physician* (Cambridge: Heffer, 1959).

37 SMHA, MS AD 1/5, 490, 526.

38 James Stuart Garner, "The Great Experiment: The Admission of Women Students to St Mary's Hospital Medical School, 1916–1925," *Medical History* 42 (1998): 65–88.

39 SMHA, MS AD 1/1, 489. Isabel Thorne, *Sketch of the Foundation and Development of the London School of Medicine for Women* (London: Women's Printing, 1915).

40 SMHA, MS AD 1/5, 135.

41 *SMHG* 14 (1908): 97.

42 SMHA, SM AD 5/2, 1.

43 Ida Mann, *Ida and the Eye*, 39–40.

44 SMHA, SM AD 5/2, 80.

45 CMAC, Moran papers, D12.

46 SMHA, SM AD 5/2, 70. See F.M.L. Thompson, ed., *The University of London and the World of Learning, 1836–1986* (London: Hambledon Press, 1990); Janet Howarth, "Women," in Brian Harrison, ed., *The History of the University of Oxford*, vol. 8: *The Twentieth Century* (Oxford: Clarendon Press, 1994), 345–75; Carol Dyhouse, *No Distinction of Sex? Women in British Universities, 1870–1939* (London: UCL Press, 1995); and Dyhouse, "Driving Ambitions: Women in Pursuit of a Medical Education, 1890–1939," *Women's History Review* 7 (1998): 321–41.

47 Garner, "The Great Experiment," 65–88.

48 The documents are sprinkled throughout the minutes and the reports of the

Medical School Committee, the Medical Committee, and the Board of Management of April and May 1924. In particular see SMHA, SM AD 35/10, 122 and 128.

49 SMHA, SM AD 5/3, 78.

50 In Maurois, *The Life of Sir Alexander Fleming*; quoted in Garner.

51 Ann Digby has argued that this first generation of women practitioners had very high ideals. Paper at the Institute for Historical Research, University of London, 1997.

52 Public Record Office (PRO), ED 24/2012, contains a sheaf of correspondence on the matter; so too does the papers of the Medical Women's Federation, CMAC.

53 SMHA, SM AD 2/8, 654–5.

54 CMAC, Moran papers, 8/2.

55 PRO, ED 24/2012.

56 *Lancet* (1936) 2: 1370–4.

57 *SMHG* 57 (1951).

58 *SMHG* 4 (1898): 16. On Rogers, see Helen Joy Power, "Sir Leonard Rogers FRS (1868–1962): Tropical Medicine in the India Medical Service" (PhD dissertation, University College London, 1993). On colonial medicine more generally, see Mark Harrison, *Public Health in British India: Anglo-Indian Preventive Medicine, 1859–1914* (Cambridge: Cambridge University Press, 1994); Waltraud Ernst and Bernard Harris, eds., *Race, Science and Medicine, 1700–1960* (London: Routledge, 1999); Poonam Bala, *Imperialism and Medicine in Bengal: A Socio-Historical Perspective* (New Delhi: Sage, 1991).

59 *SMHG* 5 (1899): 37–9

60 Ibid.: 8–11.

61 *SMHG* 19 (1913): 27–9.

62 F.S. Brereton, *The Great War and the R.A.M.C.* (London: Constable, 1919).

63 CMAC, RAMC papers, box 1089, contains a scrapbook of Goodwin's life.

64 *SMHG* 28 (1922): 115.

65 *Lancet* (1900) 2: 1525–6.

66 Meyrick Emrys-Roberts, *The Cottage Hospitals, 1859–1900* (Motcombe, Dorset: Tern Publications, 1991).

67 *SMHG* 59 (1953): 95–105.

68 *SMHG* 104, no. 2 (April 1998): 17–18.

69 *SMHG* 78, no. 2 (1972): 21–2.

70 *SMHG* 98, no. 2 (April 1992): 24–6.

71 Geoffrey Rivett, *From Cradle to Grave: Fifty Years of the NHS* (London: King's Fund, 1998), 191.

72 Brookes University Video Archives, MSVA 065, interview of Lord Porritt by Lord Cohen, 21 November 1991.

73 *SMHG* 68 (1962): 244–8.

74 Interview with Robin Abel, 14 March 2000.

75 The author's grandmother, living on a farm in Devon, made the trip, drawn by the clinic's reputation.

76 *Past and Present Nurse's League Journal* 6 (1969): 11–12.

77 *Past and Present Nurse's League Journal* 13 (1976): 15–18.

78 *SMHG* 31 (1925): 15–17.

79 Interview with John Graham Jones, 6 March 2000.

Chapter Ten

1 Gerald L. Geison, "Social and Institutional Factors in the Stagnancy of English Physiology, 1840–1870," *Bulletin of the History of Medicine* 46 (1972): 30–58; Richard D. French, *Antivivisection and Medical Science in Victorian Society* (Princeton: Princeton University Press, 1975).

2 SMHA, SM AD 2/4, 169.

3 SMHA, SM AD 2/5, 328–9.

4 Thomas Kuhn, *The Structure of Scientific Revolutions* (Chicago: Chicago University Press, 1970), 176 and passim.

5 Andrew Warwick, *Masters of Theory: A Pedagogical History of Mathematical Physics in Cambridge, 1765–1835* (Chicago: University of Chicago Press, forthcoming).

6 John Burdon Sanderson, *Handbook of the Sphygmograph: Being a Guide to Its Use in Clinical Research* (London: Robert Hardwicke, 1867).

7 Three collections of essays outline early electrocardiology: W.F. Bynum, C.J. Lawrence, and V. Nutton, eds., *The Emergence of Modern Cardiology* (London: Wellcome Institute, 1985); William Coleman and Frederic L. Holmes, eds., *The Investigative Enterprise: Experimental Physiology in Nineteenth-Century Medicine* (Berkeley: University of California Press, 1988); and Joel D. Howell, ed., *Medical Lives and Scientific Medicine at Michigan, 1891–1969* (Ann Arbor: University of Michigan Press, 1993).

8 G.W. Pickering, "In Memorium Thomas Lewis," *Clinical Science* 6 (1946–8): 3–11.

9 CMAC, GWP Pickering Papers, B3/1.

10 All three are in Sir Thomas Lewis, *Research in Medicine and Other Addresses* (London: H.K. Lewis, 1939). See Arthur Hollman, *Sir Thomas Lewis: Pioneer Cardiologist and Clinical Scientist* (London: Springer, 1996).

11 Sir Christopher C. Booth, "Clinical Research," manuscript, 44; see also his articles in the *BMJ* (1979) 1: 1469–73, and in Austoker and Bryder, *Historical Perspectives on the Role of the MRC*.

12 Lewis, *Research in Medicine*.

13 Michel Morange, *A History of Molecular Biology*, trans. Matthew Cobb (Cambridge: Harvard University Press, 1998), 114.

14 J. Stewart Cameron and Jackie Hicks, "Frederick Akbar Mahomed and His Role in the Description of Hypertension at Guy's Hospital," *Kidney International* 49 (1996): 1488–506.

15 George Pickering, *High Blood Pressure* (London: Churchill, 1968), 103.

16 Irvine H. Page, *Hypertension Research: A Memoir, 1920–1960* (New York: Pergamon Press, 1988), 109, 115.

17 Thomas Kuhn, *The Structure of Scientific Revolutions*.

18 Sir Stanley Peart, in L.A. Reynolds and E.M. Tansey, eds., *Clinical Research in Britain, 1950–1980* (London: Wellcome Trust, 2000), 23.

19 CMAC, Pickering papers, B1/51.

20 Ibid., 1, A17, autobiographical notes, 10.

21 Ibid., A16, autobiographical notes.

22 Ibid., A32.

23 Sources: SMHG 78 (1972) and personal interviews.

24 CMAC, Pickering papers, A33, 6.

25 Much of what follows is taken from Oxford Brookes University Medical Sciences Video Archives, MSVAs 82, 107, 110–12, 1993–1995, interviews of Sir Stanley Peart by Max Blythe, 1993–95, and personal interview, 13 March 2000.

26 W. Feldberg in *Dictionary of National Biography* (1961–70), 412–3.

27 Personal interview, 1997.

28 The point is forcefully advanced in Alberto Cambrosio and Peter Keating, *Exquisite Specificity: The Monoclonal Antibody Revolution* (Oxford: Oxford University Press, 1995).

29 This pattern is discernible in *Clinical Science* during the 1950s, for example.

30 Interview with Francis Diggins, 22 May 1998.

31 Interview with Stanley Peart, 13 March 2000.

32 For example, Ivor Smith, *Chromatographic and Electrophoretic Techniques* (London: William Heinemann, 1960) 1: Michel Morange, *A History of Molecular Biology*, 89. I am also grateful to John Henderson for help with this.

33 Page, *Hypertension Research*, 114.

34 J.D. Swales, ed., *Platt versus Pickering: An Episode in Recent Medical History* (London: Keynes Press, 1985).

35 Ibid., 71.

36 Nicolas Postel-Vinay, ed., *A Century of Arterial Hypertension*, trans. R. Edelstein and C. Coffin (Chichester: John Wiley & Sons, 1996), 56.

37 Pickering, *High Blood Pressure*, 256–61.

38 D.J.P. Barker and G. Rose, *Epidemiology in Medical Practice* (Edinburgh: Churchill Livingstone, 1976), 19.

39 Ibid., 20–1.

40 *BMJ* 291 (1985): 97–104; and 296 (1988): 1565–70.

41 P.S. Sever, N.R. Poulter, and K.T. Khaw, "Migration Studies and Blood Pressure: A Model for Essential Hypertension," in C.J. Mathias and P.S. Sever, eds., *Concepts in Hypertension: Festschrift for Sir Stanley Peart* (Darmstadt: Steinkopff Verlag, 1989), 55–66.

42 Personal interview with Peter Sever, 11 February 2000.

43 A.F. Lever, "Excess Renin As a Cause of Renovascular Hypertension,?" in Mathias and Sever, eds., *Concepts in Hypertension*, 2.

44 Interview with Francis Diggins, 22 May 1998.

45 Interview with H.H. Eastcott, 23 January 1999.

46 St Mary's Hospital Medical School, *The Dean's Annual Report for the Academic Year 1948–49*.

47 *Lancet* (1954) 2: 994–6.

48 Interview with H.H. Eastcott; Steven G. Friedman, *A History of Vascular Surgery* (New York: Furh Publishing, 1989); *Lancet* (1954) 2: 994–6.

49 Friedman, *A History of Vascular Surgery*, 102–07.

50 Taped reminiscences by Cherry Wise (undated).

51 Oxford Brookes Medical Sciences Video Archives, MSVAS 152–4, December 1996 interviews with Sir Roy Calne by Max Blythe.

52 *Lancet* (1969) 1: 1–5; *BMJ* (1972) 4: 139–41; (1965) 2: 1387–94; (1963) 2: 639–45.

53 For example, see Francis D. Moore, *Metabolic Care of the Surgical Patient* (Philadelphia: W.B. Saunders, 1959), 399–400.

54 *SMHG* 74 (1968), 163–4.

55 See Lara Marks, "'Not Just a Statistic': The History of USA and UK Policy over Thrombotic Disease and the Oral Contraceptive Pill, 1960s–1970s," *Social Science and Medicine* 49 (1999): 1139–55; also *Sexual Chemistry: A History of the Contraceptive Pill* (New Haven: Yale University Press, 2001).

56 Ibid.

57 Interview with Oscar Craig, 28 March 2000, and his leaving notice, *SMHG* 88 (1983): 20; Oscar Craig, *A Life in Medicine* (London: Privately published, 2000).

58 *SMHG* 93 (1988): 14–15.

59 Interview wth Ara Darzi, 30 March 2000.

60 Peter Richards, personal papers.

Chapter Eleven

1 Dominique Pestre, "Science, Political Power and the State," in John Krige and Dominique Pestre, eds., *Science in the Twentieth Century* (Amsterdam: Harwood, 1997), 69.

2 Though small compared to later sums, British spending on science wasn't low for the times: see David Edgerton, *Science, Technology and the British Industrial "Decline," 1870–1970* (Cambridge: Cambridge University Press, 1996); and "Liberal Militarism and the British State," *New Left Review* 185 (January–February 1990): 138–69.

3 A. Landsborough Thomson, *Half a Century of Medical Research* (London: HMSO, 1973), 1, 205.

4 Philip Gummett, *Scientists in Whitehall* (Manchester: Manchester University Press, 1980), 39.

5 A.H. Halsey, ed., *British Social Trends since 1900* (London: Macmillan, 1988), 269.

6 Pestre, "Science, Political Power and the State," 71; and see the essays in same volume by C. Lawrence, I. Lowy, A.M. Moulin, P.G. Abir-Am, and H. Kamminga.

7 In St Mary's Hospital Medical School, *The Dean's Annual Report for the Academic Year 1949–50.*

8 For example, Robert Olby, "The Molecular Revolution in Biology," in R.C. Olby et al., *Companion to the History of Modern Science* (London: Routledge, 1990), 505–06.

9 André Malraux, *Voices of Silence*, trans. Stuart Gilbert (1953; reprint, Granada: St Alban's, 1974).

10 Jean A.N.C. de Condorcet, *Esquisse d'un tableau historique du progrès de l'esprit humain* (1794; reprint, Paris: Editions sociales, 1971).

11 George Weisz, "Rethinking the History of Medical Specialization in Comparative Perspective," paper given at Queen's University in Kingston, Ontario, 21 November 2001.

12 SMHA, SM AD 5/5, 167, 170.

13 Ibid., 194.

14 SMHA, SM AD 5/6, 6, February 1944.

15 *SMHG* 82, no. 5 (1976): 14–15.

16 *SMHG* 67 (1961): 10–11.

17 SMHA, Inoculation Department Council, minute book.

18 A. Neuberger and R.L. Smith, in *Biographical Memoirs of the Fellows of the Royal Society* 33 (1979), 691.

19 St Mary's Hospital Medical School, *Dean's Annual Report*, 1958–59.

20 SMHA, MS AD 1/6, 68–9.

21 *SMHG* 21 (1915): 110–11; 32 (1926), 5–7.

22 *SMHG* 68 (1962): 244–8.

23 *SMHG* 37 (1931): 144–5.

24 *SMHG* 53 (1948): 20.

25 Imperial College Archives, Finance and Executive Committees of Imperial College 76 (1982–83), 19 November 1982.

26 Roy Porter, *The Greatest Benefit* (London: HarperCollins, 1997), 449.

27 E.M. Tansey and Rosemary Milligan, "The Early History of the Wellcome Research Laboratories 1894–1914," in Jonathan Liebernau, Gregory Higby, and Elaine C. Stroud, eds., *Pill Peddlars: Essays on the History of the Pharmaceutical Industry* (Madison, Wis.: American Institute of the History of Psychiatry, 1990), 91–110.; also A.R. Hall and B.A. Bembridge, *Physic and Philanthropy: A History of the Wellcome Trust, 1936–1986* (Cambridge: Cambridge University Press, 1986); interview with Peter Williams, 8 March 2000.

28 Medical Sciences Video Archives, MSVA 119, 136, 150: interviews of Peter Williams by Max Blythe, 1995–96.

29 SMHA, Academic Board, 9 December 1948.

30 SMHA, interview of W. Frankland by Alasdair Fraser and Kevin Brown (no date).

31 Interview with Alan Glynn, 5 April 2000.

32 SMHA, Medical School Council Reports 1 (1948–67), 146, 12–13.

33 *SMHG* 88, no. 1 (1982): 14–16.

34 *SMHG* 79, no. 6 (September 1973): 9–10.

35 *SMHG* 74 (1968): 183.

36 Ibid.: 184.

37 Interview with Alan Glynn, 5 April 2000.

38 Royal Society of London, Florey Papers, 98 HF 34 20:1.

39 *SMHG* 78, no. 4 (June 1973): 29–30.

40 See Pauline Mazumdar, *Species and Specificity: An Interpretation of the History of Immunology* (Cambridge: Cambridge University Press, 1995).

41 Personal communication and interview with Peter Mollison, 24 March 2000.

42 Leslie Brent, *A History of Transplantation Immunology* (London: Academic Press, 1997), 25.

43 *SMHG* 75 (1969), 199–200.

44 Brent, *A History of Transplantation Immunology*, 227 and passim.

45 *SMHG* 75 (1969): 132–4.

46 A.A. Glynn, "R.E.O. Williams and Bacteriology at St Mary's, 1960–1973," manuscript in the hands of A.A. Glynn, 1.

47 *SMHG* 69 (1964): 87.

48 Obituary by Jack Litchfield, *SMHG* 86, no. 2 (April 1981): 6–7.

49 *SMHG* 73 (1967): 21–4.

50 Interview with David Gordon, 27 April 2000.

Chapter Twelve

1 SMHA, Medical School Council, 1, 33.

2 Rosemary Stevens, *Medical Practice in Modern England: The Impact of Specialization and State Medicine* (New Haven: Yale University Press, 1966).

3 *SMHG* 53 (1947): 48.

4 *SMHG* 76, no. 4 (June 1970).

5 George Pickering, *Quest for Excellence in Medical Education: A Personal Survey* (Oxford: Oxford University Press, 1978).

6 Norman R. Eder, *National Health Insurance and the Medical Profession, 1913–1939* (London: Garland, 1982), 146–7.

7 *SMHG* 59 (1953): 127.

8 SMHA, interview with A.W. Frankland by Alasdair Fraser and Kevin Brown (no date).

9 Ibid.

10 SMHA, MS SU 1/2, 147–8.

11 *SMHG* 77, 4 (June 1971): 4–6.

12 *SMHG* 77, 5 (July 1971): 14–15.

13 *SMHG* 75 (1969): 214–15.

14 See, for example the chapter on "Mobility and Education," in A.H. Halsey, *Change in British Society from 1900 to the Present Day* (Oxford: Oxford University Press, 1994).

15 *Lancet* 2 (1951): 1049.

16 David Edgerton, "The Masculinisation of Science: Gender, Class, and Big Science in Britain around the Second World War," paper given at Cambridge, 24 September 1998.

17 SMHA, MS AD 1/2, 150.

18 Interview with Judith Hockaday, July 1998.

19 SMHA, MS Academic Board 1, 473.

20 Interview with Victoria Cattell, 1 March 2000.

21 SMHA, Medical School Council, 1, 418.

22 SMHA, Academic Board, 8 December, 305.

23 SMHA, Academic Board, October 1965 and May 1976.

24 SMHA, MS SU 1/2, 199.

25 *SMHG* 31 (1925): 130–2.

26 *SMHG* 38 (1932): 64–7.

27 *SMHG* 54 (1948): 183–9; 226–30.

28 Interview with John Graham Jones, 6 March 2000.

29 SMHA, MS SU 1/2, passim for what follows.

30 Bonney, the second secretary of the union, recalls that Frazer "felt that having an absentee Dean wasn't really to be tolerated, and he set himself up to create … not a sort of … … post for himself, but he set himself up to create an active student union (interview with George Bonney, 9 May 2000).

31 SMHA, MS AD 1/1, 199–200.

32 *SMHG* 46 (1940): 79–80.

33 *SMHG* 48 (1942): 33.

34 SMHA, MS SU 1/2, 162.

35 *SMHG* 49 (1943): 89–92.

36 Interview with George Bonney, 9 May 2000.

37 *SMHG* 66 (1960): 121–3.

38 Ibid.: 137–8, 177–8, 246–8.

39 *SMHG* 68 (1962): 2.

40 Ibid.: 61–4.

41 The distinction, adapted from Clausewitz, is elaborated in Michel de Certeau, *The Practice of Everyday Life*, trans. Steven F. Rendall (Berkeley: University of Press, California, 1984).

42 *SMHG* 68 (1962): 313–14.

43 *SMHG* 74 (1968): 180, 202–3.

44 See, for example, the correspondence between Moran and A.G. Cross, Brinton's successor as Dean in 1954, in CMAC, Moran Papers, A 7/2.

45 Denis Brinton, "Selection of Medical Students," *Lancet* (1951) 2: 1047–52.

46 Interviews with George Bonney, 9 May 2000.

47 *SMHG* 59 (1953): 164–5.

48 *SMHG* 58 (1952): 145–6.

49 *SMHG* 79, no. 8 (December 1973): 12–14.

50 *SMHG* 72 (1966): 3.

51 *SMHG* 68 (1962): 46–8.

52 *SMHG* 56 (1950): 212.

53 *SMHG* 61 (1955): 25.

54 *SMHG* 68 (1962): 209.

55 *SMHG* 74 (1968): 110.

56 *SMHG* 68 (1962): 312–13.

57 Interview with Victoria Cattell, 1 March 2000.

58 *SMHG* 69 (1963): 248.

59 Ibid.: 281.

60 *SMHG* 92, no. 3 (October 1986): 22–3.

61 *SMHG* 79, no. 3 (March–April 1973): 16–17.

62 *SMHG* 79, no. 1 (January–February 1973): 14–16.

63 By contrast Charing Cross, the Royal Free, and University College all drew more than two thousand applicants, as did Manchester, Leicester, Newcastle, Nottingham, and Sheffield. No London medical school drew less than a thousand.

64 *The Physician*, November 1985, 503–5. Peter Richards, personal papers.

65 ISCO *CareerScope* 196 (Spring 1990), 3–7. In Richards, personal papers.

66 Richards, personal papers.

67 *BMJ* 305 (1992), 1,103.

68 Richards, personal papers.

Chapter Thirteen

1   Peter Ackroyd, *London: The Biography* (London: Vintage, 2001), 526.

2   In Charles Webster, *The National Health Service: A Political History* (Oxford: Oxford University Press, 1998), 40.

3   Interview with Sir Richard Doll, March 2000.

4   See the collection by S. Lock, L.A. Reynolds, and E.M. Tansey, eds., *Ashes to Ashes: The History of Smoking and Health* (Amsterdam: Rodopi, 1998).

5   SMHA, SM AD 2/11, B732.

6   SMHA, SM AD 35/23, 18.

7   T.E. Oppé, interview, 18 May 2000, and remarks made by a clinician working at a children's hospital at the time, at Witness Seminar, 4 April 2000, on childhood asthma.

8   SMHA, SM AD 3/3, BG 1957 BG 152.

9   *Paddington Mercury*, 2 and 9 January 1970.

10 SMHA, SM AD 3/4 BG 241–3.

11 Webster, *The National Health Service*, 58.

12 Ibid., 84–5.

13 Through 1978 and 1979 the *BMJ* had a series called "Anatomy of a Consultation." Clippings are in the SMHA, MS AD 94/37.

14 Klein, *The New Politics of the National Health Service* (London: Longman, 1995, 3rd ed.), 132.

15 Jose Harris, *William Beveridge, A Biography* (Oxford: Oxford University Press, 1997).

16 Keith G. Banting, *Poverty, Politics and Policy: Britain in the 1960s* (London: Macmillan, 1979), 66–70; see also G.C. Fiegehen, P.S. Lansley, and A.D. Smith, *Poverty and Progress in Britain, 1953–73* (Cambridge: Cambridge University Press, 1977).

17 London Diocesan Conference, *The Paddington Estate* (London: Church Assembly, 1944), is the source for much of what follows.

18 Ronald Segal, *The Black Diaspora* (London: Faber & Faber, 1995), 280.

19 *SMHG* 46 (1940): 30.

20 *SMHG* 72 (1965): 80–1.

21 *Paddington Mercury*, 15 February 1963, 3 October 1969.

22 *Sunday Times*, 7 July 1963.

23 Banting, *Poverty, Politics and Policy*, 24.

24 A.H. Halsey, *Change in British Society from 1900 to the Present Day* (Oxford: Oxford University Press, 1994), 43, 131; Halsey, *British Social Trends since 1900* (London: Macmillan, 1988), 377–8.

25 Halsey, *Change in British Society*, 102.

26 Banting, *Poverty, Politics and Policy*, 68.

27 Ralf Dahrendorf, *A History of the London School of Economics and Political Science, 1895–1995* (Oxford: Oxford University Press, 1995), 382; see also the account by Titmuss's daughter, in Ann Oakley, "Making Medicine Social: The Case of the Two Dogs with Bent Legs," in Dorothy Porter, ed., *Social Medicine and Medical Sociology in the 20th Century* (Amsterdam: Rodopi, 1997), 81–96.

28 Richard M. Titmuss, *Essays on "The Welfare State"* (1958; reprint, London: George Allen & Unwin, 1976).

29 Titmuss, *Essays*, 124, 188, 197, 202.

30 *BMJ* (1942) 1: 801 and (1943) 2: 633–5.

31 R.C. Wofinden, *Health Services in England* (Bristol: John Wright & Sons, 1947), 176.

32 *SMHG* 78, no. 7 (October 1972): 8–12.

33 SMHA, Academic Board, July and October 1950.

34 Dorothy Porter, "The Decline of Social Medicine in Britain in the 1960s," in Porter, ed., *Social Medicine and Medical Sociology in the 20th Century*, 97–119.

35 Halsey, *Change in British Society*, xiv.

36 Virginia Berridge, *Health and Society in Britain since 1939* (Cambridge: Cambridge University Press, 1999), 44–5.

37 Ibid., 87.

38 Rudolph Klein, *The New Politics of the National Health Service*, 74.

39 Ibid., 75.

40 Rivett, *From Cradle to Grave*, 335.

41 London Health Planning Consortium, *Primary Health Care in Inner London* (London: London Health Planning Consortium, 1981), 3.

42 Interview with Sir Brian Jarman, 17 May 2000.

43 *BMJ* 286 (1983): 1,705–8.

44 Robin J. Talbot in *BMJ* 302 (1991): 383–6.

45 Interview with William Harris, 2 May 2000.

46 Simon Garfield, *The End of Innocence: Britain in the Time of AIDS* (London: Faber & Faber, 1994), 75–6. And see *Virginia Berridge, AIDS in the UK: The Making of a Policy, 1981–1994* (Oxford: Oxford University Press, 1996).

47 Interview with Anthony Pinching, 11 April 2000.

48 Steven Epstein, *Impure Science: AIDS, Activism, and the Politics of Knowledge* (Berkeley: University of California Press, 1996).

49 Klein, *The New Politics of the National Health Service*, 168.

50 SMHA, Medical School Committee 6 (1945), 562.

51 Kensington & Chelsea and Westminster Health Authority, Meeting of 10 May 2000, report HA (2000) 26.2.

52 James Le Fanu, *The Rise and Fall of Modern Medicine* (London: Little, Brown), 1999, 371.

53 Peter Townsend and Nick Davidson, eds., *Inequalities in Health: The Black Report* (Harmondsworth: Penguin, 1982; 1980 DHSS).

54 *Report of the Inquiry into London's Health Service, Medical Education, and Research* presented to the secretaries of state for Health and Education by Sir Bernard Tomlinson (London: HMSO, 1992).

Chapter Fourteen

1 This is a paraphrase of David Landes's description of the English countryside during the Industrial Revolution, from his *Unbound Prometheus: Technological Change and Industrial Development in Western Europe from 1750 to the Present* (Cambridge: Cambridge University Press, 1989), 69.

2 On the "hypertrophy"of medical research in the United States and its effect on education, see Kenneth M. Ludmerer, *Time to Heal: American Medical Education from the Turn of the Century to the Era of Managed Care* (Oxford: Oxford University Press, 1999).

3 *Report of the Royal Commission on Medical Education*, CMD 3569 (London: HMSO, 1968).

4 Interview with Keith Lockyer, 24 June 1998.

5 *London Medical Education – A New Framework. Report of a Working Party on Medical and Dental Teaching Resources* (London: University of London, February 1980).

6 SMHA, Academic Board, minutes for 1978–79, appendices.

7 J.P. Allan Gray, *The Central Middlesex Hospital: The First Sixty Years, 1903–1963* (London: Pitman, 1963).

8 Interview with Keith Lockyer, 24 June 1998.

9 Interview with Peter Richards, 7 January 2000.

10 Niall Fergusson, *The House of Rothschild: The World's Banker, 1849–1999* (New York: Viking, 1999), 491.

11 This was the opinion of the Development Policy Committee at St Mary's, 17 April 1985.

12 SMHA, Academic Board, minutes, letter of 23 September 1987.

13 Oxford Brookes University, Medical Sciences Video Archives, MSVA 147, interview with Kay Davies by Max Blythe, 21 November 1996.

14 Interview with John Caldwell, 5 May 2000.

15 SMHA, Academic Board, 2 October 1985, appendix, *Planning for the Late 1980s: Research Strategy Statement*.

16 SMHA, Academic Board, 6 November 1985, appendices, 60–1.

17 SMHA, Academic Board, 5 June 1985.

18 Interview with Alan Swanson, 7 April 2000.

19 Interview with Peter Richards, 7 January 2000.

20 SMHA, Academic Board, 7 May 1986, 57–8.

21 *SMHG* 95, no. 1 (January 1989): 30–1.

22 Interview with Alasdair Fraser, 13 March 2000.

23 Interview with J. Oscar Craig, 28 March 2000.

24 *SMHG* 98, no. 2 (April 1992): 45.

25 *SMHG* 99, no. 3 (October 1993): 8–10.

26 *SMHG* 101, no. 2 (April 1995): 5.

27 Interview with Christopher Edwards, 10 March 2000.

28 Interview with Neil Poulter, 10 April 2000.

29 Martha E. Keyes, "The Prion Challenge to the 'Central Dogma' of Molecular Biology, 1965–1991," *Studies in the History and Philosophy of the Biological and Biomedical Sciences* 30 (1999): 1–19; Rosalind M. Ridley and Harry F. Baker, *Fatal Protein: The Story of CJD, BSE, and Other Prion Diseases* (Oxford: Oxford University Press, 1998).

30 E-mail by Richard Sykes to staff of Imperial College, 14 December 2001; the results are available on line at http://www.rae.ac.uk/results/

31 Interview with S.N. Wickramasinghe, 17 April 2000.

32 Interview with Victoria Cattell, 1 March 2000.

33 Interview with Christopher Edwards, 10 March 2000.

Chapter Fifteen

1 In Nicholas Timmins, *The Five Giants: A Biography of the Welfare State* (London: HarperCollins, 1995), 203.

2 *SMGH* 56 (1950): 121–2.

3 *SMHG* 59 (1953): 174–5; John Keegan, *The First World War* (London: Pimlico, 1998).

4 *SMHG* 56 (1950): 120–1.

5 SMHA, interview of Alan Powditch by Alasdair Fraser, May 1997.

6 SMHA, SM AD 13/14, 76/16.

7 General Medical Council, *Good Medical Practice* (London: GMC, 1998); Mayur Lakhani, "Ten Questions about Clinical Governance," *Audit Trends* (March 1999).

8 Interviews with Christine Rose, July 1999, and Evangeline Karn, 21 September 1999.

9 Interview with Robin Touquet, 17 May 2000; S.G.T. Smith et al., "Detection of Alcohol Misusing Patients in Accident and Emergency Departments: The Paddington Alcohol Test," *Journal of Accident and Emergency Medicine* 13, 5 (September 1996): 308–12; H.L Cugnoni, I. Challoner, R. Touquet, "Not-

ting Hill Carnival 1989 - The Facts," *BMJ* 299 (1989): 1229; R. Touquet, J. Fothergill, M. Fertleman, P. McCann, "Ten Clinical Governance Safeguards for Accident and Emergency Departments," *Clinical Risk* 1 (1999): 44–9.

10 His daughter became a celebrity chef and has repeatedly spoken of his violence. She also accuses him of alcoholism, but I have found no evidence that he drank while operating.

11 *Past and Present Nurse's League Journal* 33 (1996): 9–12.

12 *SMHG* 78, no. 8 (December 1972): 22–4.

13 *SMHG* 26 (1920): 25–30.

14 Interview with Neil Poulter, 10 April 2000.

15 Interview with Jenny Large, 21 September 1999.

16 *SMHG* 97, no. 3 (October 1991): 22.

17 *SMHG* 54 (1948): 112–4.

18 *SMHG* 57 (1951): 177–81.

19 *SMHG* 56 (1950): 78–80.

20 *SMHG* 57 (1951): 122–5.

21 Simon Garfield, *The End of Innocence* (London: Faber & Faber, 1994).

22 Interview with Nick Cheshire, 7 March 2000.

23 *Past and Present Nurse's League Journal* 19 (1982): 28–35.

24 *Past and Present Nurse's League Journal* 16 (1979): 37–9.

25 Alexandra, *A Nurse's Story* (London: Privately printed, 1955), 51.

26 *Past and Present Nurse's League Journal* 19 (1982): 20–1.

27 *Past and Present Nurses' League Journal* 36 (1999): 8–14.

28 Interview with Jenny Large, 21 September 1999.

29 *SMHG* 71 (1965): 49.

30 Ibid., 49.

31 *SMHG* 73 (1967): 153–5.

32 Interview with Christine Rose, July 1999.

33 *SMHG* 4 (1934): 28–30.

34 Anne Marie Rafferty, *The Politics of Nursing Knowledge* (London: Routledge, 1996), 53; Brian Abel-Smith, *A History of the Nursing Profession* (London: Heinemann, 1960).

35 SMHA, SM AD 2/6, 164.

36 SMHA, SM AD 35/21, 44.

37 SMHA, SM AD 35/24, 22 May 1958.

38 SMHA, SM AD 35/25, 9 May 1960.

39 Interview with Stanley Holder, 1 December 1999.

40 Rafferty, *The Politics of Nursing Knowledge*, 1.

41 Interview with Justin Gaffney, 23 February 2000.

42 Interview with Tess Cann, 1 March 2000.

43 Ibid.

44 *SMHG* 6 (1900): 108–11.

45 *SMHG* 57 (1951): 88.

46 *SMHG* 62 (1956): 139–41.

47 Interview with Jenny Large, 21 September 1999.

48 *Past and Present Nurse's League Journal* 19 (1982): 28–35.

49 Information on the Rothschilds is from Niall Ferguson, *The House of Rothschild: The World's Banker, 1849–1999* (New York: Viking, 1999).

50 SMHA, SM AD 2/4, 223–4. See Michael Ignatieff, *The Needs of Strangers* (London: Chatto & Windus, 1984).

51 *SMHG* 69 (1963), 273–4.

52 The Dixon Team Inquiry Report (April 1999).

53 June Opie, *Over My Dead Body* (London: Methuen, 1957).

54 Philip Rieff, *The Triumph of the Therapeutic* (Chicago: Chicago University Press, 1966); and see the essays by Thomas Osborne, Alan Peterson, and Sarah Nettleton in Alan Peterson and Robin Bunton, eds., *Foucault, Health and Medicine* (London: Routledge, 1997). The case is most forcefully and philosophically stated in Thomas Mann's novel *The Magic Mountain* (1924).

Index